Severe Asthma

Editor

ROHIT K. KATIAL

IMMUNOLOGY AND ALLERGY CLINICS OF NORTH AMERICA

www.immunology.theclinics.com

Consulting Editor
STEPHEN A. TILLES

August 2016 • Volume 36 • Number 3

ELSEVIER

1600 John F. Kennedy Boulevard • Suite 1800 • Philadelphia, Pennsylvania, 19103-2899
http://www.theclinics.com

IMMUNOLOGY AND ALLERGY CLINICS OF NORTH AMERICA Volume 36, Number 3
August 2016 ISSN 0889-8561, ISBN-13: 978-0-323-45971-6
Editor: Jessica McCool
Developmental Editor: Kristen Helm

Immunology and Allergy Clinics of North America (ISSN 0889–8561) is published quarterly by Elsevier Inc., 360 Park Avenue South, New York, NY 10010-1710. Months of issue are February, May, August, and November. Periodicals postage paid at New York, NY and additional mailing offices. Subscription prices are $320.00 per year for US individuals, $508.00 per year for US institutions, $100.00 per year for US students and residents, $395.00 per year for Canadian individuals, $220.00 per year for Canadian students, $644.00 per year for Canadian institutions, $445.00 per year for international individuals, $644.00 per year for international institutions, $220.00 per year for international students. To receive student/resident rate, orders must be accompanied by name of affiliated institution, date of term, and the *signature* of program/residency coordinator on institution letterhead. Orders will be billed at individual rate until proof of status is received. Foreign air speed delivery is included in all *Clinics* subscription prices. All prices are subject to change without notice. **POSTMASTER**: Send address changes to *Immunology and Allergy Clinics of North America*, Elsevier Health Sciences Division, Subscription Customer Service, 3251 Riverport Lane, Maryland Heights, MO 63043. **Customer Service: 1-800-654-2452 (U.S. and Canada); 314-447-8871 (outside U.S. and Canada). Fax: 314-447-8029. E-mail: journalscustomerservice-usa@elsevier.com (for print support); journalsonlinesupport-usa@elsevier.com (for online support).**

Reprints. For copies of 100 or more, of articles in this publication, please contact the Commercial Reprints Department, Elsevier Inc., 360 Park Avenue South, New York, New York 10010-1710. Tel. 212-633-3874, Fax: 212-633-3820, E-mail: reprints@elsevier.com.

Immunology and Allergy Clinics of North America is covered in MEDLINE/PubMed (Index Medicus), Current Contents/Life Sciences, Science Citation Index, ISI/BIOMED, Chemical Abstracts, and EMBASE/Excerpta Medica.

Contributors

CONSULTING EDITOR

STEPHEN A. TILLES, MD
Executive Director, ASTHMA Inc. Clinical Research Center; Partner, Northwest Asthma and Allergy Center; Clinical Professor of Medicine, University of Washington, Seattle, Washington

EDITOR

ROHIT K. KATIAL, MD, FACAAI, FAAAAI, FACP
Professor of Medicine, Department of Allergy and Immunology; Associate Vice President of Clinical Research and Industry Relationships; Co-director of The Asthma Institute at National Jewish Health, Helen Wohlberg and Herman Lambert Chair in Pharmacokinetics, National Jewish Health, Denver, Colorado

AUTHORS

FERNANDO ALEMAN, MD
Division of Respirology, St Joseph's Healthcare Hamilton, McMaster University, Hamilton, Ontario, Canada

BRUCE G. BENDER, PhD
Professor, Pediatric Behavioral Health, National Jewish Health, Denver, Colorado

GENERY D. BOOSTER, PhD
Assistant Professor, Pediatric Behavioral Health, National Jewish Health, Denver, Colorado

TARA F. CARR, MD
Assistant Professor, Division of Pulmonary, Allergy, Critical Care, and Sleep Medicine, University of Arizona, Tucson, Arizona

NEHA M. DUNN, MD
Department of Allergy and Immunology, National Jewish Health, Denver, Colorado

DEBRA DYER, MD
Professor, Department of Radiology, National Jewish Health, Denver, Colorado

LINDSAY K. FINKAS, MD
Instructor, Division of Allergy and Clinical Immunology, Department of Medicine, National Jewish Health, Denver, Colorado

BART HILVERING, MD
Department of Respiratory Medicine; Nuffield Department of Medicine, University of Oxford, Oxford, United Kingdom; Laboratory of Translational Immunology, Department of Respiratory Medicine, University Medical Center Utrecht, Utrecht, The Netherlands

FLAVIA C.L. HOYTE, MD
Division of Allergy and Clinical Immunology, Department of Medicine, National Jewish Health, Denver, Colorado; Division of Allergy and Clinical Immunology, Department of Internal Medicine, University of Colorado Hospital, Aurora, Colorado

BRIDGETTE L. JONES, MD, MSc, FAAAAI, FAAP
Divisions of Pediatric Pharmacology and Therapeutic Innovation; Allergy, Asthma and Clinical Immunology, Associate Professor, Department of Pediatrics, Children's Mercy Hospitals and Clinics, University of Missouri Kansas City School of Medicine, Kansas City, Missouri

DAVID A. KAMINSKY, MD
Division of Pulmonary and Critical Care Medicine, University of Vermont College of Medicine, Burlington, Vermont

ROHIT K. KATIAL, MD, FACAAI, FAAAAI, FACP
Professor of Medicine, Department of Allergy and Immunology; Associate Vice President of Clinical Research and Industry Relationships; Co-director of The Asthma Institute at National Jewish Health, Helen Wohlberg and Herman Lambert Chair in Pharmacokinetics, National Jewish Health, Denver, Colorado

TILMAN KOELSCH, MD
Assistant Professor, Department of Radiology, National Jewish Health, Denver, Colorado

MONICA KRAFT, MD
Professor, Division of Pulmonary, Allergy, Critical Care, and Sleep Medicine, University of Arizona, Tucson, Arizona

HUI FANG LIM, MBBS, MRCP(UK)
Assistant Professor of Medicine, Department of Respiratory Medicine, National University of Singapore, Singapore, Singapore

DAVID LYNCH, MD
Professor, Department of Radiology, National Jewish Health, Denver, Colorado

RICHARD MARTIN, MD
Professor and Chair, Department of Medicine, National Jewish Health, Denver, Colorado

LUCAS MIKULIC, MD
Division of Pulmonary and Critical Care Medicine, University of Vermont Medical Center, Burlington, Vermont

PARAMESWARAN NAIR, MD, PhD, FRCP, FRCPC
Frederick E. Hargreave Teva Innovation Professor of Medicine, Division of Respirology, St Joseph's Healthcare Hamilton, McMaster University, Hamilton, Ontario, Canada

ALYSSA A. OLAND, PhD
Assistant Professor, Pediatric Behavioral Health, National Jewish Health, Denver, Colorado

JACQUELINE O'TOOLE, DO
Department of Medicine, University of Vermont Medical Center, Burlington, Vermont

REYNOLD A. PANETTIERI Jr, MD
Vice Chancellor, Clinical and Translational Science; Director, Rutgers Institute for Translational Medicine and Science; Professor of Medicine, Robert Wood Johnson Medical School; Emeritus Professor of Medicine, University of Pennsylvania, Philadelphia, Pennsylvania

IAN D. PAVORD, FMedSci, DM, FRCP
Professor, Department of Respiratory Medicine; Nuffield Department of Medicine, University of Oxford, Oxford, United Kingdom

NIRUPAMA PUTCHA, MD, MHS
Assistant Professor of Medicine, Division of Pulmonary and Critical Care Medicine, Johns Hopkins University School of Medicine, Baltimore, Maryland

JOHN CALEB RICHARDS, MD
Assistant Professor, Department of Radiology, National Jewish Health, Denver, Colorado

LINDA ROGERS, MD, FCCP
Associate Professor of Medicine, Clinical Director, Adult Asthma Program, Mount Sinai-National Jewish Health Respiratory Institute, Icahn School of Medicine at Mount Sinai, New York, New York

LANNY J. ROSENWASSER, MD
Division of Allergy, Asthma and Clinical Immunology, Department of Pediatrics, Children's Mercy Hospitals and Clinics, University of Missouri Kansas City School of Medicine, Kansas City, Missouri

RAHUL SHRIMANKER, MRCP
Department of Respiratory Medicine; Nuffield Department of Medicine, University of Oxford, Oxford, United Kingdom

XIAO CHLOE WAN, MD
Clinical Fellow, Division of Pulmonary, Critical Care, Sleep and Allergy, University of California, San Francisco, San Francisco, California

EILEEN WANG, MD, MPH
Division of Allergy and Clinical Immunology, Department of Medicine, National Jewish Health, Denver, Colorado; Division of Allergy and Clinical Immunology, Department of Internal Medicine, University of Colorado Hospital, Aurora, Colorado

ROBERT A. WISE, MD
Professor of Medicine, Division of Pulmonary and Critical Care Medicine, Johns Hopkins University School of Medicine, Baltimore, Maryland

PRESCOTT G. WOODRUFF, MD, MPH
Professor of Medicine, Division of Pulmonary, Critical Care, Sleep and Allergy, Department of Medicine and Cardiovascular Research Institute, University of California, San Francisco, San Francisco, California

Contents

The epidemiology and physiology of severe asthma are inherently linked because of varying phenotypes and expressions of asthma throughout the population. To understand how to better treat severe asthma, we must use both population data and physiologic principles to individualize therapies among groups with similar expressions of this disease.

A significant body of work in the genetics of asthma currently exists. However, current knowledge has not been clarifying in understanding the pathophysiology of asthma and therapeutic treatment of the disease. Severe asthma in adults and children is a significant burden in relation to disproportionate disease morbidity, mortality, and health utilization. This disease phenotype is not well understood; current effective treatment regimens are limited. Genetic studies may lead to improved understanding of the pathophysiology of severe asthma and identification of relevant subsets, which allow more targeted and effective therapies and the realization of Precision Medicine in asthma.

Asthma is the most common chronic illness among children in the United States and can impact nearly all aspects of functioning. Most research suggests that children with severe asthma display more emotional and behavioral problems than their healthy peers. These psychological difficulties are associated with increased risk for functional impairments and problematic disease course. Multidisciplinary teams that assess and treat these psychosocial factors using psychoeducational and behavioral interventions are important for children whose asthma is poorly controlled. Future research should examine the ways in which stress, emotions, and immune functions interact, so as to develop more preventative interventions.

Gastroesophageal reflux and obstructive sleep apnea syndrome are conditions that practitioners have been encouraged to evaluate and treat as part of a comprehensive approach to achieving asthma control. In this review, the author looks at the evidence linking these two conditions as factors that may impact difficult-to-control asthma and looks critically at the evidence suggesting that evaluation and treatment of these conditions when present impacts asthma control.

Asthma is an inflammatory condition of both the small and large airways. Recently the small airways have gained attention as studies have shown significant inflammation in the small airways in all severities of asthma. This inflammation has correlated with peripheral airway resistance and as a result, noninvasive methods to reliably measure small airways have been pursued. In addition, recent changes in asthma inhalers have led to alterations in drug formulations and the development of extrafine particle inhalers that improve delivery to the distal airways.

Chronic bacterial infection is implicated in both the development and severity of asthma. The atypical bacteria *Mycoplasma pneumoniae* and *Chlamydophila pneumoniae* have been identified in the airways of asthmatics and correlated with clinical features such as adult onset, exacerbation risks, steroid sensitivity, and symptom control. Asthmatic patients with evidence of bacterial infection may benefit from antibiotic treatment directed towards these atypical organisms. Examination of the airway microbiome may identify microbial communities that confer risk for or protection from severe asthma.

Patients with severe asthma and concomitant chronic rhinosinusitis often have severe, refractory upper and lower airway inflammation. This inflammation has been proposed to be similar throughout the upper and lower airways leading to the unified airways concept. This article reviews chronic rhinosinusitis with and without nasal polyps, and the subgroup with aspirin-exacerbated respiratory disease, while focusing on the relationship with asthma. Additionally, diagnosis and treatment with current and newer therapies are discussed.

The debate about whether asthma and chronic obstructive pulmonary disease (COPD) are distinct clinical syndromes is not new; there is heightened interest in understanding the group of individuals with obstructive lung disease who seem to have elements of both conditions because recent studies have demonstrated increased risk for respiratory events and exacerbations. We describe the clinical characteristics of this subtype of disease and suggest 4 working definitions of individuals who would fall into the asthma–COPD overlap category. Understanding the mechanisms underlying these subtypes will hopefully lead into a better understanding of therapeutic strategies that can target specific pathobiologic pathways.

Asthma is one of the most common diseases of the lung. Asthma manifests with common, although often subjective and nonspecific, imaging features at radiography and high-resolution computed tomography. The primary role of imaging is not to make a diagnosis of asthma but to identify complications, such as allergic bronchopulmonary aspergillosis, or mimics of asthma, such as hypersensitivity pneumonitis. This article reviews the imaging features of asthma as well as common complications and mimics.

Biomarkers have been critical for studies of disease pathogenesis and the development of new therapies in severe asthma. In particular, biomarkers of type 2 inflammation have proven valuable for endotyping and targeting new biological agents. Because of these successes in understanding and marking type 2 inflammation, lack of knowledge regarding non–type 2 inflammatory mechanisms in asthma will soon be the major obstacle to the development of new treatments and management strategies in severe asthma. Biomarkers can play a role in these investigations as well by providing insight into the underlying biology in human studies of patients with severe asthma.

Asthma is a heterogeneous disease that can be classified into different clinical endotypes, depending on the type of airway inflammation, clinical severity, and response to treatment. This article focuses on the eosinophilic endotype of asthma, which is defined by the central role that eosinophils play in the pathophysiology of the condition. It is characterized by persistently elevated sputum and/or blood eosinophils and by a significant response to treatments that suppress eosinophilia. Eosinophil activity in the airway may be more important than their numbers and this needs to be investigated. Transciplomic or Metabolomic signatures may also be useful to identify this endotype.

Although 2 T-helper type 2 inflammation evokes airway hyperresponsiveness and narrowing, neutrophilic or pauci-immune asthma accounts for significant asthma morbidity. Viruses, toxicants, environmental tobacco smoke exposure, and bacterial infections induce asthma exacerbations mediated by neutrophilic inflammation or by structural cell (pauci-immune) mechanisms. Therapeutic challenges exist in the management of neutrophilic and pauci-immune phenotypes because both syndromes manifest steroid insensitivity. The recognition that neutrophil subsets exist and their functions are unique poses exciting opportunities to develop precise therapies. The conventional thought to target neutrophil activation or migration globally may explain why current drug development in neutrophilic asthma remains challenging.

Severe asthma is a complex and heterogeneous disease. The European Respiratory Society and American Thoracic Society guidelines define severe asthma for patients 6 years or older as "asthma which requires treatment with high-dose inhaled corticosteroids...plus a second controller or systemic corticosteroids to prevent it from becoming 'uncontrolled' or which remains 'uncontrolled' despite this therapy." This article reviews available traditional therapies, data behind their uses in severe asthma, and varying recommendations. As various asthma endotypes and phenotypes are better understood and characterized, targeted therapies should help improve disease outcomes, efficacy, and cost-effectiveness.

Asthma is characterized by typical symptoms, variable airway obstruction and airway inflammation. Most patients with asthma are well controlled when treated with inhaled corticosteroids. However, around 10% have severe asthma, and remain symptomatic and/or at risk of asthma attacks despite maximum inhaled therapy. Identification of eosinophilic airways inflammation is particularly important as biological agents blocking interleukin (IL)-5, IL-13 and both IL-4 and 13 are effective treatments in this sub-group. The future will be identification of potentially responsive patients on the basis of biomarkers rather than arbitrary physiological patterns of disease, and targeted treatment with specific cytokine blockade.

IMMUNOLOGY AND ALLERGY CLINICS OF NORTH AMERICA

THE CLINICS ARE AVAILABLE ONLINE!
Access your subscription at:
www.theclinics.com

Foreword

Severe Asthma: Chipping Away at the Unmet Need

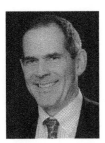

Stephen A. Tilles, MD
Consulting Editor

Only two decades ago, patients with severe, poorly controlled asthma were plentiful, and their treatment often included daily oral prednisone, theophylline, and a short-acting β-agonist dosed every 6 hours. The subsequent availability of high-potency inhaled corticosteroids, long-acting inhaled β-agonists, leukotriene modifiers, and monoclonal anti-IgE upgraded our treatment arsenal dramatically. In fact, because of these advances, many asthma patients currently enjoy a markedly improved quality of life with fewer medication side effects. However, while the total number of severe, poorly controlled asthma patients may be smaller than it once was, there is still a significant unmet need that has encouraged continued innovation to help these patients. In this issue of *Immunology and Allergy Clinics of North America*, Rohit Katial has assembled an impressive group of prominent authors to provide cutting-edge reviews on a wide range of topics relating to severe asthma. Topics include pathophysiology, genetics, immunological and radiographic diagnostics, comorbidities and, importantly, a comprehensive range of therapeutic approaches from biopharmaceutical targets to Traditional Chinese Medicine. This *Immunology and Allergy Clinics of North America* issue is a "must-have" reference for all practicing asthma specialists.

Stephen A. Tilles, MD
ASTHMA Inc. Clinical Research Center
Northwest Asthma and Allergy Center
University of Washington
9725 Third Avenue NE
Suite 500
Seattle, WA 98115, USA

E-mail address:
stilles@nwasthma.com

http://dx.doi.org/10.1016/j.iac.2016.05.002
0889-8561/16/$ – see front matter © 2016 Published by Elsevier Inc.
immunology.theclinics.com

Preface

Severe Asthma: A Heterogeneous Disease

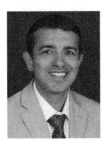

Rohit K. Katial, MD, FACAAI, FAAAAI, FACP
Editor

Severe asthma is a heterogeneous disease characterized by variable airflow obstruction with cough, dyspnea, and wheezing. Such patients are at risk of exacerbations, which may lead to hospitalization, and in rare circumstances, death. Over the past decades, the prevalence of severe asthma has been estimated to be around 5% to 10% of the total asthmatic population. However, the exact prevalence is not known because of the lack of an accurate and consistent definition of severe asthma. In the literature, a distinction is sometimes made between "difficult-to-control asthma" and "severe refractory asthma." In patients with difficult-to-control asthma, the lack of asthma control is generally due to other factors than asthma itself, such as nonadherence to treatment or comorbidities. On the other hand, in patients with severe refractory asthma, the disease remains uncontrolled despite addressing and removing all possible factors that might aggravate the underlying disease. Management of severe asthma is associated with a high and disproportionate consumption of health care resources. In addition, there exists a substantial unmet clinical need. Therefore, much research is currently ongoing on topics such as assessment and evaluation, phenotyping, and novel treatment modalities for severe asthma.

The majority of patients with asthma can be treated effectively with the currently available medications. However, a proportion of patients labeled as "severe refractory asthma" remain a challenge for the treating clinician. Recently, monoclonal antibodies targeting interleukin-4 receptor, interleukin-5, and interleukin-13 have demonstrated efficacy by reducing exacerbations when administered in addition to standard therapies in severe asthma. Highlighting the importance of phenotyping, these therapeutics have enhanced efficacy in subjects selected based on elevated eosinophils or T helper 2–associated markers. Therefore, it becomes imperative for the clinician dealing with these difficult patients to have a more complete understanding of this group's heterogeneity in order to target therapy appropriately. This issue on severe asthma provides a

Immunol Allergy Clin N Am 36 (2016) xv–xvi
http://dx.doi.org/10.1016/j.iac.2016.05.001
0889-8561/16/$ – see front matter © 2016 Published by Elsevier Inc.

immunology.theclinics.com

comprehensive review covering genetics, physiology, biomarkers, comorbidities, phenotypes, psychosocial factors, as well as traditional and emerging therapies.

Rohit K. Katial, MD, FACAAI, FAAAAI, FACP
National Jewish Health
1400 Jackson Street
Denver, CO 80206, USA

E-mail address:
katialr@njhealth.org

Epidemiology and Pulmonary Physiology of Severe Asthma

Jacqueline O'Toole, DO[a], Lucas Mikulic, MD[b],
David A. Kaminsky, MD[c],*

KEYWORDS

- Demographics • Phenotype • Health care utilization • Pulmonary function
- Lung elastic recoil • Ventilation heterogeneity • Gas trapping
- Airway hyperresponsiveness

KEY POINTS

- The definition of severe asthma is still a work in progress.
- The severity of asthma is predictive of higher health care utilization.
- Cluster analysis is useful in characterizing severe asthma phenotypes.
- Airway hyperresponsiveness in severe asthma is a result of abnormal airflow, lung recoil, ventilation, and gas trapping.
- Patients with severe asthma may have a reduced perception of dyspnea.

INTRODUCTION

Severe asthma is a characterized by a complex set of clinical, demographic, and physiologic features. In this article, we review both the epidemiology and pulmonary physiology associated with severe asthma.

DEMOGRAPHICS OF SEVERE ASTHMA

Asthma has long been recognized as a worldwide noncommunicable disease of importance. Within the population of individuals with asthma, there is a subgroup of individuals at high risk for complications, exacerbations, and a poor quality of life.

The authors have nothing to disclose.
[a] Department of Medicine, University of Vermont Medical Center, 111 Colchester Avenue, Burlington, VT 05401, USA; [b] Division of Pulmonary and Critical Care Medicine, University of Vermont Medical Center, Given D208, 89 Beaumont Avenue, Burlington, VT 05405, USA; [c] Division of Pulmonary and Critical Care Medicine, University of Vermont College of Medicine, Given D213, 89 Beaumont Avenue, Burlington, VT 05405, USA
* Corresponding author.
E-mail address: David.kaminsky@uvm.edu

Immunol Allergy Clin N Am 36 (2016) 425–438
http://dx.doi.org/10.1016/j.iac.2016.03.001
0889-8561/16/$ – see front matter

These individuals are classified with severe asthma and they account for 5% to 15% of individuals with asthma in the United States and the world.[1,2] Severe asthma, as defined by the American Thoracic Society and European Respiratory Society (ATS/ERS) clinical practice guidelines, is asthma requiring treatment with high-dose inhaled corticosteroids (ICS) and a second controller during the prior year, and/or oral steroids for at least half of the prior year to prevent symptoms from becoming uncontrolled.[1] Severe asthma also can be described as uncontrolled despite reliance on ICS or frequent oral steroid use.[3] Most of these population numbers are based on questionnaires investigating reported symptoms, particularly the presence of wheezing to assess global asthma burden. Wheezing notoriously overdiagnoses asthma, so may create a slightly higher prevalence than the population truly represents. According to information from the Centers for Disease Control and Prevention (CDC) and Environmental Protection Agency, in 2011, there were 25.9 million individuals in the United States, including 7.1 million children, diagnosed with asthma.[4] In a similar effort in 2013, the CDC found asthma prevalence of 7.3% in America with 8.3% prevalence in children and 7% prevalence in adults. In the black population in the United States there was an almost 50% increase in asthma diagnoses over the past 10 years. Epidemiologic research is ongoing to investigate environmental and social influences on race patterns in asthma prevalence.[5] Evidence also shows that although poverty level does not significantly affect the frequency of asthma attacks among children, adults with incomes less than 250% of the federal poverty level were more likely to report asthma attacks than those with incomes over 450% of the poverty level.[6] Asthma also accounts for a significant number of deaths both in the United States and worldwide. In 2007 alone, there were 3447 deaths in the United States attributed to asthma.[7] Data collected in 2010 as part of the National Hospital Ambulatory Medical Care Survey identified asthma exacerbations as the primary visit diagnosis for more than 15 million office visits and outpatient medical center visits along with 2 million emergency department (ED) visits.[8]

In The Epidemiology and Natural history of asthma: Outcomes and treatment Regimens (TENOR) cohort of patients with severe asthma, gender was distributed differently between older and younger populations.[9] For the adult patients, 71% were women compared with 43% of adolescents and 34% of children. This is similar to the findings of Zein and colleagues,[2] who observed that after adolescence there is a shift from male-predominant severe asthma to female.

COHORT CHARACTERISTICS OF SEVERE ASTHMA

Over the past 20 years, there have been large cohorts constructed to observe trends in therapies and patient outcomes related to asthma. These were created to better understand high-risk individuals and what traits may contribute to more severe asthma or difficult to control asthma. The 2 largest studies in the United States are the previously mentioned TENOR cohort,[9] and the Severe Asthma Research Program (SARP).[10] In both studies, most patients were enrolled by specialists rather than by identifying asthma based on questionnaires completed by the patient.

The TENOR cohort demonstrated that the presence of a recent exacerbation within 3 months of introduction to the study was the strongest predictor of future asthma exacerbation in individuals older than 12.[9] This remained high when adjusted for patient demographics. Recent exacerbation was defined as an ED visit or overnight hospitalization. Increased risk also remained significant if patients required oral corticosteroids in the 3 months preceding baseline evaluation (**Box 1**). Other factors suggesting high risk included prior pneumonia, intubation, and postbronchodilator

---

Box 1
Predictors of asthma severity as demonstrated in Severe Asthma Research Program (SARP) and The Epidemiology and Natural history of asthma: Outcomes and treatment Regimens (TENOR) cohorts

- Emergency visit or hospital stay within prior 3 months
- Use of oral corticosteroids within prior 3 months
- Prior pneumonia or intubation
- Postbronchodilator forced vital capacity (FVC) less than 70% predicted
- Prebronchodilator FEV1 diminished
- Lower than normal level of blood basophils
- Asthma symptoms with routine physical activity
- Fewer number of positive skin tests

Children

- Nonwhite
- More than 3 allergic triggers

---

forced vital capacity (FVC) less than 70% predicted. Additional predictors of exacerbations in children included nonwhite ethnicity and presence of more than 3 allergic triggers.[11]

In adults older than 65, the older patients had lower health care utilization, better reported quality of life, and fewer control issues despite the presence of worse lung function when compared with those younger than 65. In this study, it was unclear if this was related to better compliance and more extensive medication regimens. Overall, the severe asthma classification primarily included adults older than 18 years, those with weight gain over time, black race, persistent airflow limitation, and aspirin-sensitive asthma.[9]

The SARP cohort was created after the 2000 National Heart, Lung, and Blood Institute workshop on severe asthma to investigate characteristics of those with severe asthma and create more succinct diagnostic criteria.[10] This study enrolled patients from major sites in the United States and from 1 European site. The analysis of this cohort revealed various patterns based on objective (pulmonary function, skin prick testing, and immunoglobulin [Ig]E levels) and self-reported questionnaire assessments. The characteristics that independently increased the likelihood of having severe asthma were the presence of diminished prebronchodilator forced expiratory volume in 1 second (FEV1), which carried a 36% increase in likelihood of severe asthma with every 5% decrease in percent predicted FEV1, history of pneumonia, lower number of blood basophils, asthma symptoms during routine physical activity, and lower numbers of positive skin allergy tests. In the population younger than 12 years old included in SARP, the duration of asthma, baseline lung function, and the number of controller medications required were most consistently predictive of the asthma phenotype.[12]

The most frequently reported symptoms among the severe asthma group in the SARP cohort were cough and shortness of breath. This cohort did show that daily cough, chest tightness, and nighttime symptoms were associated with higher health care utilization, suggesting greater impact on individuals' lives than those with different symptoms.[10]

FINANCIAL IMPACT

Severe asthma accounts for a greater proportion of costs and health care utilization compared with controlled asthma. The TENOR data demonstrated that costs increase directly with number of control issues.[13] This mimics a prospective study done in 1996 in France for 1 year following costs related to asthma and severity of asthma.[14] In the 3 months before enrollment in TENOR cohort, 10% of individuals had at least 1 hospitalization or ED visit for asthma for adults, adolescents, and children. Also reported was 50% of adults and 40% of adolescents had oral corticosteroid bursts and unplanned primary care appointments in that time frame for asthma symptoms. High-dose ICS were used in 56% of children and 26% of adolescents at onset of this study. There were consistently high rates of reliance on the health care system despite use of high-dose ICS in these patients. In the TENOR cohort, 53% of adults and 44% of adolescents who were on long-term controllers required oral corticosteroid (OCS) bursts in the 3 months before study initiation.[11] In this same cohort, patients with controlled asthma had fewer work and school absences, and asthma costs increased directly with number of control problems. In the TENOR group, the average cost throughout the 3-year study for uncontrolled asthma was $14,212 compared with $6452 for controlled asthma per patient.[11] Additionally, according to the CDC, asthma accounted for $56 billion in medical costs including lost school and work days, and early death in 2007; $50 billion of that was accounted for by direct medical costs. Over the span of 2002 to 2007, cost was estimated at $3300 per person per year in health care expenses.[7]

DISEASE HETEROGENEITY OF SEVERE ASTHMA

Asthma is a heterogeneous disease with many potential targets for improvement in control. One set of variables related to severity and control involves environment and exposures. Sheehan and Phipatankul[15] completed a review looking at asthma control and environmental factors. This review showed that children with comorbid severe allergic rhinitis were more likely to have uncontrolled asthma. Additionally, this review highlighted the growing argument that exposure and sensitization to mouse allergen is more predictive of severe asthma than cockroach antigen.[16] It is also interesting to note that although the public limitation of tobacco use has translated to some decreases in childhood hospitalizations related to tobacco exposure, there is also a trend toward increased indoor pollutants as homes become more insulated to promote energy efficiency.[15] Otherwise, tobacco use and exposure are related to more severe symptoms and worse control along with diminished response to ICS.[15] Additional trends shown to be associated with more severe asthma include smoking and second-hand smoke exposure. It is found that those with severe sinus disease, gastroesophageal reflux disease, and obstructive sleep apnea also have a tendency to experience more severe asthma exacerbations. Adults with sensitization to aspergillus have an association with more severe asthma onset as adults.[1]

Because of the heterogeneity across this disease category, clusters of similar characteristics are becoming identified as more descriptive phenotypes to guide management. This may prove to be more helpful in guiding therapy than classification based on level of control alone. From the SARP data set, 5 clusters of asthma were identified as having similar characteristics.[17] The first 2 clusters involved individuals with atopic asthma. Atopic or eosinophilic asthma is currently one of the most commonly recognized asthma phenotypes. As many as 50% to 60% of asthma cases can be attributed to atopy.[18] IgE mediates the allergic response in asthma, and individuals with asthma have higher levels of IgE than their counterparts without asthma. In the TENOR cohort,

IgE levels were found to be higher in men compared with women and in children and adolescents compared with adults and correlated to severity of asthma in younger individuals.[11] IgE levels were also higher in smokers compared with former or never smokers and adults with childhood-onset asthma compared with the adult-onset asthma population. IgE levels were also higher in nonwhite individuals compared with white individuals. When corrected for education level only, there remained a significant difference in IgE levels between black and nonblack groups. Among African American participants in SARP, there was an increase in number of mast cells with higher IgE levels bound to these mast cells.[19] Atopic asthma was divided into younger, mostly female individuals with childhood-onset atopic asthma and normal lung function and older subjects, 66% of whom were women with primarily childhood-onset, atopic asthma. In the older subjects there is a trend of predominantly normal prebronchodilator lung function or lung function that had reversed to normal over the course of the study period. These individuals relied more on medications than the group younger at diagnosis.[17] This phenotype was also described by Haldar and colleagues[20] in a subset of individuals with refractory asthma and poor medication compliance. The early-onset atopic group in this descriptive study also required high doses of corticosteroid therapy similar to the SARP cluster 2.

The third SARP cluster of individuals was predominantly female, older age, and obese, with a body mass index (BMI) higher than 30 kg/m^2. These individuals had late-onset asthma and were less likely to be atopic. Although they have shorter duration of their asthma history, they were more likely to have diminished pulmonary function at baseline.[17] This phenotype has been an increasingly important focus of research and characterized elsewhere. These individuals tend to have worse control, poor response to controller medication, and disease complicated by presence of obesity-related comorbidities and metabolic issues.[21] Obesity-related asthma has also been described to have decreased airway inflammation suggesting adipokines play a role in mediating disease.[22] The exact mechanism of how obesity influences asthma remains unclear but is an important research area.

An additional cluster consisted of individuals with a long duration of disease and a severe reduction in baseline pulmonary function. This was divided into 2 groups based on ability to reverse lung function after bronchodilator, as well as different degrees of atopy and age of onset of disease. Nearly half also required 3 or more OCS bursts over the prior year, with 70% of this cohort having some aspect of daily symptoms and poor quality of life.[17] Additionally, in the TENOR cohort, it was observed that black patients had a higher frequency of ED visits and more problems with asthma control. There was also a pattern of worse quality of life and more reliance on 3 or more control medications. This did not change statistically when adjusted for socioeconomics, disease severity, BMI, allergen sensitivity, or medication adherence. This suggests there is a genetic component trending data this way. As of yet, the exact mechanism remains unclear, but IgE levels and TH2-related alleles are both areas of investigation.[9,23]

PULMONARY PHYSIOLOGY OF SEVERE ASTHMA

Severe asthma includes asthma phenotypes of a wide variety. Although much has been learned about severe asthma from studying large cohorts of patients, we also need to investigate the pathophysiology of severe asthma to help discriminate among the various phenotypes and better understand and address this large public health issue. These physiologic abnormalities can be categorized as alterations in airflow, airway resistance, lung recoil, gas trapping, ventilation heterogeneity, airway hyperresponsiveness, and perception of dyspnea (**Fig. 1**). In the following sections we examine each of these areas as they relate to severe asthma.

AIRFLOW

The most important hallmark of the physiologic definition of asthma is variable and reversible airflow limitation. Of all the pulmonary function tests, FEV1 is the most reliable indicator of the severity of airflow limitation, but it correlates poorly with severity of disease.[24] Although asthma is characterized as severe when FEV1 is less than 60% predicted,[25] other criteria can define severe asthma even with normal lung function.[10,26] Patients with severe asthma may have incomplete or poorly reversible airflow limitation,[27] and reversibility does not appear to influence survival.[28] When reversibility does occur, it appears to be due mainly to an increase in FVC, suggesting a reduction in gas trapping.[29] A recent study has shown that gas trapping (elevated residual volume/total lung capacity (RV/TLC)) was present in 48% of patients with poorly controlled asthma.[30] Severe asthma is also characterized by reduced fluctuations in low lung function (peak flow), suggesting less ability of the airway tree to respond to therapy.[31] Patients with severe asthma have accelerated loss of lung function over time compared with patients with mild to moderate asthma and healthy controls, which is related to increased airway wall thickness by computed tomography (CT) imaging.[32]

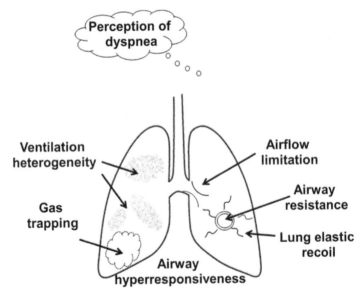

Fig. 1. Physiologic abnormalities in severe asthma. Multiple physiologic abnormalities occur in severe asthma. Like all asthma, severe asthma is characterized by airflow limitation that may be reversible. Airflow limitation is caused by variable contributions of increased airway resistance and reduced lung elastic recoil. In addition, airway narrowing results in ventilation heterogeneity throughout the lung, which may become extreme and result in airway closure with consequent gas trapping. All of these factors may contribute to the development of airway hyperresponsiveness. In addition, patients with severe asthma or poorly controlled asthma that have had near fatal events also have a reduced perception of dyspnea, making it extremely dangerous for them to develop severe lung dysfunction without sufficient awareness in time to seek medical care.

AIRWAY RESISTANCE

The fundamental mechanisms behind airflow limitation are loss of elastic recoil and increased airway resistance upstream from the equal pressure point that occurs during forced expiration.[33,34] Airway resistance (Raw) is increased by any process that narrows the airway lumen, which may include airway smooth muscle constriction, airway wall thickening, luminal mucus and inflammation, and loss of elastic recoil.

Raw is usually measured clinically during body plethysmography; however, measuring overall Raw may not detect subtle abnormalities in the lung periphery, where the total cross-sectional area of the airways is so large that this area only contributes approximately 10% of total airway resistance.[35] One method that may yield insight into this "silent zone" is the forced oscillation technique (FOT), which, because it probes the lung across different frequencies of imposed airflow, is able to differentiate proximal from distal contributions to lung mechanics and measure the contributions to lung impedance by resistance and reactance.[36]

The FOT has revealed that small airway dysfunction plays a crucial role in the pathophysiology of severe asthma.[26,37] For example, Lutchen and colleagues[38] showed that the response to methacholine in asthma results in a heterogeneous constriction pattern, which derives from airway closure that is poorly responsive to deep inflation. Alfieri and colleagues[39] evaluated the response to methacholine in patients with asthma by using FEV1 and FOT. Small airway dysfunction by FOT was more associated with excessive bronchoconstriction (fall in FVC), than with sensitivity to methacholine (fall in FEV1), implicating small airway closure in the response. Shi and colleagues[40] showed that indexes of peripheral airway dysfunction by FOT are more common in children with poor asthma control, and may predict loss of control. In adults, asthma control is associated with changes in lung reactance, reflecting residual peripheral airway dysfunction related to ventilation heterogeneity, airway closure, and gas trapping.[41]

LOSS OF ELASTIC RECOIL

In addition to increased Raw, airflow limitation may also be due to loss of elastic recoil. This has usually been associated with emphysema, but the loss of lung recoil has been noted in previous studies of patients with asthma.[42,43] Typically, the pressure-volume curve of the lung in individuals with asthma is shifted up, but has a normal slope, reflecting that the elastic properties of the lung are normal.[43] Yet some studies have shown that patients with asthma have a loss of elastic recoil when compared with healthy subjects.[44] This is in the absence of any abnormalities by CT imaging or diffusing capacity of the lung for carbon monoxide (DLCO) to suggest the presence of emphysema, and has been dubbed "pseudophysiologic emphysema."[42] The mechanism for the loss of recoil is unknown, but recently autopsy examination has revealed mild centrilobular emphysema not apparent by CT.[45] Loss of recoil would have profound consequences for airway narrowing, as the loss of interdependence between airways and parenchyma would allow excessive airway narrowing during bronchoconstriction.[44] This has been seen in near-fatal asthma[44] and in patients with asthma–chronic obstructive pulmonary disease overlap syndrome.[45] The mechanism of the loss of interdependence is unknown, but may be due to peribronchial inflammation,[46] remodeling of the outer airway wall,[47] or loss of surrounding alveolar attachments,[48] all of which may uncouple the airway wall from the tethering forces of the lung tissue and allow unopposed airway narrowing or closure.

Another interesting aspect of lung function in asthma related to lung recoil is the response to deep inhalation. Healthy subjects and individuals with asthma exposed to an acute bronchoconstricting stimulus typically bronchodilate in response to a deep breath.[37] However, in spontaneous obstruction of patients with asthma, a deep breath results in bronchoconstriction.[37] The mechanisms involved in these effects are unclear, but may relate to relative hysteresis of airway and lung parenchyma, airway smooth muscle contractile properties, and altered forces of interdependence.[49] The ability to bronchodilate in response to a deep breath is less with increasing severity of asthma,[50] and failure of a deep breath to protect against bronchoconstriction is associated with airways hyperresponsiveness.[51] The failure to bronchodilate in response to a deep breath may be a fundamental defect in severe asthma that inhibits the ability of deep breaths to defend against severe airway narrowing.[52]

GAS TRAPPING

In addition to the FEV1 being a key indicator of airflow limitation, the FVC also is important in asthma. First, because the FVC is measured during a forced expiration, it may be reduced by gas compression and early airway closure. In severe asthma, Wenzel and colleagues[53] showed that there is a reduced FVC/slow vital capacity (SVC) ratio in a group of individuals with severe asthma with persistent eosinophilia who were at higher risk for near-fatal events, suggesting a higher propensity to airway closure during forced expiration. Gibbons and colleagues[54] described how falls in FVC following methacholine reflect excessive bronchoconstriction, reflecting extreme airway narrowing or airway closure in the lung periphery. Sorkness and colleagues[29] further developed this concept, evaluating the FVC as a surrogate for gas trapping, and the FEV1/FVC ratio as a marker of airflow limitation in individuals with severe and nonsevere asthma. They found that compared with individuals with nonsevere asthma, individuals with severe asthma had lower FEV1, lower FVC, and higher RV/TLC, even if no airflow limitation was seen on spirometry, reflecting a higher degree of gas trapping in the severe asthma group. Using the single breath nitrogen washout technique, airway closure has been shown to be associated with recurrent exacerbations in severe asthma.[55] In addition, airtrapping on CT imaging is also associated with severity of asthma, asthma-related hospitalizations, and need for mechanical ventilation among patients with severe asthma.[56]

In addition to an elevated RV/TLC and consequent lower FVC, patients with severe asthma may have an elevated functional residual capacity (FRC),[30] which may be due, in part, to gas trapping. In addition, as FRC relates directly to the balance of recoil forces between lung and chest wall, the mechanism may also relate to a prolonged respiratory system time constant from increased airway resistance, with a consequent reduction in the time available for the lungs to empty.[57] There is also evidence for increased inspiratory muscle activity during expiration, resulting in a higher FRC that allows for tidal breathing at a lower airway resistance.[57,58]

VENTILATION HETEROGENEITY

Ventilation heterogeneity refers to the unevenness of ventilation seen by gas distribution tests, frequency dependence of resistance or reactance by the FOT, and by imaging studies. Ventilation heterogeneity likely contributes to severe asthma because of the increased work of breathing expected, the derangements in gas exchange, and its association with airway hyperresponsiveness (AHR).[59,60] Increased ventilation heterogeneity, as reflected by an elevated Phase III slope during a single breath nitrogen washout, is seen in patients with poorly controlled asthma.[61] Studies performing multiple breath nitrogen washout (MBNW) have revealed that severe asthma is characterized by ventilation heterogeneity in the lung periphery measured by abnormalities in the convection (conducting airways) and diffusion-dependent (acinar airways) components of the Phase III slope. In severe asthma, Thompson and colleagues[62] found that FEV1 correlated with acinar ventilation heterogeneity. However, neither acinar nor conductive ventilation heterogeneity was associated with gas trapping, which the investigators hypothesized was therefore due to widespread airway closure in many parts of the lung. Similarly, Farah and colleagues[63] showed that poor asthma control is associated with small airways disease by MBNW and treatment with ICS improves these abnormalities and asthma control.

Imaging studies also evaluate ventilation heterogeneity in the lung. Xenon ventilation CT and hyperpolarized xenon or helium lung MRI ventilation are 2 techniques that can be used to quantify ventilation heterogeneity. For example, Samee and colleagues[64] and Altes and colleagues[65] showed that patients with severe asthma have more ventilation defects, as seen by hyperpolarized MRI. In an elegant correlative study, Gonem and colleagues[66] demonstrated that acinar ventilation heterogeneity by MBNW corresponds to acinar ventilation defects by hyperpolarized MRI and airtrapping by CT, especially in individuals with severe asthma.

AIRWAY HYPERRESPONSIVENESS AND PERCEPTION OF DYSPNEA

Perhaps the most important physiologic characteristic of asthma is AHR, which develops as a consequence of multiple mechanisms.[67] Because severe asthma is associated with these mechanisms, including reduced FEV1, increased airway resistance, loss of recoil, gas trapping, and airway closure, it is no surprise that patients with severe asthma tend to have more AHR,[68] although the relationship between severity of AHR and asthma is variable.[69]

There is a subgroup of patients with severe asthma with marked AHR who are at greater risk of fatal bronchoconstriction. This group has been described as brittle asthma, and is often constituted by highly atopic, young, female patients with a predominant neutrophilic response, in whom symptoms appear to develop suddenly in a matter of hours.[70] Another group of patients with near-fatal asthma is characterized by a predominant eosinophilic inflammatory response that develops over days. This group, which constitutes 80% to 85% of patients with severe asthma, appears to have a decreased perception of dyspnea.[71] Kikuchi and colleagues[72] showed that patients with a history of near-fatal asthma had a decreased perception of dyspnea to both resistive loaded breathing and to hypoxia. Magadle and colleagues[73] demonstrated that patients with asthma with a low perception of dyspnea were older, more often women with a longer duration of asthma, had low daily use of B2 agonist, and more ED visits, admissions to hospital, and death. To date, different mechanisms have been proposed for poor perception, either genetic or acquired, such as adaptation to chronic hypoxic states and blunted respiratory response to hypoxemia.[70,72–74]

The FOT has also been used to explore the relationship between mechanical lung impedance and the sensation of dyspnea in response to bronchial provocation. A study performed by Antonelli and colleagues[75] revealed that dyspnea to methacholine had 2 distinctive patterns depending on the level of bronchoconstriction. With mild bronchoconstriction, dyspnea was associated with measures of airway narrowing and loss of bronchodilation to deep breath, whereas with moderate to severe bronchoconstriction, it was related to ventilation heterogeneity and lung volume recruitment. These responses perhaps suggest a more proximal effect of mild bronchoconstriction, and a more peripheral effect of moderate to severe bronchoconstriction. In support of this, Van der Wiel and colleagues[76] showed that small airways dysfunction, as assessed by FOT, was associated with an increase in dyspnea during methacholine challenge, and with the severity of bronchoconstriction as assessed by the dose response slope.

SUMMARY

Asthma involves multiple abnormalities in the physiologic function of the lung. It appears that severe asthma is particularly characterized by changes in the lung periphery that result in increased airway closure and gas trapping, loss of airway parenchymal interdependence, and increased ventilation heterogeneity, all of which contribute to increased AHR. In addition, severe asthma associated with near-fatal events is characterized by reduced perception of dyspnea. All of these components may contribute to not only the baseline severity of asthma, but also the propensity for loss of asthma control and near-fatal exacerbations.

REFERENCES

1. Chung K, Wenzel S, Brozek J, et al. International ERS/ATS guidelines on definition, evaluation and treatment of severe asthma. Eur Respir J 2014;43:343–73.
2. Zein J, Dweik R, Comhair S, et al. Asthma is more severe in older adults. PLoS One 2015;10:e0133490.
3. Thomson C, Welsh C, Carno M, et al. ATS Clinical Practice Guideline: summary for clinicians. Ann Am Thorac Soc 2014;11:996–7.
4. National Center for Health Statistics, CDC. Environmental Protection Agency fact sheet. National health interview survey data on lifetime asthma prevalence 2011. Available at: www.CDC.gov. Accessed August 1, 2015.
5. Wright R, Suglia S, Levy J, et al. Transdisciplinary research strategies for understanding socially patterned disease: the Asthma Coalition on Community, Environment, and Social Stress (ACCESS) project as a case study. Cien Saude Colet 2008;13:1729–41.
6. Moorman J, Person C, Zahran H. Asthma attacks among persons with current asthma—United States, 2001-2010. CDC health disparities and inequalities report—US 2013. MMWR Morb Mortal Wkly Rep 2013;62:93–7.
7. Centers for Disease Control and Prevention. Vital signs asthma. 2011. Available at: www.cdc.gov/nchs. Accessed August 2, 2015.
8. National hospital ambulatory medical care survey: 2010 emergency department summary tables. 2010. Available at: http://www.cdc.gov/nchs/data/ahcd/nhamcs_emergency/2010_ed_web_tables.pdf. Accessed August 2, 2015.
9. Chipps B, Haselkorn T, TENOR Study Group. Key findings and clinical implications from the epidemiology and natural history of asthma: outcomes and treatment regimens (TENOR) study. J Allergy Clin Immunol 2012;130:332–43.
10. Moore W, Bleecker E, Curran-Everett D, et al. Characterization of the severe asthma phenotype by the NHLBI severe asthma research program. J Allergy Clin Immunol 2007;119:405–13.
11. Chipps B, Zeiger R, Dorenbaum A, et al. Assessment of asthma control and asthma exacerbations in the epidemiology and natural history of asthma: outcomes and treatment regimens (TENOR) observational cohort. Curr Respir Care Rep 2012;1:259–69.
12. Fitzpatrick A, Teague G, Meyers D, et al. Heterogeneity of severe asthma in childhood: confirmation by cluster analysis of children in the National Institutes of Health/National Heart, Lung, and Blood Institute Severe Asthma Research Program. J Allergy Clin Immunol 2010;127:382–9.

13. Sullivan S, Rasouliyan L, Russo P, et al. Extent, patterns, and burden of uncontrolled disease in severe or difficult to treat asthma. Allergy 2007;62:126–33.

14. Godard P, Chanez P, Siraudin L, et al. Costs of asthma are correlated with severity: a 1-yr prospective study. Eur Respir J 2002;19:61–8.

15. Sheehan W, Phipatankul W. Difficult to control asthma: epidemiology and its link with environmental factors. Curr Opin Allergy Clin Immunol 2015;15:397–401.

16. Ownby D. Will the real inner city allergen please standup? J Allergy Clin Immunol 2013;132:836–7.

17. Moore W, Meyers D, Wenzel S, et al. Identification of asthma phenotypes using cluster analysis in the severe asthma research program. Am J Respir Crit Care Med 2010;181:315–23.

18. Arbes S, Calatroni A, Mitchell H, et al. Age-dependent interaction between atopy and eosinophils in asthma cases: results from NHANES 2005-2006. Clin Exp Allergy 2013;43:544–50.

19. Jarjour N, Erzurum S, Bleecker E, et al. Severe asthma: lessons learned from the National Heart, Lung, and Blood Institute Severe Asthma Research Program. Am J Respir Crit Care Med 2012;185:356–62.

20. Haldar P, Pavord I, Shaw D, et al. Cluster analysis and clinical asthma phenotypes. Am J Respir Crit Care Med 2008;178:218–24.

21. Lugugo N, Kraft M, Dixon A. Does obesity produce a distinct asthma phenotype? Pulmonary physiology and pathophysiology of disease. J Appl Physiol 2010;108: 729–33.

22. Sideleva O, Suratt B, Black K, et al. Obesity and asthma an inflammatory disease of adipose tissue not the airway. Am J Respir Crit Care Med 2012;186:598–605.

23. Gamble C, Talbott E, Israel E, et al. Racial differences in biologic predictors of severe asthma: data from the severe asthma research program. J Allergy Clin Immunol 2010;126(6):1149–55.

24. Teeter J, Bleecker E. Relationship between airway obstruction and respiratory symptoms in adult asthmatics. Chest 1998;113:272–7.

25. Busse WW, Camargo CA, Boushey HA, et al. Expert Panel Report 3: Guidelines for the diagnosis and management of asthma - Summary Report 2007. Washington, DC: US Department of Health and Human Services, National Institutes of Health, National Heart, Lung, and Blood Institute; 2007.

26. Wenzel S. Physiologic and pathologic abnormalities in severe asthma. Clin Chest Med 2006;27:29–40.

27. The ENFUMOSA Group. The ENFUMOSA cross-sectional European multicentre study of the clinical phenotype of chronic severe asthma. Eur Respir J 2003; 22:470–7.

28. Hansen E, Phanareth K, Laursen L, et al. Reversible and irreversible airflow obstruction as predictor of overall mortality in asthma and chronic obstructive pulmonary disease. Am J Respir Crit Care Med 1999;159:1267–71.

29. Sorkness R, Bleecker E, Busse W, et al. Lung function in adults with stable but severe asthma: air trapping and incomplete reversal of obstruction with bronchodilation. J Appl Physiol 2008;104:394–403.

30. Perez T, Chanez P, Dusser D, et al. Prevalence and reversibility of lung hyperinflation in adult asthmatics with poorly controlled disease and significant dyspnea. Allergy 2016;71(1):108–14.

31. Thamrin C, Nydegger R, Stern G, et al. Associations between fluctuations in lung function and asthma control in two populations with differing asthma severity. Thorax 2011;66:1036–42.

32. Witt C, Sheshadri A, Carsltrom L, et al. Longitudinal changes in airway remodeling and air trapping in severe asthma. Acad Radiol 2014;21:986–93.

33. Mead J, Turner J, Macklem P, et al. Significance of the relationship between lung recoil and maximum expiratory flow. J Appl Physiol 1967;22:95–108.

34. Pride N, Permutt S, Riley R, et al. Determination of maximum expiratory flow from the lungs. J Appl Physiol 1967;23:646–62.

35. Macklem P, Mead J. Resistance of central and peripheral airways measured by a retrograde catheter. J Appl Physiol 1967;22:395–401.

36. Bates J, Irvin C, Farre R, et al. Oscillation mechanics of the respiratory system. Compr Physiol 2011;1:1233–72.

37. Papa G, Pellegrino G, Pellegrino R. Asthma and respiratory physiology: putting lung function into perspective. Respirology 2014;19:960–9.

38. Lutchen K, Jensen A, Atileh H, et al. Airway constriction pattern is a central component of asthma severity. The role of deep inspirations. Am J Respir Crit Care Med 2001;164:207–15.

39. Alfieri V, Aiello M, Pisi R, et al. Small airway dysfunction is associated to excessive bronchoconstriction in asthmatic patients. Respir Res 2014;15:86.

40. Shi Y, Aledia A, Galant S, et al. Peripheral airway impairment measured by oscillometry predicts loss of asthma control in children. J Allergy Clin Immunol 2013; 131:718–23.

41. Kelly V, Sands S, Harris S, et al. Respiratory system reactance is an independent determinant of asthma control. J Appl Physiol 2013;115:1360–9.

42. Gelb A, Licuanan J, Shinar C. Unsuspected pseudophysiologic emphysema in chronic persistent asthma. Am J Respir Crit Care Med 2000;162:1778–82.

43. Woolcock A, Read J. The static elastic properties in the lungs in asthma. Am Rev Respir Dis 1968;98:788–94.

44. Gelb A, Schein A, Nussbaum E, et al. Risk factors for near-fatal asthma. Chest 2004;126:1138–46.

45. Gelb A, Yamamoto A, Verbeken E, et al. Unraveling the pathophysiology of the asthma-COPD overlap syndrome. Chest 2015;148:313–20.

46. Macklem P. Mechanical factors determining maximum bronchoconstriction. Eur Respir J Suppl 1989;6:516s–9s.

47. Dolhnikoff M, da Silva L, de Araujo B, et al. The outer wall of small airways is a major site of remodeling in fatal asthma. J Allergy Clin Immunol 2009;123:1090–7.

48. Mauad T, Silva L, Santos M, et al. Abnormal alveolar attachments with decreased elastic fiber content in distal lung in fatal asthma. Am J Respir Crit Care Med 2004;170:857–62.

49. Pellegrino R, Violante B, Brusasco V. Maximal bronchoconstriction in humans. Relationship to deep inhalation and airway sensitivity. Am J Respir Crit Care Med 1996;153:115–21.

50. Scichilone N, Marchese R, Soresi S, et al. Deep inspiration-induced changes in lung volume decrease with severity of asthma. Respir Med 2007;101:951–6.

51. Scichilone N, Permutt S, Togias A. The lack of the bronchoprotective and not the bronchodilatory ability of deep inspiration is associated with airway hyperresponsiveness. Am J Respir Crit Care Med 2001;163:413–9.

52. Skloot G, Permutt S, Togias A. Airway hyperresponsiveness in asthma: a problem of limited smooth muscle relaxation with inspiration. J Clin Invest 1995;96:2393–403.

53. Wenzel S, Schwartz L, Langmack E, et al. Evidence that severe asthma can be divided pathologically into two inflammatory subtypes with distinct physiologic and clinical characteristics. Am J Respir Crit Care Med 1999;160:1001–8.

54. Gibbons W, Sharma A, Lougheed D, et al. Detection of excessive bronchoconstriction in asthma. Am J Respir Crit Care Med 1996;153:582–9.
55. in't Veen J, Beekman A, Bel E, et al. Recurrent exacerbations in severe asthma are associated with enhanced airway closure during stable episodes. Am J Respir Crit Care Med 2000;161:1902–6.
56. Busacker A, Newell J, Keefe T, et al. A multivariate analysis of risk factors for the air-trapping asthmatic phenotype as measured by quantitative CT analysis. Chest 2009;135:48–56.
57. Cormier Y, Lecours R, Legris C. Mechanisms of hyperinflation in asthma. Eur Respir J 1990;3:619–24.
58. Martin J, Powell E, Shore S, et al. The role of respiratory muscles in the hyperinflation of bronchial asthma. Am Rev Respir Dis 1980;121:441–7.
59. Chapman D, Berend N, Horlyck K, et al. Does increased baseline ventilation heterogeneity following chest wall strapping predispose to airway hyperresponsiveness? J Appl Physiol 2012;113:25–30.
60. Kaminsky D, Daud A, Chapman D. Relationship between the baseline alveolar volume-to-total lung capacity ratio and airway responsiveness. Respirology 2014;19:1046–51.
61. Bourdin A, Paganin F, Prefaut C, et al. Nitrogen washout slope in poorly controlled asthma. Allergy 2006;61:85–9.
62. Thompson B, Douglass J, Ellis M, et al. Peripheral lung function in patients with stable and unstable asthma. J Allergy Clin Immunol 2013;131:1322–8.
63. Farah C, King G, Brown N, et al. The role of the small airways in the clinical expression of asthma in adults. J Allergy Clin Immunol 2012;129:381–7.
64. Samee S, Altes T, Powers P, et al. Imaging the lungs in asthmatic patients using hyperpolarized helium-3 magnetic resonance: assessment of response to methacholine and exercise challenge. J Allergy Clin Immunol 2003;111:1205–11.
65. Altes T, Mugler J, Ruppert K, et al. Clinical correlates of lung ventilation defects in asthmatic children. J Allergy Clin Immunol 2016;137(3):789–96.e7.
66. Gonem S, Hardy S, Buhl N, et al. Characterization of acinar airspace involvement in asthmatic patients using inert gas washout and hyperpolarized 3helium magnetic resonance. J Allergy Clin Immunol 2015;137(2):417–25.
67. Berend N, Salome C, King G. Mechanisms of airway hyperresponsiveness in asthma. Respirology 2008;13:624–31.
68. Porsbjerg C, Rasmussen L, Nolte H, et al. Association of airway hyperresponsiveness with reduced quality of life in patients with moderate to severe asthma. Ann Allergy Asthma Immunol 2007;98:44–50.
69. Weiss S, VAN ML, Zeiger R. Relationship between airway hyperresponsiveness and asthma severity in the childhood asthma management program. Am J Respir Crit Care Med 2000;162:50–6.
70. Restrepo R, Peters J. Near-fatal asthma: recognition and management. Curr Opin Pulm Med 2008;14:13–23.
71. in't Veen J, Smits H, Ravensberg A, et al. Impaired perception of dyspnea in patients with severe asthma. Am J Respir Crit Care Med 1998;158:1134–41.
72. Kikuchi Y, Okabe S, Tamura G, et al. Chemosensitivity and reception of dyspnea in patients with a history of near-fatal asthma. N Engl J Med 1994; 330:1329–34.
73. Magadle R, Berar-Yanay N, Weiner P. The risk of hospitalization and near-fatal and fatal asthma in relation to perception of dyspnea. Chest 2002; 121:329–33.

74. Eckert D, Catcheside P, McEvoy R. Blunted sensation of dyspnoea and near fatal asthma. Eur Respir J 2004;24:197–9.
75. Antonelli A, Crimi E, Gobbi A, et al. Mechanical correlates of dyspnea in bronchial asthma. Physiol Rep 2013;1:e00166.
76. van der Weil E, Postma D, van der Molen T, et al. Effects of small airway dysfunction on the clinical expression of asthma: a focus on asthma symptoms and bronchial hyper-responsiveness. Eur J Allergy Clin Immunol 2014;69: 1681–8.

Linkage and Genetic Association in Severe Asthma

Bridgette L. Jones, MD, MSc[a,b,*], Lanny J. Rosenwasser, MD[b]

KEYWORDS

- Asthma • Genetics • Severe • GWAS • Linkage • Genotype • Endotype
- Phenotype

KEY POINTS

- The pathogenesis of severe asthma is poorly understood, which leads to difficulty in management of the disease.
- Genetic variation has been associated with severe asthma in children and adults.
- Genetic association studies may lead to improved understanding of severe asthma pathophysiology and therapeutic treatments.

INTRODUCTION

Severe asthma is defined in the National Heart, Lung, and Blood Institute 2007 guidelines by the frequency of symptoms, β2-agonist use, limitations on daily activities, and exacerbations requiring systemic steroids.[1] The American Thoracic Society (ATS) defines severe asthma as "asthma which requires treatment with high dose inhaled corticosteroids (ICS) plus a second controller (and/or systemic CS) to prevent it from becoming 'uncontrolled' or which remains 'uncontrolled' despite this therapy" (European Respiratory Society/ATS Guidelines on Definition, Evaluation, and Treatment of Severe Asthma). It is estimated that severe asthma occurs in approximately less than 10% of patients with asthma. However, the burden of severe asthma on health care use and expenditures and loss of school/work days are disproportionate compared with milder asthma types.

The authors have no commercial or financial conflicts of interest to disclose.
[a] Division of Pediatric Pharmacology and Therapeutic Innovation, Department of Pediatrics, Children's Mercy Hospitals and Clinics, University of Missouri Kansas City School of Medicine, 2401 Gillham Road, Kansas City, MO 64108, USA; [b] Division of Allergy, Asthma and Clinical Immunology, Department of Pediatrics, Children's Mercy Hospitals and Clinics, University of Missouri Kansas City School of Medicine, 2401 Gillham Road, Kansas City, MO 64108, USA
* Corresponding author. 2401 Gillham Road, Kansas City, MO 64108.
E-mail address: bljones@cmh.edu

Immunol Allergy Clin N Am 36 (2016) 439–447
http://dx.doi.org/10.1016/j.iac.2016.03.002   immunology.theclinics.com
0889-8561/16/$ – see front matter © 2016 Elsevier Inc. All rights reserved.

Overall, severe asthma is poorly understood, although considerable work has been done in the area. The natural history and progression of the disease have not been clearly elucidated. Some patients tend to have severe symptoms in childhood that persist and may worsen in adulthood. Other patients may exhibit a milder disease phenotype in childhood and progress to a more severe phenotype in adulthood. It is also not well understood as to what the primary contributors or triggers are for development of the severe asthma phenotype. Potential triggers or contributors of severe asthma include environment exposures (eg, air pollution), virus exposure, hormonal changes, and comorbid conditions. As phenotypes of asthma related to underlying disease pathophysiology have been more readily recognized, specific pathophysiologic phenotypes have also been associated with severe asthma. Eosinophilic asthma has been described to exist in up to one-half of adult patients with severe asthma, whereby eosinophils persist in the airway despite high-dose inhaled and systemic steroid exposure.[2] Aspirin-induced asthma, characterized by nasal polyps, aspirin sensitivity, and asthma, is another phenotype that has been associated with severe asthma. Prevalence rates of aspirin-induced asthma among adults with severe asthma have been reported at approximately 14%.[3] Neutrophilic asthma has also been associated with severe asthma. Studies have demonstrated that patients with severe asthma often have a neutrophil predominance in their sputum. Neutrophilic asthma has been observed in patients experiencing an exacerbation and also associated with fatal asthma exacerbations.[4] A Pauci-inflammatory phenotype has also been described whereby typical inflammatory cells are not observed on bronchoscopy. Little is known about this possible phenotype, and some have suggested that the lack of inflammatory cells may be the result of corticosteroid treatment rather than a distinct phenotype.[5]

Genetic association studies may lead to better understanding of the severe asthma phenotype regarding biological pathways involved and may also lead to improved treatments. Severe asthma is likely multifactorial, which is the result of specific environmental exposures or triggers in a genetically susceptible host. For example, in some children with a specific genetic makeup, exposure to a specific virus during a specific time in physiologic development may lead to severe asthma. Furthermore, an adult with a specific genetic signature exposed to a certain cumulative environmental exposure may lead to the development of severe asthma. Genetic variation is also important to consider when discussing the variation in observed natural history of the disease and therapeutic response. The purpose of this review is to describe some of the potentially relevant genetic variants that have been associated with severe asthma, which may lead to better understanding of the disease phenotype and improved treatment in the future. Genome-wide association studies (GWAS) and candidate gene studies have been important in identifying potential variants and disease pathways to focus on in relation to severe asthma pathogenesis, clinical features, and potentially, treatment response in children and adults.

GENETIC VARIANTS ASSOCIATED WITH SEVERE ASTHMA
17q21 Region

Sequence variation on chromosome 17q21 was initially identified in relation to risk of early-onset childhood asthma and risk of asthma associated with tobacco smoke exposure within GWAS. Among 12 single-nucleotide polymorphisms (SNPs) identified in their analysis to be associated with asthma risk, 7 of them were located in the 17q21 region, indicating that this gene region is likely of importance in the disease.[6] One variant, rs7216389, located in the intronic region of GSDMB, has been associated with expression of a nearby gene *ORMDL3* whereby the gene is reported to be involved in encoding transmembrane proteins in the endoplasmic reticulum. However, the complete function and potential affect in asthma are not understood. The rs7216389 SNP association with early-onset asthma has been replicated within several European and Asian cohorts.[7,8] Furthermore, rs7216389 has been associated with a severe type of early-onset asthma in children, and in the initial study where the region was identified, children included were of more severe asthma phenotype (step 3 or worse).[9] Another study in children also identified an association between the SNP and asthma, asthma exacerbations, school absence, and oral steroid use, suggesting a more severe and/or uncontrolled phenotype association.[10] A subsequent study also found that the SNP was associated with severe asthma classification among patients with childhood onset of asthma.[11] Other studies also have found that rs721389 is associated with symptoms of severe asthma in children, such as exacerbation requiring oral steroids or hospitalization. In a cohort of children in Copenhagen, the hazard ratio (2.73) for development of acute exacerbation requiring oral steroids or hospitalization was almost 3 times among those with homozygous recessive genotype (rs721389 TT) compared with those with heterozygous or homozygous wild-type genotype.[12] The 17q21 region has shown that it is indeed important in severe asthma. Further exploration of the functional significance of observed variants is needed to elucidate the biological impact of genetic variation in this region and potentially lead to improved interventions for those with genetic variation in the region.

Interleukin-33/IL1RL1

Multiple genetic variants within *IL33* and *IL1RL1* have been identified to be associated with asthma via GWAS and candidate gene studies conducted among primarily Caucasian participants.[13] The interleukin-33 (IL-33)/ILqRL1 pathway has been implicated in the regulation of several cytokines and to be involved in the TH_2 inflammatory response. *IL33*, located on chromosome 9, contains numerous SNPs, which have been mainly identified in noncoding regions and are in strong linkage disequilibrium. *IL1RL1*, on chromosome 2q12, possesses several synonymous and nonsynonymous variants also exhibiting strong linkage among SNPs. Many identified variants within the IL-33/IL1RL1 pathway have varying consequences, such as alterations in gene expression and amino acid changes and are functionally unclear.[14] In vitro studies have shown that IL-33 expression in lung specimens was associated with severe asthma.[15] Other translational studies in children have revealed increased cellular expression of IL-33 in association with increased reticular basement membrane thickness in specimens obtained from children with severe therapy-resistant asthma.[16] The group has also conducted further studies in children confirming the association between IL-33 levels and the severe asthma clinical phenotype.[17] Also, for *IL1RL1*, an SNP (rs1921622) was associated with severe RSV bronchiolitis, requiring mechanical ventilation, in a Dutch neonatal cohort.[18] A GWAS study in a Danish cohort revealed an association between SNPs (rs928413 and rsrs1558641) in *IL33/IL1RL1* gene regions and severe asthma exacerbations as defined by number of hospitalizations.[19] This work suggests that it is an important region for pediatric asthma and especially severe asthma in children. More recent work has also been conducted in adults enrolled in the Severe Asthma Research Program, which has also observed an association between the gene region and asthma severity. This work has also begun to elucidate some of the potential functionally relevance of this gene region as expression of the IL33 receptor, *ST2L*, and severe asthma.[20] However, further work is needed to replicate findings in adults and children and to determine the therapeutic and clinical significance.

Tumor Growth Factor-β

Tumor growth factor-β (TGF-β) is a profibrotic inflammatory cytokine and is involved airway remodeling in the lung. The cytokine exerts affects in the lung, resulting in structural changes, such as subepithelial fibrosis, airway smooth muscle remodeling, and microvascular changes. Several TGF-β SNPs have been associated with asthma severity in children and adults.[21–23] Studies in adults have also revealed potential additive effects of TGF-β variation and tobacco smoke, resulting in severe asthma. Genetic variants in the gene have been associated with irreversible airway obstruction among men who were chronic smokers.[24] Investigators have demonstrated an association between rs1800469 (C-509T) and increased serum TGF-β levels and worsening asthma severity among Taiwanese adults, and another SNP in the promoter region of the gene was also associated with asthma in this cohort.[25] The TGF-β C-509T SNP has been the most consistently replicated variant associated with severe asthma. Other SNPs have also been associated with the disease phenotype; however, they are less replicated. One study found an association between TGF-β rs6957 and more severe airway abnormality. Participants with this variant genotype exhibited increased airway hyperresponsiveness and airflow obstruction, increased subepithelial eosinophil and macrophage counts, and increased basement membrane thickness. Another TGF-β SNP, rs4803455, has also been associated with an accelerated decline in FEV1 (forced expiratory volume in 1 second).[26] Another study also investigated the association between asthma and severe asthma for 4 variants among Caucasian adults (C-509T, T869 C, 915C, 72insC). The investigators only observed an association with these variants when comparing stratified cohorts of severe asthma versus mild asthma phenotype.[27] Another study conducted in both children and adults identified an association between TGF-β1 T869 C and severe asthma classification. However, the investigators did not find an association between the C-509T TGF-β1 SNP and the disease phenotype in this overall younger cohort of participants from Brazil.[28] These studies indicated that the C-509T SNP may be most important in adult-onset severe asthma. As TGF-β has a known functional role in the pathophysiology of asthma and especially one that is plausible to contribute to severe asthma, further work in the area may include potential therapeutic interventions directed toward the pathway, which may have the most significance among those with variant genotypes associated with severe disease.

CHI3L1

Chitin has been described as the second most abundant polysaccharide found in nature after cellulose. Chitin is a major component of several allergen inducers/triggers, such as fungi and house dust mites. Therefore, exposure to the polysaccharide has been shown to illicit inflammatory responses in the lung. Chitin-degrading enzymes, chitinases, are present within the body, including in the human lung, and are involved in the innate immune response to chitin. Chitinase-like proteins, which bind but do not cleave chitin, have been linked to asthma.[29] CH13L1/YKL-40 is a chitinase-like protein that has been demonstrated to have increased serum levels in correlation with asthma severity, and airway remodeling in patients with asthma.[30] A study conducted in children found that YKL-40 serum levels were associated with asthma severity whereby children with higher levels were more likely to have therapy-resistant asthma.[31] These data indicate that chitin regulation is important in disease pathogenesis especially among more severe phenotypes. Genetic variation has been identified within CH13L1, which may also be associated with disease and severity. In a GWAS, investigators identified a CHI3L1 promoter SNP (−131C → G), which was associated with elevated serum YKL-40 levels, asthma, bronchial hyperresponsiveness, and decline in lung function in a Hutterite population of European descent. The same SNP also was predictive of asthma and YKL-40 serum levels during the first 5 years of life in a replication birth cohort.[32] Others have also identified an association between *CHI3L1* genetic variation (rs1538372 and rs10399931) and asthma risk in a Taiwanese population.[33] These genetic variants deserve further exploration especially among those with elevated environmental exposure to chitin and allergic asthma phenotypes.

OTHER POTENTIAL VARIANTS

Other variants have also been identified via GWAS in association with asthma, which may have future implications for severe asthma. With further studies to replicate initial associations with asthma, relevance to severe asthma in children and adults may be revealed (**Table 1**).

Current Controversies/Limitations

As discussed, several potentially important genes and gene regions have been identified that likely influence the severe asthma phenotype. Major limitations in the current knowledge regarding the impact of genetics in severe asthma include (1) lack of study in diverse racial/ethnic populations; and (2) limited understanding of functional significance among several identified genes/gene regions.

Although African Americans suffer disproportionate asthma prevalence, morbidity, and mortality relative to other racial groups, they are significantly understudied within genetic association studies of asthma along with other racial/ethnic groups (eg, Hispanics). The first GWAS study among participants of African ancestry (African American and African Caribbean) was reported in 2010. Investigators identified an association between gene variants and asthma that had not been previously identified in European populations (*ADRA1B, PRNP, DPP10*); however, individual SNP analyses within these genes were not able to be replicated in African American replication cohorts. The investigators point out some of the barriers in genetic studies of African Americans, which include inadequate gene chips for identification of relevant SNPs among African Americans and inadequate statistical capabilities for rare variants.[34] Other understudied and highly affected ethnic groups include those of Hispanic descent whereby similar limitations also exist.

Table 1
Other gene regions to consider in the study of severe asthma

Chromosome	SNP(s)	Gene/Gene Region	Cohort	Reference
5	rs11741137 rs2069885 rs1859430	*IL-9*	Majority Caucasian and Cost Rican Children	35
7	rs6967330	*CDHR3*	Danish children	19
10	rs6585018 rs1322997 rs3410444	*PDCD4*	German children	36
1	rs2786098	*DENND1B*	European and African American children	13
16	rs8832 rs1029489	*IL-4/IL13* pathway	Majority non-Hispanic white	37

Strides should be made to overcome technological and statistical barriers so as to improve the current knowledge of genetics among these groups, leading to better understanding of disease and therapeutic interventions especially for these highly affected groups.

Although several genetic polymorphisms have been identified to be associated with asthma and the severe asthma phenotype, none have had a meaningful clinical impact, allowing inclusion of genetic information in the day-to-day clinical evaluation of asthma; this has been one common criticism of current asthma-related genetic knowledge. Revelation of gene regions (eg, *ORMDL3*, IL33/ILqRL1) associated with asthma has provided important clues about unexplored areas related to disease pathophysiology; however, the functional significance of many of these genes/gene regions is not well understood, which limits the clinical utility for these findings. Future work is needed to explore the functional relevance of identified variants and their impact on disease pathophysiology. This work will also be important in designing therapeutic interventions to target identified disease-causing defects leading to one of the ultimate goals of personalized asthma care (**Fig. 1**).

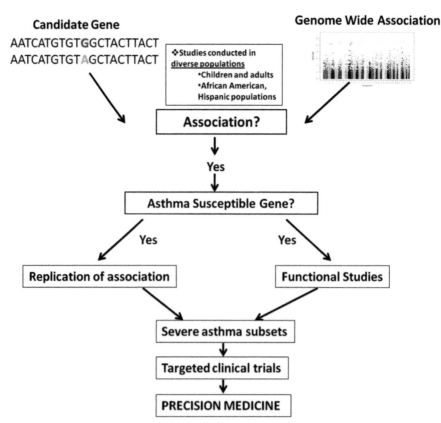

Fig. 1. Paradigm of genetic investigation in severe asthma. (*Adapted from* Meng JF, Rosenwasser L. Unraveling the genetic basis of asthma and allergic diseases. Allergy Asthma Immunol Res 2010;2(4):216.)

FUTURE CONSIDERATIONS/SUMMARY

Severe asthma is a poorly understood phenotype that has led to difficulties in managing the disease and limited effective therapeutic interventions. Genetic studies discussed in this review have revealed novel genes and pathways in association with the disease. Further work in these areas and further exploration of genetic association and linkage in severe asthma will be important to better understanding the pathophysiology of this phenotype and to developing successful therapeutic treatments.

REFERENCES

1. National Asthma Education and Prevention Program. Expert panel report 3 (EPR-3): guidelines for the diagnosis and management of asthma–summary report 2007. J Allergy Clin Immunol 2007;120(5 Suppl):S94–138.
2. Wenzel SE, Schwartz LB, Langmack EL, et al. Evidence that severe asthma can be divided pathologically into two inflammatory subtypes with distinct physiologic and clinical characteristics. Am J Respir Crit Care Med 1999;160(3):1001–8.
3. Mascia K, Haselkorn T, Deniz YM, et al. Aspirin sensitivity and severity of asthma: evidence for irreversible airway obstruction in patients with severe or difficult-to-treat asthma. J Allergy Clin Immunol 2005;116(5):970–5.
4. Jatakanon A, Uasuf C, Maziak W, et al. Neutrophilic inflammation in severe persistent asthma. Am J Respir Crit Care Med 1999;160(5 Pt 1):1532–9.
5. Wenzel SE. Severe asthma in adults. Exp Lung Res 2005;31(Suppl 1):22.
6. Moffatt MF, Kabesch M, Liang L, et al. Genetic variants regulating ORMDL3 expression contribute to the risk of childhood asthma. Nature 2007;448(7152):470–3.
7. Karunas AS, Iunusbaev BB, Fedorova I, et al. Genome-wide association study of bronchial asthma in the Volga-Ural region of Russia. Mol Biol (Mosk) 2011;45(6):992–1003 [in Russian].
8. Leung TF, Sy HY, Ng MC, et al. Asthma and atopy are associated with chromosome 17q21 markers in Chinese children. Allergy 2009;64(4):621–8.
9. Halapi E, Gudbjartsson DF, Jonsdottir GM, et al. A sequence variant on 17q21 is associated with age at onset and severity of asthma. Eur J Hum Genet 2010;18(8):902–8.
10. Tavendale R, Macgregor DF, Mukhopadhyay S, et al. A polymorphism controlling ORMDL3 expression is associated with asthma that is poorly controlled by current medications. J Allergy Clin Immunol 2008;121(4):860–3.
11. Binia A, Khorasani N, Bhavsar PK, et al. Chromosome 17q21 SNP and severe asthma. J Hum Genet 2011;56(1):97–8.
12. Bisgaard H, Bonnelykke K, Sleiman PM, et al. Chromosome 17q21 gene variants are associated with asthma and exacerbations but not atopy in early childhood. Am J Respir Crit Care Med 2009;179(3):179–85.
13. Moffatt MF, Gut IG, Demenais F, et al. A large-scale, consortium-based genome-wide association study of asthma. N Engl J Med 2010;363(13):1211–21.
14. Grotenboer NS, Ketelaar ME, Koppelman GH, et al. Decoding asthma: translating genetic variation in IL33 and IL1RL1 into disease pathophysiology. J Allergy Clin Immunol 2013;131(3):856–65.
15. Prefontaine D, Lajoie-Kadoch S, Foley S, et al. Increased expression of IL-33 in severe asthma: evidence of expression by airway smooth muscle cells. J Immunol 2009;183(8):5094–103.

16. Saglani S, Lui S, Ullmann N, et al. IL-33 promotes airway remodeling in pediatric patients with severe steroid-resistant asthma. J Allergy Clin Immunol 2013;132(3): 676–85.e3.

17. Castanhinha S, Sherburn R, Walker S, et al. Pediatric severe asthma with fungal sensitization is mediated by steroid-resistant IL-33. J Allergy Clin Immunol 2015; 136(2):312–22.e7.

18. Faber TE, Schuurhof A, Vonk A, et al. IL1RL1 gene variants and nasopharyngeal IL1RL-a levels are associated with severe RSV bronchiolitis: a multicenter cohort study. PLoS One 2012;7(5):e34364.

19. Bonnelykke K, Sleiman P, Nielsen K, et al. A genome-wide association study identifies CDHR3 as a susceptibility locus for early childhood asthma with severe exacerbations. Nat Genet 2014;46(1):51–5.

20. Traister RS, Uvalle CE, Hawkins GA, et al. Phenotypic and genotypic association of epithelial IL1RL1 to human TH2-like asthma. J Allergy Clin Immunol 2015; 135(1):92–9.

21. Che Z, Zhu X, Yao C, et al. The association between the C-509T and T869C polymorphisms of TGF-beta1 gene and the risk of asthma: a meta-analysis. Hum Immunol 2014;75(2):141–50.

22. Hobbs K, Negri J, Klinnert M, et al. Interleukin-10 and transforming growth factor-beta promoter polymorphisms in allergies and asthma. Am J Respir Crit Care Med 1998;158(6):1958–62.

23. Meng J, Thongngarm T, Nakajima M, et al. Association of transforming growth factor-beta1 single nucleotide polymorphism C-509T with allergy and immunological activities. Int Arch Allergy Immunol 2005;138(2):151–60.

24. Liebhart J, Polak M, Dabrowski A, et al. The G/G genotype of transforming growth factor beta 1 (TGF-beta1) single nucleotide (+915G/C) polymorphism coincident with other host and environmental factors is associated with irreversible bronchoconstriction in asthmatics. Int J Immunogenet 2008;35(6):417–22.

25. Chiang CH, Chuang CH, Liu SL, et al. Genetic polymorphism of transforming growth factor beta1 and tumor necrosis factor alpha is associated with asthma and modulates the severity of asthma. Respir Care 2013;58(8):1343–50.

26. Ierodiakonou D, Postma DS, Koppelman GH, et al. TGF-beta1 polymorphisms and asthma severity, airway inflammation, and remodeling. J Allergy Clin Immunol 2013;131(2):582–5.

27. Pulleyn LJ, Newton R, Adcock IM, et al. TGFbeta1 allele association with asthma severity. Hum Genet 2001;109(6):623–7.

28. de Faria I, de Faria E, Toro A, et al. Association of TGF-β1, CD14, IL-4, IL-4R and ADAM33 gene polymorphisms with asthma severity in children and adolescents. J Pediatr (Rio J) 2008;84(3):203–10.

29. Mack I, Hector A, Ballbach M, et al. The role of chitin, chitinases, and chitinase-like proteins in pediatric lung diseases. Mol Cell Pediatr 2015;2(1):3.

30. Chupp GL, Lee CG, Jarjour N, et al. A chitinase-like protein in the lung and circulation of patients with severe asthma. N Engl J Med 2007;357(20):2016–27.

31. Konradsen JR, James A, Nordlund B, et al. The chitinase-like protein YKL-40: a possible biomarker of inflammation and airway remodeling in severe pediatric asthma. J Allergy Clin Immunol 2013;132(2):328–35.e5.

32. Ober C, Tan Z, Sun Y, et al. Effect of variation in CHI3L1 on serum YKL-40 level, risk of asthma, and lung function. N Engl J Med 2008;358(16):1682–91.

33. Tsai Y, Ko Y, Huang M, et al. CHI3L1 polymorphisms associate with asthma in a Taiwanese population. BMC Med Genet 2014;15:86.

34. Mathias RA, Grant AV, Rafaels N, et al. A genome-wide association study on African-ancestry populations for asthma. J Allergy Clin Immunol 2010;125(2): 336–46.e4.
35. Sordillo JE, Kelly R, Bunyavanich S, et al. Genome-wide expression profiles identify potential targets for gene-environment interactions in asthma severity. J Allergy Clin Immunol 2015;136(4):885–92.e2.
36. Binia A, Van Stiphout N, Liang L, et al. A polymorphism affecting MYB binding within the promoter of the PDCD4 gene is associated with severe asthma in children. Hum Mutat 2013;34(8):1131–9.
37. Slager RE, Otulana BA, Hawkins GA, et al. IL-4 receptor polymorphisms predict reduction in asthma exacerbations during response to an anti-IL-4 receptor alpha antagonist. J Allergy Clin Immunol 2012;130(2):516–22.e4.

Psychosocial Factors in Severe Pediatric Asthma

Genery D. Booster, PhD*, Alyssa A. Oland, PhD, Bruce G. Bender, PhD

KEYWORDS

- Asthma • Children • Adolescents • Parents • Psychosocial

KEY POINTS

- Most research suggests that children with severe asthma display more emotional and behavioral problems than their healthy peers.
- Psychological difficulties are associated with increased risk for functional impairments and problematic disease course.
- Caregivers of children with asthma are at increased risk for emotional difficulties, which may have a significant impact on their ability to manage their child's asthma.
- Multidisciplinary teams that assess and treat these psychological factors are important for children whose asthma is poorly controlled.

Asthma is the most common chronic illness among children in the United States, affecting an estimated 6.8 million (9.4%) children.[1] A more complete understanding of pediatric asthma involves the integration of genetic, immunological, and psychosocial factors that may affect symptom presentation, chronicity, and illness management.[2] Increasingly, the health and functioning of children with asthma has been examined within a larger social-ecological framework (**Fig. 1**)[3] that includes parents, extended family, caregivers, and psychosocial providers, as well as the child's medical care team.[4] The purpose of this report was to examine the psychological variables that impact asthma management and severity, and to provide a rationale for a multidisciplinary approach to patient care.

RELATIONSHIP BETWEEN ASTHMA AND BEHAVIORAL DISTURBANCE
Epidemiological Associations

Although the literature regarding psychiatric comorbidities and behavioral problems among children with asthma is somewhat conflicting,[5–12] most research suggests that children with asthma display more emotional and behavior problems than their

Disclosure Statement: The authors have nothing to disclose.
Pediatric Behavioral Health, National Jewish Health, 1400 Jackson Street, Denver, CO 80206, USA
* Corresponding author.
E-mail address: boosterg@NJHealth.org

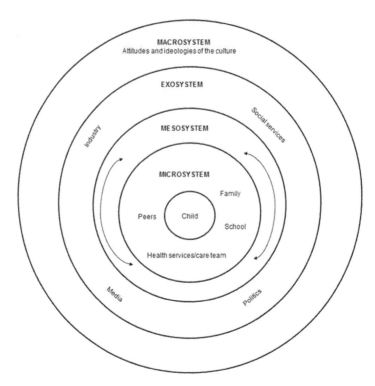

Fig. 1. Social-ecological framework.

healthy peers.[5,13–23] A meta-analysis of emotional and behavioral functioning in children with asthma concluded that they display more behavioral difficulties than do healthy children, with a stronger effect size for internalizing behaviors such as anxiety and affective symptoms ($d = 0.73$) than for externalizing behaviors, such as symptoms of inattention, hyperactivity, and oppositional behaviors ($d = 0.40$).[5]

Internalizing symptoms
Estimates of the prevalence of internalizing disorders, such as anxiety and affective disorders, range from 5% to 43% of children with asthma, which is significantly above the prevalence in the general pediatric population.[13–16,21,23,24] In addition, parents of children with asthma report significantly more internalizing symptoms in their children compared with parents of healthy controls.[13,18,20,25–27] Importantly, increased asthma severity has been associated with greater behavioral and emotional difficulties, which may account for the wide range in epidemiological results. Studies directly comparing children with mild or intermittent asthma with those with persistent and severe asthma have found significantly higher rates of internalizing difficulties among children with severe asthma.[5,13,15,28,29] When compared with healthy controls, children with mild and/or remitted asthma have not shown heightened vulnerability to psychological disorders compared with healthy children.[8,15] These results suggest that children with severe asthma, but not those with mild to moderate asthma, may be especially at risk for comorbid internalizing difficulties.

In addition to differences in asthma severity, there is preliminary evidence of differential prevalence of self-reported internalizing symptoms by asthma phenotype. Two studies comparing children with atopic asthma with those with nonatopic (or nonallergic) asthma found significantly higher rates of internalizing difficulties in girls with nonatopic asthma. Specifically, girls with nonatopic asthma were 3 times more likely to have comorbid depressive[22] and emotional[30] symptoms compared with healthy children, whereas atopic asthma was not associated with emotional symptoms.[30] Such findings may vary depending on methods of subject selection and psychological measures, and future research is needed to corroborate these findings.

Externalizing symptoms
Although less well documented than internalizing symptoms, multiple studies suggest that children with asthma may be at increased risk for externalizing behavioral problems, and in particular, attention problems.[11,28] One study found a more than twofold increase in parent-reported attention problems in children with symptomatic asthma.[11] As with internalizing difficulties, the association between asthma and externalizing behavioral problems has been shown to increase with asthma severity.[13,15,28] This association may be especially important, as management of severe asthma requires careful attention to symptoms and organization of medical routines.

Psychosocial Risk Factors for Poor Outcomes

Child psychopathology
Aggregate evidence indicates that psychological difficulties are associated with increased risk for functional impairments and problematic disease course. Children with both asthma and an internalizing disorder, for example, demonstrate increased physical and functional impairments,[16,24,31] greater frequency and severity of reported asthma symptoms,[30,32–34] more missed school days,[33] increased use of rescue medications,[35] more frequent urgent and emergent care use,[34] poorer pulmonary functioning,[34] and increased frequency of emotional triggers for asthma,[36] even when controlling for disease severity.[24,32,36] An association between psychological distress and nonadherence to treatment regimens further undermines illness control.[37]

Although research clearly demonstrates the functional impact of psychological distress in children with asthma, the mechanisms behind this association are less clear. There is some evidence that psychological symptoms may affect subjective reporting of symptoms, as some research suggests that psychological distress may not predict more objective measures of asthma, such as prednisone bursts.[33] There is also some evidence that children's illness perceptions (eg, that asthma negatively impacts their life and is hard to control) may partially mediate the relationship between anxiety and asthma symptoms.[38]

Caregiver functioning
In addition to increased child psychopathology, accumulating evidence suggests that caregivers of children with asthma are at increased risk for emotional difficulties. Recent research indicates that these caregivers show significantly higher rates of depression,[26,35,39–44] anxiety,[35,40] and posttraumatic stress disorder,[24] with prevalence rates as high as 63% among parents of children with severe asthma.[39] A recent meta-analysis examining internalizing symptoms in caregivers of children with asthma found a large effect size for both anxious and depressive symptoms, with a stronger relationship between parental psychopathology and asthma in those with medically confirmed asthma and those recruited from clinical settings,[40] suggesting that caregivers of children with severe asthma may be at particular risk.[39]

Importantly, caregivers' psychological functioning may have a significant impact on their ability to manage their child's asthma. Maternal depressive symptoms, for example, have been associated with increased difficulties using proper inhaler technique, forgetting medication doses, greater exposure to tobacco smoke, less understanding about medication use, lower self-efficacy, and less confidence in their abilities to control their child's asthma symptoms.[26,44,45] In addition, maternal depressive symptoms have been associated with increased use of quick relief medications,[42] more frequent emergency room visits,[43,46] increased frequency of asthma attacks,[26] and repeated child hospitalizations,[32] even after controlling for baseline asthma morbidity.[32,43]

Family functioning
In accordance with a social-ecological framework (see **Fig. 1**), family functioning and parent-child relationships have been increasingly examined as dynamics that can affect severe pediatric asthma. Wood and colleagues,[47,48] in particular, have presented a Biobehavioral Family Model (**Fig. 2**) hypothesizing that family emotional climate, quality of parent-parent relations, parent-child relational security, and biobehavioral reactivity (eg, emotion regulation) may collectively serve as a risk or protective factor for asthma disease severity in children, and a number of recent studies provide preliminary evidence to support this theory. Structural equation models have shown that an observed negative family emotional climate significantly predicts child depression, which in turn predicts asthma disease severity[47] and emotional triggers for asthma.[36] Relational stress pathways predicting asthma symptoms remained significant, even when adherence was controlled for in the model.[47] Furthermore, family affective responsiveness and parental stress have been shown to significantly predict medication adherence.[49,50] In sum, the psychological status of children and their parents can serve to either foster or impede the management of the child's asthma. In children whose asthma is poorly controlled, the medical team should consider interventions that address these psychological factors.

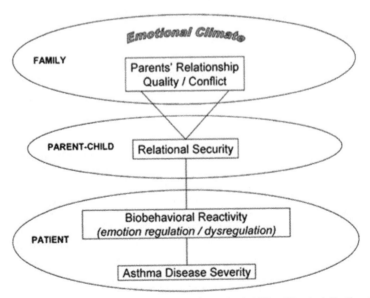

Fig. 2. Biobehavioral family model. (*From* Wood BL, Lim J, Miller BD, et al. Testing the biobehavioral family model in pediatric asthma: pathways of effect. Fam Proc 2008;47(1):22; with permission.)

Life stress

Acute and chronic stressors, both independently and in conjunction, have been significantly associated with asthma exacerbations.[51] Accordingly, children and adolescents exposed to severe and chronic stressors, such as those living in low-income urban communities, have been at disproportionate risk for severe asthma.[52,53] Although the mechanisms behind this association are not fully understood, preliminary research suggests that children exposed to chronic stress may show a heightened inflammatory profile. Children with asthma from low-income backgrounds, for example, have been shown to have increased numbers of cytokines from peripheral blood lymphocytes stimulated in vitro compared with children from high socioeconomic backgrounds, suggesting disadvantaged children may respond to exacerbating factors with greater activation of the immune system.[54] Similarly, children with asthma who experienced higher levels of chronic family stress showed a heightened inflammatory profile (increased production of immune markers included in production of asthma-related cytokines, including interleukin [IL]-4, IL-5, and interferon gamma) at times when they experienced a stressful event. Importantly, these stress-related changes did not occur in children with lower levels of chronic family stress, or in healthy controls. This combination of acute and chronic stress was also associated with increased asthma symptoms[55] and may be especially relevant for the management of children with severe, chronic asthma.

BEHAVIORAL INTERVENTIONS FOR CHILDREN WITH SEVERE ASTHMA AND THEIR FAMILIES

Given the complex nature of the etiology, course, and management of severe asthma and the relationship of psychosocial factors in disease management and exacerbations, pediatric psychologists are uniquely positioned to provide valuable consultation to health care providers as well as assessment and intervention to families. Psychosocial interventions for asthma may include educational programs, behavioral interventions, cognitive-behavioral therapy, family interventions, community-based interventions, and the use of technology. To date, there is limited and inconclusive evidence on the efficacy of psychological interventions for asthma[56] and for problematic severe asthma.[57] Additionally, there have been concerns regarding methodological shortcomings in many of the studies to date, including small sample sizes, use of convenience samples, inconsistency in outcome measures, and a lack of randomized controlled designs.[57] Nonetheless, emerging evidence indicates that behavioral interventions can improve the quality of life and medical outcomes for children with asthma.

Patient and Family Education

Self-management training and education are well-established and essential parts of treatment for patients with asthma throughout their course of care.[58] Strengths of patient and family psychoeducation programs include cost-effectiveness, inclusion of problem-solving strategies, and that clinical interview tools, such as the Family Asthma Management System Scale (FAMSS),[59] can be used to individualize intervention.[60] Reviews of the efficacy of educational programs for pediatric patients with asthma have found that they improved knowledge and confidence,[61,62] reduced subsequent emergency department visits or hospital admissions,[61,63] improved adherence,[64,65] and resulted in significant gains in lung function, fewer school days missed, and less activity restriction.[63] Additionally, a meta-analysis exploring the efficacy of family psychoeducational programs found that they improved asthma symptoms.[66] Further, a randomized controlled trial indicated that small interactive group education was effective in reducing emergency room visits and courses of oral corticosteroids and improving quality of life.[67]

Lack of access to effective interventions can be a barrier for patients and families, particularly for high-risk patients. As such, there has been focus on providing school-based and emergency room–based interventions. A review of school-based asthma education programs found that they resulted in improved knowledge, self-efficacy, and self-management behaviors in children,[62] and use of school-based medication supervision resulted in improved asthma control.[68] Research has suggested that including parents, even when the intervention is school-based, and providing parental support, can be beneficial. For example, school-based interventions that include parents, compared with those that did not include parents, resulted in improved parent self-efficacy for asthma attack prevention and management.[69] Provision of ongoing parental support also resulted in improved adolescent asthma management.[70] Additionally, research exploring the efficacy of emergency room–based interventions found that follow-up in an emergency department embedded clinic resulted in significantly reduced unscheduled asthma care visits and increased adherence.[71]

With emerging communication technology advances, there are a growing number of avenues through which education can be received by patients and families. A review of various interactive computerized education programs found improved knowledge and symptoms.[72,73] Additionally, use of an Internet-based asthma education and monitoring program[72] and use of electrical device monitoring combined with structured feedback[74,75] were shown to result in improved child adherence. Further, a multimedia Web-based asthma management program tailored to urban high school students resulted in reduced symptoms, school absences, activity restrictions, and hospitalizations.[76] Improving medication adherence long term, however, may require more intensive interventions. One study, for example, found that peer support and mp3-delivered peer asthma messages were not sufficient to improve outcomes among low-income minority adolescents with persistent asthma.[77]

Meta-analysis results indicate that educational interventions, without additional therapeutic supports, have variable effects on child adherence[78,79] and are not by themselves sufficient for improving asthma management and health outcomes.[80–82] As such, research has explored the efficacy of education interventions combined with additional interventions. For example, incorporating cognitive, behavioral, and psychosocial interventions into a school-based education program resulted in reduced asthma severity,[83] and asthma psychoeducation combined with family therapy resulted in a significant reduction in child airway inflammation, improved child adjustment to asthma, and increased parental efficacy with regard to asthma management.[84] Similarly, a parent-child teamwork intervention combined with psychoeducation resulted in improved adherence, reduced parent-child conflict, and significant health improvements, such as improved small airway functioning, reduced report of asthma symptoms, and reduced activity restrictions.[85] Multisystemic therapy, which is an intensive home and community-based family intervention,[60] was used with African American adolescents with moderate to severe asthma and resulted in improved asthma management and lung function.[86]

Cognitive-Behavioral Interventions

Several studies have also explored the benefit of behavioral and cognitive-behavioral (CBT) interventions. Cognitive-behavioral approaches focus on identifying and modifying unhelpful thoughts and behaviors relevant to a problematic behavior. For example, research has shown that a CBT stress management intervention combined with patient education resulted in improved lung function, reduced stress, and reduced depression.[87] A study exploring the use of a 3-month intervention that included education, self-management, and behavioral strategies found that the intervention resulted in significant improvements in knowledge and attitude, peak-flow readings, and methacholine challenge test results and significant reductions in emergency room visits.[88] Additionally, behavioral strategies have been shown to result in reduced school absences and use of as-needed medications[89] and improved adherence.[90] Further, parent behavioral counseling and cotinine feedback resulted in significant reductions in child secondhand smoke exposure *only* in families with children with severe asthma (vs children with mild-moderate asthma).[91]

As research has demonstrated strong evidence for a link between stress and asthma, there has also been a focus on the efficacy of self-regulation therapies. Some positive findings have emerged for self-regulation therapies, such as biofeedback, relaxation, and active coping for patients with asthma.[92] Lehrer[92] cautioned that relaxation methods may have adverse immediate effects, such as relaxation-induced bronchoconstriction, if used during an acute asthma flare. He also raised concern that the use of relaxation therapies has not been adequately researched in patients with emotionally induced asthma attacks, high levels of anxiety, or panic disorder.

Taken together, results to date indicate that interventions that combine education with cognitive, behavioral, self-regulation, and/or family components may be of benefit for patients with severe asthma. It is proposed that a comprehensive multidisciplinary approach to teaching asthma self-management skills, involvement of the community in program design, and an increased focus on evaluation and treatment of family stress, interactions, and relationships[60,93]; family conflict; parental stress; parenting styles; and child behavior[93] can produce greater benefit and outcomes for children with asthma. Given the health risks in pediatric patients with severe asthma, research is particularly needed specifically focusing on this population.

FUTURE CONSIDERATIONS

Although significant medical and psychological advances have been made in recent years, much work remains to be done both in our understanding of the contribution of psychosocial factors and in the development and testing of multidisciplinary interventions. The literature examining the impact of psychosocial factors in severe asthma is fraught with methodological inconsistencies that temper any conclusions made regarding the body of literature. Researchers have used a variety of techniques and assessment methods to examine psychosocial factors, ranging from child and parent reports to direct clinical observation. Additionally, studies have also used differing methods to assess the presence of asthma, ranging from parent report of symptoms to complex medical confirmation. That associations between psychological symptoms and asthma diagnosis have been shown to differ depending on the method of assessment, cloud full understanding of available evidence.[94] Utilization of more objective measures of asthma symptoms, as well as multimethod assessment of psychopathology, would help clarify these complex relationships. Further, additional examination of asthma onset within a bio-psychosocial framework, and research examining the complex interactions among stress, emotions, immune function, and asthma exacerbations could provide the basis for development of more preventative interventions.

REFERENCES

1. Bloom BC, Cohen RA. Summary health statistics for U.S. children: national health interview survey, 2006. Hyattsville (MD): National Center for Health Statistics; 2007.
2. American Academy of Allergy, Asthma and Immunology (AAAAI). Allergic disorders: promoting best practices. Milwaukee (WI): American Academy of Allergy, Asthma and Immunology (AAAAI); 2000.
3. Bronfenbrenner U. The ecology of human development. Cambridge (MA): Harvard University Press; 1979.
4. Kazak AE. Family systems practice in pediatric psychology. J Pediatr Psychol 2002;27:133–43.
5. McQuaid EL, Kopel SJ, Nassau JH. Behavioral adjustment in children with asthma: a meta-analysis. J Dev Behav Pediatr 2001;22:430–9.
6. Wolf JM, Miller GE, Chen E. Parent psychological states predict changes in inflammatory markers in children with asthma and healthy children. Brain Behav Immun 2008;22:433–41.
7. Ortega AN, Huertas SE, Canino G, et al. Childhood asthma, chronic illness, and psychiatric disorders. J Nerv Ment Dis 2002;190:275–81.
8. Bender BG, Annett RD, Ikle D, et al. Relationship between disease and psychological adaptation in children in the childhood asthma management program and their families. Arch Pediatr Adolesc Med 2000;154:706–13.
9. Berz J, Murdock KK, Koinis Mitchell D. Children's asthma, internalizing problems, and social functioning: an urban perspective. J Child Adolesc Psychiatr Nurs 2005;18:181–97.
10. Markson S, Fiese BH. Family rituals as a protective factor for children with asthma. J Pediatr Psychol 2000;25:471–9.
11. Arif AA. The association between symptomatic asthma and neurobehavioral comorbidities among children. J Asthma 2010;47:792–6.
12. Calam R, Gregg L, Goodman R. Psychological adjustment and asthma in children and adolescents: the UK nationwide mental health survey. Psychosom Med 2005;67:105–10.
13. Vila G, Nollet-Clemencon C, de Blic J, et al. Asthma severity and psychopathology in tertiary care department for children and adolescents. Eur Child Adolesc Psychiatry 1998;7:137–44.
14. Vila G, Nollet-Clemecon C, Vera M, et al. Prevalence of DSM-IV disorders in children and adolescents with asthma versus diabetes. Can J Psychiatry 1999;44:562–9.
15. Goodwin RE, Fergusson DM, Horwood LJ. Asthma and depressive and anxiety disorders among young persons in the community. Psychol Med 2004;34:1465–74.
16. Katon W, Lozano P, Russo J, et al. The prevalence of DSM-IV anxiety and depressive disorders in youth with asthma compared with controls. J Adolesc Health 2007;41:455–63.
17. Feldman JM, Ortega AN, McQuaid EL, et al. Comorbidity between asthma attacks and internalizing disorders among Puerto Rican children at one-year follow-up. Psychosomatics 2006;47:333–9.
18. Gillaspy SR, Hoff AL, Mullins LL, et al. Psychological distress in high-risk youth with asthma. J Pediatr Psychol 2002;27:363–71.
19. Goodwin RD, Robinson M, Sly PD, et al. Severity and persistence of asthma and mental health: a birth cohort study. Psychol Med 2013;43:1313–22.

20. Teyhan A, Galobardes B, Henderson J. Child allergic symptoms and mental well-being: the role of maternal anxiety and depression. J Pediatr 2014;165:592–9.
21. Bussing R, Burket RC, Kelleher ET. Prevalence of anxiety disorders in a clinic-based sample of pediatric asthma patients. Psychosomatics 1996;37:108–0115.
22. Bahreinian S, Ball GD, Colman I, et al. Depression is more common in girls with nonatopic asthma. Chest 2011;140:1138–45.
23. Ortega AN, McQuaid EL, Canino G, et al. Comorbidity of asthma and anxiety and depression in Puerto Rican children. Psychosomatics 2004;45:93–9.
24. Kean EM, Kelsay K, Wambolt F, et al. Posttraumatic stress in adolescents with asthma and their parents. J Am Acad Child Adolesc Psychiatry 2006;45:78–86.
25. Klinnert MD, Nelson HS, Price MR, et al. Onset and persistence of childhood asthma: predictors from infancy. Pediatrics 2001;108:e69–75.
26. Feldman JM, Perez EA, Canino G, et al. The role of caregiver major depression in the relationship between anxiety disorders and asthma attacks in island Puerto Rican youth and young adults. J Nerv Ment Dis 2011;199:313–8.
27. Meuret AE, Ehrenreich JT, Pincus DB, et al. Prevalence and correlates of asthma in children with internalizing psychopathology. Depress Anxiety 2006;23:502–8.
28. Blackman A, Gurka MJ. Developmental and behavioral comorbidities of asthma in children. J Dev Behav Pediatr 2007;28:92–9.
29. Kohlboeck G, Koletzko S, Bauer CP, et al. Association of atopic and non-atopic asthma with emotional symptoms in school children. Pediatr Allergy Immunol 2013;24:230–6.
30. Richardson LP, Lozano P, Russo J, et al. Asthma symptom burden: relationship to asthma severity and anxiety and depression symptoms. Pediatrics 2006;118:1042–51.
31. McCauley E, Katon W, Russo J, et al. Impact of anxiety and depression on functional impairment in adolescents with asthma. Gen Hosp Psychiatry 2007;29:214–22.
32. Weil CM, Wade SL, Bauman LJ, et al. The relationship between psychosocial factors and asthma morbidity in inner-city children with asthma. Pediatrics 1999;104:1274–80.
33. Bender BG, Zhang L. Negative affect, medication adherence, and asthma control in children. J Allergy Clin Immunol 2008;122:490–5.
34. Fiese BH, Winter MA, Wambolt FS, et al. Do family mealtime interactions mediate the association between asthma symptoms and separation anxiety? J Child Psychol Psychiatry 2010;51:144–51.
35. Feldman JM, Steinberg D, Kutner H, et al. Perception of pulmonary function and asthma control: the differential role of child versus caregiver anxiety and depression. J Pediatr Psychol 2013;38:1091–100.
36. Wood BL, Lim JH, Miller BD, et al. Family emotional climate, depression, emotional triggering of asthma, and disease severity in pediatric asthma: examination of pathways of effect. J Pediatr Psychol 2007;32:542–51.
37. Bender BG. Risk taking, depression, adherence, and symptom control in adolescents and young adults with asthma. Am J Respir Crit Care Med 2006;173:953–7.
38. McGrady ME, Cotton S, Rosenthol SL, et al. Anxiety and asthma symptoms in urban adolescents with asthma: the mediating role of illness perceptions. J Clin Psychol Med Settings 2010;17:349–56.
39. Leao LL, Zhang L, Sousa PLR, et al. High prevalence of depression amongst mothers of children with asthma. J Asthma 2009;46:388–91.

40. Easter G, Sharpe L, Hunt CJ. Systematic review and meta-analysis of anxious and depressive symptoms in caregivers of children with asthma. J Pediatr Psychol 2015;40:623–32.

41. Szabo A, Mezei G, Kovari E, et al. Depressive symptoms amongst asthmatic children's caregivers. Pediatr Allergy Immunol 2010;21:e667–73.

42. Kub J, Jennings JM, Donithan M, et al. Life events, chronic stressors, and depressive symptoms in low-income urban mothers with asthmatic children. Public Health Nurs 2009;26:297–306.

43. Bartlett SJ, Kolodner K, Butz AM, et al. Maternal depressive symptoms and emergency department use among inner-city children with asthma. Arch Pediatr Adolesc Med 2001;155:347–53.

44. Lim JH, Wood BL, Miller BD. Maternal depression and parenting in relation to child internalizing symptoms and asthma disease activity. J Fam Psychol 2008; 22:264–73.

45. Martinez KG, Perez EA, Ramirez R, et al. The role of caregivers' depressive symptoms and asthma beliefs on asthma outcomes among low-income Puerto Rican children. J Asthma 2009;46:136–41.

46. Brown ES, Gan V, Jeffress J, et al. Psychiatric symptomatology and disorders in caregivers of children with asthma. Pediatrics 2006;118:e1715–20.

47. Wood BL, Lim J, Miller BD, et al. Testing the biobehavioral family model in pediatric asthma: pathways of effect. Fam Process 2008;47:21–40.

48. Lim JH, Wood BL, Miller BD, et al. Effects of paternal and maternal depressive symptoms on child internalizing symptoms and asthma disease activity: mediation by interparental negativity and parenting. J Fam Psychol 2011;25:137–46.

49. Bender B, Milgrom H, Rand C, et al. Psychological factors associated with medication nonadherence in asthmatic children. J Asthma 1998;35:347–53.

50. DeMore M, Adams C, Wilson N, et al. Parenting stress, difficult child behavior, and use of routines in relation to adherence in pediatric asthma. Child Health Care 2005;34:245–59.

51. Sandberg S, Paton JY, Ahola S, et al. The role of acute and chronic stress in asthma attacks in children. Lancet 2000;356:982–7.

52. Claudio L, Tulton L, Doucette J, et al. Socioeconomic factors and asthma hospitalization rates in New York City. J Asthma 1999;36:343–50.

53. Frederico JM, Liu AH. Overcoming childhood asthma disparities of the inner-city poor. Pediatr Clin North Am 2003;50:655–75.

54. Chen E, Fisher E, Bacharier LB, et al. Socioeconomic status, stress, and immune markers in adolescents with asthma. Psychosom Med 2003;65:984–92.

55. Marin TJ, Chen E, Munch JA, et al. Double-exposure to acute stress and chronic family stress is associated with immune changes in children with asthma. Psychosom Med 2009;71:378–84.

56. Eccleston C, Palermo TM, Fisher E, et al. Psychological interventions for parents of children and adolescents with chronic illness. Cochrane Database Syst Rev 2012;(8):CD009660.

57. Yorke J, Fleming SL, Shuldham C. A systematic review of psychological interventions for children with asthma. Pediatr Pulmonol 2007;42(2):114–24.

58. Ritz T, Meuret AE, Trueba AF, et al. Psychosocial factors and behavioral medicine interventions in asthma. J Consult Clin Psychol 2013;81(2):231–50.

59. Kilnnert MD, McQuaid EL, Gavin LA. Assessing the family asthma management system. J Asthma 1997;34:77–88.

60. Celano MP. Family processes in pediatric asthma. Curr Opin Pediatr 2006;18(5): 539–44.

61. Boyd M, Lasserson TJ, Mckean MC, et al. Interventions for educating children who are at risk of asthma-related emergency department attendance. Cochrane Database Syst Rev 2009;(2):CD001290.

62. Coffman JM, Cabana MD, Yelin EH. Do school-based asthma education programs improve self-management and health outcomes? Pediatrics 2009; 124(2):729–42.

63. Guevara JP, Wolf FM, Grum CM, et al. Effects of educational interventions for self management of asthma in children and adolescents: systematic review and meta-analysis. BMJ 2003;326(7402):1308–9.

64. Morton RW, Everard ML, Elphick HE. Adherence in childhood asthma: the elephant in the room. Arch Dis Child 2014;99(10):949–53.

65. Otsuki M, Eakin MN, Rand CS, et al. Adherence feedback to improve asthma outcomes among inner-city children: a randomized trial. Pediatrics 2009;124(6): 1513–21.

66. Bernard-bonnin AC, Stachenko S, Bonin D, et al. Self-management teaching programs and morbidity of pediatric asthma: a meta-analysis. J Allergy Clin Immunol 1995;95(1 Pt 1):34–41.

67. Watson WT, Gillespie C, Thomas N, et al. Small-group, interactive education and the effect on asthma control by children and their families. CMAJ 2009;181(5): 257–63.

68. Gerald LB, Mcclure LA, Mangan JM, et al. Increasing adherence to inhaled steroid therapy among schoolchildren: randomized, controlled trial of school-based supervised asthma therapy. Pediatrics 2009;123(2):466–74.

69. Terpstra JL, Chavez LJ, Ayala GX. An intervention to increase caregiver support for asthma management in middle school-aged youth. J Asthma 2012;49(3): 267–74.

70. Yang TO, Sylva K, Lunt I. Parent support, peer support, and peer acceptance in healthy lifestyle for asthma management among early adolescents. J Spec Pediatr Nurs 2010;15(4):272–81.

71. Teach SJ, Crain EF, Quint DM, et al. Improved asthma outcomes in a high-morbidity pediatric population: results of an emergency department-based randomized clinical trial. Arch Pediatr Adolesc Med 2006;160(5):535–41.

72. Bussey-Smith KL, Rossen RD. A systematic review of randomized control trials evaluating the effectiveness of interactive computerized asthma patient education programs. Ann Allergy Asthma Immunol 2007;98(6):507–16.

73. Chan DS, Callahan CW, Hatch-pigott VB, et al. Internet-based home monitoring and education of children with asthma is comparable to ideal office-based care: results of a 1-year asthma in-home monitoring trial. Pediatrics 2007; 119(3):569–78.

74. Burgess SW, Sly PD, Devadason SG. Providing feedback on adherence increases use of preventive medication by asthmatic children. J Asthma 2010; 47(2):198–201.

75. Spaulding SA, Devine KA, Duncan CL, et al. Electronic monitoring and feedback to improve adherence in pediatric asthma. J Pediatr Psychol 2012;37(1):64–74.

76. Joseph CL, Peterson E, Havstad S, et al. A Web-based, tailored asthma management program for urban African-American high school students. Am J Respir Crit Care Med 2007;175(9):888–95.

77. Mosnaim G, Li H, Martin M, et al. Adherence to inhaled corticosteroids in minority adolescents with asthma: a randomized, controlled trial. J Allergy Clin Immunol Pract 2013;1:485–93.

78. Dean AJ, Walters J, Hall A. A systematic review of interventions to enhance medication adherence in children and adolescents with chronic illness. Arch Dis Child 2010;95(9):717–23.
79. Haynes RB, Ackloo E, Sahota N, et al. Interventions for enhancing medication adherence. Cochrane Database Syst Rev 2008;(2):CD000011.
80. Clark NM, Griffiths C, Keteyian SR, et al. Educational and behavioral interventions for asthma: who achieves which outcomes? A systematic review. J Asthma Allergy 2010;3:187–97.
81. Crocker DD, Kinyota S, Dumitru GG, et al. Effectiveness of home-based, multi-trigger, multicomponent interventions with an environmental focus for reducing asthma morbidity: a community guide systematic review. Am J Prev Med 2011; 41(2 Suppl 1):S5–32.
82. Kahana S, Drotar D, Frazier T. Meta-analysis of psychological interventions to promote adherence to treatment in pediatric chronic health conditions. J Pediatr Psychol 2008;33(6):590–611.
83. Kintner E, Cook G, Allen A, et al. Feasibility and benefits of a school-based academic and counseling program for older school-age students with asthma. Res Nurs Health 2012;35(5):507–17.
84. Ng SM, Li AM, Lou VW, et al. Incorporating family therapy into asthma group intervention: a randomized waitlist-controlled trial. Fam Process 2008;47(1):115–30.
85. Duncan CL, Hogan MB, Tien KJ, et al. Efficacy of a parent-youth teamwork intervention to promote adherence in pediatric asthma. J Pediatr Psychol 2013;38(6): 617–28.
86. Naar-king S, Ellis D, King PS, et al. Multisystemic therapy for high-risk African American adolescents with asthma: a randomized clinical trial. J Consult Clin Psychol 2014;82(3):536–45.
87. Long KA, Ewing LJ, Cohen S, et al. Preliminary evidence for the feasibility of a stress management intervention for 7- to 12-year-olds with asthma. J Asthma 2011;48(2):162–70.
88. Chen SH, Huang JL, Yeh KW, et al. Interactive support interventions for caregivers of asthmatic children. J Asthma 2013;50(6):649–57.
89. Dahl J, Gustafsson D, Melin L. Effects of a behavioral treatment program on children with asthma. J Asthma 1990;27(1):41–6.
90. Kamps JL, Rapoff MA, Roberts MC, et al. Improving adherence to inhaled corticosteroids in children with asthma: a pilot of a randomized clinical trial. Child Health Care 2008;37(4):261–77.
91. Wilson SR, Farber HJ, Knowles SB, et al. A randomized trial of parental behavioral counseling and cotinine feedback for lowering environmental tobacco smoke exposure in children with asthma: results of the LET'S Manage Asthma trial. Chest 2011;139(3):581–90.
92. Lehrer PM. Emotionally triggered asthma: a review of research literature and some hypotheses for self-regulation therapies. Appl Psychophysiol Biofeedback 1998;23(1):13–41.
93. Clarke SA, Calam R. The effectiveness of psychosocial interventions designed to improve health-related quality of life (HRQOL) amongst asthmatic children and their families: a systematic review. Qual Life Res 2012;21(5):747–64.
94. Klinnert MD, McQuaid EL, McCormick D, et al. A multimethod assessment of behavioral and emotional adjustment of children with asthma. J Pediatr Psychol 2000;25:35–46.

Role of Sleep Apnea and Gastroesophageal Reflux in Severe Asthma

 CrossMark

Linda Rogers, MD

KEYWORDS

- Asthma • Obstructive sleep apnea • Gastroesophageal reflux
- Continuous positive airway pressure • Comorbidity

KEY POINTS

- Treatment of gastroesophageal reflux (GER) with proton pump inhibitors (PPIs) has a limited impact on symptoms and lung function in patients with asthma and symptomatic GER.
- Treatment with PPI of GER identified by pH probe in the absence of GER symptoms does not improve asthma control.
- The impact of treatment of severe GER on asthma has not been fully explored in existing clinical trials.
- Multiple potential mechanisms suggest a relationship between obstructive sleep apnea syndrome (OSA) and asthma, but the directionality of cause and effect is unclear.
- Limited data suggest that treatment of OSA may improve asthma, but further exploration of clinical outcomes and mechanism of benefit are warranted.

INTRODUCTION

Historically, asthma guidelines recommend assessing and treating comorbid conditions in order to achieve asthma control. Recent guidelines from the European Respiratory Society/American Thoracic Society propose the term difficult to control asthma for those in whom treatment of comorbid conditions will presumably improve asthma control.[1] In this review, the author reviews evidence linking obstructive sleep apnea syndrome (OSA) and gastroesophageal reflux (GER) to "difficult to control" asthma and looks critically at the evidence base supporting that evaluation and treatment of these conditions impacts asthma control.

Disclosure: The author does not have any disclosures pertaining to the topic in this review.
Department of Medicine, Mount Sinai-National Jewish Health Respiratory Institute, Icahn School of Medicine at Mount Sinai, One Gustave L. Levy Place, Box 1232, New York, NY 10029, USA
E-mail address: linda.rogers@mssm.edu

Immunol Allergy Clin N Am 36 (2016) 461–471
http://dx.doi.org/10.1016/j.iac.2016.03.008
0889-8561/16/$ – see front matter © 2016 Elsevier Inc. All rights reserved.

IS THERE A LINK BETWEEN ASTHMA AND GASTROESOPHAGEAL REFLUX?

The prevalence of GER may be present at a higher rate in those with asthma than what would be expected based on general population prevalence of GER alone. Diagnosis of GER by pH probe in those with asthma with or without typical reflux symptoms has identified prevalence rates of 40% to 60%.[2-4] Despite coexistence of these conditions, it is unclear whether GER impacts asthma control or whether asthma increases the likelihood of GER.

DOES GASTROESOPHAGEAL REFLUX IMPACT ASTHMA CONTROL OR DOES ASTHMA CONTRIBUTE TO GASTROESOPHAGEAL REFLUX?

A classic hypothesis linking asthma and GER involves the direct microaspiration of acidic gastric contents into the lower airways triggering epithelial damage, neurogenic inflammation, and bronchoconstriction.[5-8] Because of shared embryologic origin and innervation of the esophagus and airways via the vagus nerve, reflux in the upper esophagus can trigger bronchoconstriction without direct aspiration. These two hypotheses have been referred to as *reflux theory* and *reflex theory* and are illustrated in **Fig. 1**. Nonacid reflux with bile acids and pepsin has been associated with GER symptoms, although a relationship with extraesophageal manifestations of GER is less clear.[3] Findings suggestive of laryngopharyngeal reflux by laryngoscopy or bronchoscopy is common in refractory asthma and may potentially impact asthma via reflux or reflex pathways.[9]

   Contrarians have argued that the presence of asthma impacts lower esophageal sphincter (LES) tone and, thus, promotes GER rather than GER triggering asthma.[10] Swings in intrathoracic pressure and/or descent of the diaphragm due to hyperinflation may reverse the normal thoracoabdominal pressure gradient, drawing the LES into the chest and altering its barrier function. Asthma may lower LES tone and promote GER via direct effects of beta agonists and theophylline.[11]

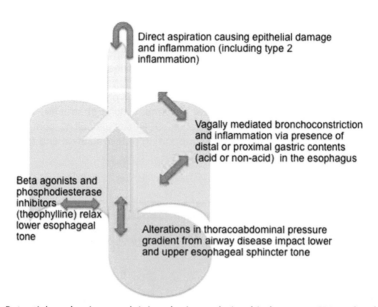

Fig. 1. Potential mechanisms explaining the interrelationship between GER and asthma.

DOES TREATMENT OF GASTROESOPHAGEAL REFLUX WITH PROTON PUMP INHIBITORS HELP CONTROL ASTHMA?

GER as a proposed cause of poorly controlled nonallergic or intrinsic asthma has been proposed for more than 50 years.[9,12–14] Several randomized clinical trials performed in the 1980s to 1990s examining the effect of GER treatment on asthma had significant methodological limitations, including small sample size, use of H_2 blockers alone, failure to use clinically effective doses of proton-pump inhibitors, and short duration of followup.[15–21] In 2003, a systematic review pooled a small group of modest-sized randomized controlled trials, but a significant treatment effect was not identified.[22] Since 2005, several large randomized placebo-controlled clinical trails directly examining this issue were conducted; the largest ones are presented in **Table 1**.

Littner and colleagues[23] performed a 24-week study of symptomatic GER and asthma treated with proton pump inhibitors (PPIs). Although reduced exacerbations and improved quality of life were noted in the PPI-treated patients, there was no difference in the primary outcome of daily symptoms. Kiljander and colleagues[24] studied patients with asthma and nocturnal symptoms, GER symptoms, or both and found no effect of PPI treatment on most asthma-related end points but found modest effects on peak flow in those with nocturnal asthma and GER. In the Study of Acid Reflux and Asthma (SARA) of participants with GER symptoms less than twice weekly, 24 weeks of high-dose PPIs did not impact the primary end point of episodes of poor asthma control, a composite score including step-up of treatment, lung function, urgent care, and exacerbations requiring steroids, despite the presence of GER by pH probe 40% of participants.[4] The same investigators also looked at the specific role of proximal reflux by use of dual pH probe testing and found no difference in lung function or asthma symptoms with PPI treatment of proximal reflux, although greater oral corticosteroid use and worse asthma-related quality of life were observed in those with proximal reflux.[25] In the Study of Acid Reflux in Children with Asthma, testing and treatment of clinically occult GER did not improve asthma control in children with uncontrolled asthma despite the presence of GER by pH probe in 43% of children. Moreover, a higher rate of adverse effects was noted in PPI-treated children, including increased respiratory tract infections.[26] The modest benefit observed in studies of patients with symptomatic GER does not exclude some benefit in these patients or a potential impact of treatment of severe or uncontrolled GER in asthma, a group excluded from the SARA study as the they would have an indication for treatment based on gastrointestinal issues alone.[23,24,26,27] A more recent systematic review looking at this issue in adults identified 11 trials containing 2524 patients and found a small effect of PPI on morning peak flow that was statistically significant but of unclear clinical significance (mean difference 8.68 L/min [95% confidence interval, 2.35–15.02]).[28] There was no effect on symptom scores, evening peak flow, asthma quality of life questionnaire (AQLQ), or forced expiratory volume in 1 second. Interestingly, a large case control study using the National Veterans Affairs and Centers for Medicare and Medicaid Services Databases found that a GER diagnosis was associated with a decreased risk of asthma-related events across all ages by 13% to 28%.[29]

UNRESOLVED ISSUES SURROUNDING THE RELATIONSHIP BETWEEN GASTROESOPHAGEAL REFLUX AND ASTHMA

The failure of PPIs to significantly impact asthma measures in existing clinical trials does not completely exclude a possible role of acid or nonacid reflux in asthma. In a systematic review, lifestyle modification including weight loss and elevation of the head of the bed impacted GER.[30] It is possible that use of PPI in the absence of

Table 1
Large randomized placebo-controlled trials of proton-pump inhibitor therapy in asthma and suspected comorbid gastroesophageal reflux

Author	Treatment Group (n)	Control Group (n)	GER Symptoms/GER Diagnosis	PPI Dosage	Duration	Results of Primary End Point	Other Outcomes
Kiljander et al,[18] 1999	52	52	Yes pH probe (GER 53%)	Omeprazole 20 mg 1 × daily	8 wk	Not described	Improved nocturnal symptoms and FEV_1 [a]
Littner et al,[23] 2005	99	108	Yes Symptoms (pH probe optional)	Lansoprazole 30 mg 2 × daily	24 wk	Asthma symptom diaries: no difference	Reduced exacerbations and improved quality of life
Kiljander et al,[24] 2006	387	383	With and without GER symptoms[b]	Esomeprazole 40 mg 2 × daily	16 wk	Modestly improved PEF in those with GER and nocturnal asthma	No difference in symptoms or exacerbations
Mastronarde et al,[4] 2009	200	193	No pH probe GER 40%	Esomeprazole 40 mg 2 × daily	24 wk	No difference in episodes of poor asthma control[c]	No difference in lung function or other measures
Kiljander et al,[27] 2010	632	328	Yes GER symptoms >2 d/wk	Esomeprazole 40 mg 1–2 × daily	26 wk	Modest improved PEF in both esomeprazole groups	Modest improvement in FEV_1 and AQLQ
Holbrook et al,[26] 2012	157	149	No pH probe subgroup (n = 115) GER 43%	Lansoprazole 15 or 30 mg daily	24 wk	ACQ: no change	No change in lung function or episodes of poor asthma control

Abbreviations: ACQ, asthma control questionnaire; AQLQ, asthma quality of life questionnaire; FEV_1, forced expiratory volume in 1 second; PEF, peak expiratory flow; PPI, proton pump inhibitor.
[a] Crossover study.
[b] Study participants stratified by the presence of GER symptoms and/or nocturnal asthma.
[c] Episodes of poor asthma control defined by a decrease of 30% or more in the morning peak expiratory flow rate on 2 consecutive days, as compared with the patients' best rate during the run-in period; an urgent visit, defined as an unscheduled health care visit for asthma symptoms; or the need for a course of oral prednisone for treatment of asthma.

lifestyle modification accounted for lack of benefits in clinical trials. Patients with severe GER or motility disorders were largely excluded from these clinical trials, and a potential benefit of treatment in these patients cannot be excluded. PPIs do not address nonacid reflux including bile acids and pepsin; whereas impedance monitoring can detect nonacid reflux, controversy persists regarding optimal therapy for nonacid reflux.[3] Lastly, the possible risks of PPIs include enteric and respiratory infections (including *Clostridium difficile*), osteoporosis, B12 deficiency, electrolyte abnormalities, malabsorption, and diarrhea; thus, long-term treatment with these agents may not be justified given modest effects in asthma in the absence of significant gastrointestinal indications.[31]

The American College of Gastroenterology's current guidelines do not recommend surgery for those with presumed extraesophageal manifestations of GER that do not respond to PPI.[32] Nevertheless, several uncontrolled case series suggest a benefit of surgery for concomitant asthma and GER.[3,33] A systematic review of antireflux surgery in asthma found that surgery may improve asthma symptoms but not pulmonary function.[34] A 2-year unblinded randomized controlled trial comparing medical and surgical reflux therapies suggested superiority of surgery compared with medical therapy, with 75.0% of surgical patients showing an improvement in nocturnal asthma symptoms compared with 9.1% and 4.2% of patients on medical therapy and controls, respectively.[35]

A case series of sequential treatment with high-dose PPI followed by fundoplication in patients with asthma who were carefully evaluated at baseline, after PPI treatment and after fundoplication, found an improvement in cough and dyspnea after fundoplication in the absence of changes in objective measures, such as fraction of exhaled nitric oxide, spirometry, and bronchial hyperreactivity.[36] Use of prokinetic agents have also been advocated in refractory GER, but to date there is no high-quality evidence supporting this practice.[37] A new minimally invasive procedure for GER treatment, Stretta, uses catheter-applied radiofrequency energy to the LES, muscle, and gastric cardia to ameliorate GER. The role of this procedure in GER-associated asthma remains to be determined.

In summary, current evidence suggests that the presence of GER symptoms should largely drive how GER is treated when present along with uncontrolled asthma. Current evidence does not support investigation for occult GER as a cause of uncontrolled asthma in children or adults because treatment does not clearly improve asthma outcomes. Large placebo-controlled trials of symptomatic GER in asthma have shown modest effects on symptoms and lung function. A role of the treatment of severe GER in uncontrolled asthma and the impact of prokinetic agents, antireflux surgery, and novel radiofrequency procedures on asthma control in those with comorbid GER remain unclear.

WHAT IS THE RELATIONSHIP BETWEEN OBSTRUCTIVE SLEEP APNEA SYNDROME AND ASTHMA?

OSA is highly prevalent in difficult-to-treat asthma, with rates of more than 85% reported in some case series.[38,39] As large studies using polysomnography are expensive and not always feasible, population-based studies of OSA and asthma are largely based on symptom reports, diagnosis codes, and standardized questionnaires. The accuracy of prevalence rates in these studies has been questioned, as nocturnal dyspnea and wheeze from asthma can overlap significantly with symptoms of OSA.[40,41] In the population-based Wisconsin Sleep Cohort Study, participants without OSA by polysomnography at baseline were more likely to develop polysomnographically identified OSA after 8 years if they had a diagnosis of asthma.[42]

Epidemiologic studies suggest that OSA may be associated with uncontrolled asthma. In those with severe asthma, OSA by polysomnography is linked to frequent asthma exacerbations.[43,44] In children with severe asthma, 63% have concomitant OSA.[45,46] A population-based study in China found that OSA was twice as common in those with asthma than in controls, and those with more than one emergency department visit for asthma had the highest likelihood of OSA.[47] Julien and colleagues[38] found that patients with more severe asthma had a higher apnea-hypopnea index and more severe OSA compared with those with milder asthma. The presence of both GER and OSA was associated with poor control of asthma in local residents and responders to the World Trade Center terrorist attack.[48] In the Severe Asthma Research Program Cohort, those with a high risk of OSA based on standardized questionnaires had more asthma symptoms, greater β_2-agonist use, and greater health care utilization for asthma.[49]

PATHOPHYSIOLOGY OF THE INTERRELATIONSHIP BETWEEN ASTHMA AND OBSTRUCTIVE SLEEP APNEA SYNDROME

The relationship between asthma and OSA may be bidirectional as illustrated in **Fig. 2**. There may be a direct impact of one condition on the other or their relationship may be mediated via common comorbidities, including GER, rhinitis, and obesity. Allergic and nonallergic rhinitis, present in most patients with asthma, cause increased nasal resistance to breathing during sleep and negative oropharyngeal pressure during inspiration and may predispose to upper airway collapse.[50]

OSA may affect resting lung volumes during sleep, cause direct effects on smooth muscle and airway hyperreactivity, or trigger localized upper airway or systemic inflammation. Vagal stimulation from upper airway collapse may trigger bronchial hyperreactivity.[51] Tissue vibration with snoring, repeated upper airway obstructive events causing mechanical trauma, and cyclical hypoxemia with apneic events may trigger a local and/or systemic inflammatory response with cytokines, including interleukins 6 and 8 (IL-6, IL-8), vascular endothelial growth factor, tumor necrosis factor alpha (TNF-α), and C-reactive protein (CRP).[52–54] In an animal model, chronic intermittent hypoxia skewed an allergic immune response toward a more Th-1-predominant

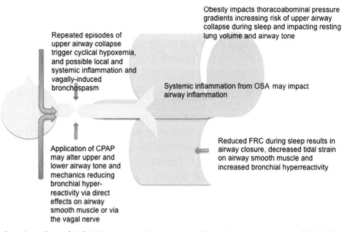

Obesity impacts thoracoabominal pressure gradients increasing risk of upper airway collapse during sleep and impacting resting lung volume and airway tone

Repeated episodes of upper airway collapse trigger cyclical hypoxemia, and possible local and systemic inflammation and vagally-induced bronchospasm

Systemic inflammation from OSA may impact airway inflammation

Application of CPAP may alter upper and lower airway tone and mechanics reducing bronchial hyper-reactivity via direct effects on airway smooth muscle or via the vagal nerve

Reduced FRC during sleep results in airway closure, decreased tidal strain on airway smooth muscle and increased bronchial hyperreactivity

Fig. 2. Mechanisms by which OSA or continuous positive airway pressure (CPAP) may impact asthma. FRC, functional residual capacity.

cellular phenotype.[55] In humans, a recent study identified increased neutrophilic airway inflammation in patients with asthma and OSA.[55]

A cardinal feature of asthma is an intrinsic defect in airway smooth muscle function.[56] A reduction of periodic stretching of airway smooth muscle can lead to bronchial hyperreactivity, and hyperinflation and maintenance of elevated end inspiratory lung volumes is a mechanism of defense against this in asthma.[57] This effect is diminished with the reduction of functional residual capacity that occurs during sleep, resulting in a loss of airway parenchymal interdependence and loss of the ability of deep inspiration to dilate airways.[58] This mechanism may be at play in obesity-related asthma as well as in comorbid OSA and asthma. This mechanism may also have potential therapeutic implications, as the use of continuous positive airway pressure (CPAP) might impact this intrinsic smooth muscle dysfunction of asthma even in the absence of OSA.

DOES TREATMENT WITH CONTINUOUS POSITIVE AIRWAY PRESSURE WITH OR WITHOUT OBSTRUCTIVE SLEEP APNEA SYNDROME IMPACT ASTHMA CONTROL?

Several unblinded cohort studies of CPAP in those with asthma and OSA suggested improvement in symptoms, reduced rescue β-agonist use, and improved peak flow rates.[51,59–61] Three months of CPAP in patients with moderate to severe persistent asthma reduced serum inflammatory markers, including CRP, TNF, and IL-6.[62]

CPAP is currently being explored as a treatment of asthma in the absence of OSA. In several animal models, chronic lung inflation via CPAP reduces airway smooth muscle contractility in vivo and in vitro, including in a rabbit model of allergic airway inflammation.[63,64] Lin and colleagues[65] observed a decrease in methacholine responsiveness when treating participants with documented bronchial hyperreactivity in the absence of clinical asthma with nasal CPAP. In a pilot sham-controlled study of adults with mild asthma, use of nocturnal CPAP (8–10 cm H_2O) was associated with a 2.7-fold increase in the provocative concentration of methacholine resulting in a 20% decrease in forced expiratory volume in 1 second compared with control.[66] This study led to a subsequent randomized controlled trial involving 194 participants designed to assess 12 weeks of treatment with CPAP 1 cm H_2O (sham CPAP), 5 cm H_2O (medium level CPAP), or 10 cm H_2O (high-level CPAP) on bronchial hyperreactivity in asthma. This trial will be one of the largest prospective clinical trials looking at the impact of CPAP on asthma and may shed important light on mechanisms by which CPAP might improve asthma but will not directly examine the role of OSA as an asthma comorbidity and whether CPAP improves asthma when both conditions are present. Moreover, concerns regarding the ability of those with uncontrolled asthma with or without a diagnosis of sleep apnea to tolerate CPAP remain.[67]

In summary, there is a gathering body of evidence that asthma predisposes to development of OSA and that this likelihood increases with increasing asthma severity.

Similarly, asthma and commonly related conditions, including GER, rhinitis, and obesity, may increase the likelihood of development of OSA. There are several plausible mechanisms by which asthma and OSA may be related and by which each condition may impact the outcome of the other. There is a lack of controlled, prospective clinical trials supporting the contention that treatment of OSA impacts asthma outcomes. An exploration of the impact of CPAP treatment of asthma, specifically targeting treatment of bronchial hyperreactivity even in the absence of OSA, may potentially lead to a nonpharmacologic adjunct in management of asthma and may help promote understanding of disease mechanisms that have not been the target of pharmacologic therapy. Similar to the relationship between asthma and GER, symptomatic GER and OSA warrant treatment in and of themselves when present as comorbid conditions with asthma regardless of the likelihood of impact on asthma; a better understanding of whether this in turn impacts asthma control, particularly in severe asthma, remains to be determined.

REFERENCES

1. Chung KF, Wenzel SE, Brozek JL, et al. International ERS/ATS guidelines on definition, evaluation and treatment of severe asthma. Eur Respir J 2014;43:343–73.
2. Harding SM, Guzzo MR, Richter JE. The prevalence of gastroesophageal reflux in asthma patients without reflux symptoms. Am J Respir Crit Care Med 2000;162: 34–9.
3. Naik RD, Vaezi MF. Extra-esophageal gastroesophageal reflux disease and asthma: understanding this interplay. Expert Rev Gastroenterol Hepatol 2015;9: 969–82.
4. American Lung Association Asthma Clinical Research Centers, Mastronarde JG, Anthonisen NR, et al. Efficacy of esomeprazole for treatment of poorly controlled asthma. N Engl J Med 2009;360:1487–99.
5. Hamamoto J, Kohrogi H, Kawano O, et al. Esophageal stimulation by hydrochloric acid causes neurogenic inflammation in the airways in guinea pigs. J Appl Physiol (1985) 1997;82:738–45.
6. Mansfield LE, Hameister HH, Spaulding HS, et al. The role of the vague nerve in airway narrowing caused by intraesophageal hydrochloric acid provocation and esophageal distention. Ann Allergy 1981;47:431–4.
7. Mansfield LE, Stein MR. Gastroesophageal reflux and asthma: a possible reflex mechanism. Ann Allergy 1978;41:224–6.
8. Spaulding HS Jr, Mansfield LE, Stein MR, et al. Further investigation of the association between gastroesophageal reflux and bronchoconstriction. J Allergy Clin Immunol 1982;69:516–21.
9. Good JT Jr, Kolakowski CA, Groshong SD, et al. Refractory asthma: importance of bronchoscopy to identify phenotypes and direct therapy. Chest 2012;141: 599–606.
10. Turbyville JC. Applying principles of physics to the airway to help explain the relationship between asthma and gastroesophageal reflux. Med Hypotheses 2010; 74:1075–80.
11. Crowell MD, Zayat EN, Lacy BE, et al. The effects of an inhaled beta(2)-adrenergic agonist on lower esophageal function: a dose-response study. Chest 2001;120:1184–9.
12. Mays EE. Intrinsic asthma in adults. Association with gastroesophageal reflux. JAMA 1976;236:2626–8.
13. Overholt RH, Voorhees RJ. Esophageal reflux as a trigger in asthma. Dis Chest 1966;49:464–6.
14. Goodall RJ, Earis JE, Cooper DN, et al. Relationship between asthma and gastro-oesophageal reflux. Thorax 1981;36:116–21.
15. Boeree MJ, Peters FT, Postma DS, et al. No effects of high-dose omeprazole in patients with severe airway hyperresponsiveness and (a)symptomatic gastro-oesophageal reflux. Eur Respir J 1998;11:1070–4.
16. Ford RM. Asthma in Australia. Aust N Z J Med 1994;24:71.

17. Harding SM, Richter JE, Guzzo MR, et al. Asthma and gastroesophageal reflux: acid suppressive therapy improves asthma outcome. Am J Med 1996;100: 395–405.
18. Kiljander TO, Salomaa ER, Hietanen EK, et al. Gastroesophageal reflux in asthmatics: a double-blind, placebo-controlled crossover study with omeprazole. Chest 1999;116:1257–64.
19. Levin TR, Sperling RM, McQuaid KR. Omeprazole improves peak expiratory flow rate and quality of life in asthmatics with gastroesophageal reflux. Am J Gastroenterol 1998;93:1060–3.
20. Meier JH, McNally PR, Punja M, et al. Does omeprazole (Prilosec) improve respiratory function in asthmatics with gastroesophageal reflux? A double-blind, placebo-controlled crossover study. Dig Dis Sci 1994;39:2127–33.
21. Teichtahl H, Kronborg IJ, Yeomans ND, et al. Adult asthma and gastrooesophageal reflux: the effects of omeprazole therapy on asthma. Aust N Z J Med 1996;26:671–6.
22. Gibson PG, Henry RL, Coughlan JL. Gastro-oesophageal reflux treatment for asthma in adults and children. Cochrane Database Syst Rev 2003;(2):CD001496.
23. Littner MR, Leung FW, Ballard ED 2nd, et al. Lansoprazole Asthma Study G. Effects of 24 weeks of lansoprazole therapy on asthma symptoms, exacerbations, quality of life, and pulmonary function in adult asthmatic patients with acid reflux symptoms. Chest 2005;128:1128–35.
24. Kiljander TO, Harding SM, Field SK, et al. Effects of esomeprazole 40 mg twice daily on asthma: a randomized placebo-controlled trial. Am J Respir Crit Care Med 2006;173:1091–7.
25. DiMango E, Holbrook JT, Simpson E, et al. Effects of asymptomatic proximal and distal gastroesophageal reflux on asthma severity. Am J Respir Crit Care Med 2009;180:809–16.
26. Writing Committee for the American Lung Association Asthma Clinical Research Centers, Holbrook JT, Wise RA, et al. Lansoprazole for children with poorly controlled asthma: a randomized controlled trial. JAMA 2012;307:373–81.
27. Kiljander TO, Junghard O, Beckman O, et al. Effect of esomeprazole 40 mg once or twice daily on asthma: a randomized, placebo-controlled study. Am J Respir Crit Care Med 2010;181:1042–8.
28. Chan WW, Chiou E, Obstein KL, et al. The efficacy of proton pump inhibitors for the treatment of asthma in adults: a meta-analysis. Arch Intern Med 2011;171: 620–9.
29. Sumino K, O'Brian K, Bartle B, et al. Coexisting chronic conditions associated with mortality and morbidity in adult patients with asthma. J Asthma 2014;51: 306–14.
30. Kaltenbach T, Crockett S, Gerson LB. Are lifestyle measures effective in patients with gastroesophageal reflux disease? An evidence-based approach. Arch Intern Med 2006;166:965–71.
31. Owen C, Marks DJ, Banks M. The dangers of proton pump inhibitor therapy. Br J Hosp Med 2014;75:C108–12.
32. Katz PO, Gerson LB, Vela MF. Guidelines for the diagnosis and management of gastroesophageal reflux disease. Am J Gastroenterol 2013;108:308–28 [quiz: 29].
33. Rothenberg S, Cowles R. The effects of laparoscopic Nissen fundoplication on patients with severe gastroesophageal reflux disease and steroid-dependent asthma. J Pediatr Surg 2012;47:1101–4.

34. Field SK, Gelfand GA, McFadden SD. The effects of antireflux surgery on asthmatics with gastroesophageal reflux. Chest 1999;116:766–74.
35. Sontag SJ, O'Connell S, Khandelwal S, et al. Asthmatics with gastroesophageal reflux: long term results of a randomized trial of medical and surgical antireflux therapies. Am J Gastroenterol 2003;98:987–99.
36. Kiljander T, Rantanen T, Kellokumpu I, et al. Comparison of the effects of esomeprazole and fundoplication on airway responsiveness in patients with gastrooesophageal reflux disease. Clin Respir J 2013;7:281–7.
37. Glicksman JT, Mick PT, Fung K, et al. Prokinetic agents and laryngopharyngeal reflux disease: prokinetic agents and laryngopharyngeal reflux disease: a systematic review. Laryngoscope 2014;124:2375–9.
38. Julien JY, Martin JG, Ernst P, et al. Prevalence of obstructive sleep apnea-hypopnea in severe versus moderate asthma. J Allergy Clin Immunol 2009;124: 371–6.
39. Yigla M, Tov N, Solomonov A, et al. Difficult-to-control asthma and obstructive sleep apnea. J Asthma 2003;40:865–71.
40. Janson C, De Backer W, Gislason T, et al. Increased prevalence of sleep disturbances and daytime sleepiness in subjects with bronchial asthma: a population study of young adults in three European countries. Eur Respir J 1996;9:2132–8.
41. Larsson LG, Lindberg A, Franklin KA, et al. Symptoms related to obstructive sleep apnoea are common in subjects with asthma, chronic bronchitis and rhinitis in a general population. Respir Med 2001;95:423–9.
42. Teodorescu M, Barnet JH, Hagen EW, et al. Association between asthma and risk of developing obstructive sleep apnea. JAMA 2015;313:156–64.
43. ten Brinke A, Sterk PJ, Masclee AA, et al. Risk factors of frequent exacerbations in difficult-to-treat asthma. Eur Respir J 2005;26:812–8.
44. Teodorescu M, Polomis DA, Hall SV, et al. Association of obstructive sleep apnea risk with asthma control in adults. Chest 2010;138:543–50.
45. Kheirandish-Gozal L, Dayyat EA, Eid NS, et al. Obstructive sleep apnea in poorly controlled asthmatic children: effect of adenotonsillectomy. Pediatr Pulmonol 2011;46:913–8.
46. Shanley LA, Lin H, Flores G. Factors associated with length of stay for pediatric asthma hospitalizations. J Asthma 2015;52:471–7.
47. Shen TC, Lin CL, Wei CC, et al. Risk of obstructive sleep apnea in adult patients with asthma: a population-based cohort study in Taiwan. PLoS One 2015;10: e0128461.
48. Jordan HT, Stellman SD, Reibman J, et al. Factors associated with poor control of 9/11-related asthma 10-11 years after the 2001 World Trade Center terrorist attacks. J Asthma 2015;52:630–7.
49. Teodorescu M, Broytman O, Curran-Everett D, et al. Obstructive sleep apnea risk, asthma burden, and lower airway inflammation in adults in the Severe Asthma Research Program (SARP) II. J Allergy Clin Immunol Pract 2015;3:566–75.e1.
50. Kalpaklioglu AF, Kavut AB, Ekici M. Allergic and nonallergic rhinitis: the threat for obstructive sleep apnea. Ann Allergy Asthma Immunol 2009;103:20–5.
51. Guilleminault C, Quera-Salva MA, Powell N, et al. Nocturnal asthma: snoring, small pharynx and nasal CPAP. Eur Respir J 1988;1:902–7.
52. Aihara K, Oga T, Chihara Y, et al. Analysis of systemic and airway inflammation in obstructive sleep apnea. Sleep Breath 2013;17:597–604.
53. Vgontzas AN, Papanicolaou DA, Bixler EO, et al. Elevation of plasma cytokines in disorders of excessive daytime sleepiness: role of sleep disturbance and obesity. J Clin Endocrinol Metab 1997;82:1313–6.

54. Yokoe T, Minoguchi K, Matsuo H, et al. Elevated levels of C-reactive protein and interleukin-6 in patients with obstructive sleep apnea syndrome are decreased by nasal continuous positive airway pressure. Circulation 2003;107:1129–34.
55. Broytman O, Braun RK, Morgan BJ, et al. Effects of chronic intermittent hypoxia on allergen-induced airway inflammation in rats. Am J Respir Cell Mol Biol 2015; 52:162–70.
56. Skloot G, Permutt S, Togias A. Airway hyperresponsiveness in asthma: a problem of limited smooth muscle relaxation with inspiration. J Clin Invest 1995;96: 2393–403.
57. Brown RH, Pearse DB, Pyrgos G, et al. The structural basis of airways hyperresponsiveness in asthma. J Appl Physiol (1985) 2006;101:30–9.
58. Irvin CG, Pak J, Martin RJ. Airway-parenchyma uncoupling in nocturnal asthma. Am J Respir Crit Care Med 2000;161:50–6.
59. Chan CS, Woolcock AJ, Sullivan CE. Nocturnal asthma: role of snoring and obstructive sleep apnea. Am Rev Respir Dis 1988;137:1502–4.
60. Ciftci TU, Ciftci B, Guven SF, et al. Effect of nasal continuous positive airway pressure in uncontrolled nocturnal asthmatic patients with obstructive sleep apnea syndrome. Respir Med 2005;99:529–34.
61. Lafond C, Series F, Lemiere C. Impact of CPAP on asthmatic patients with obstructive sleep apnoea. Eur Respir J 2007;29:307–11.
62. Karamanli H, Ozol D, Ugur KS, et al. Influence of CPAP treatment on airway and systemic inflammation in OSAS patients. Sleep Breath 2014;18:251–6.
63. Xue Z, Yu Y, Gao H, et al. Chronic continuous positive airway pressure (CPAP) reduces airway reactivity in vivo in an allergen-induced rabbit model of asthma. J Appl Physiol (1985) 2011;111:353–7.
64. Xue Z, Zhang L, Liu Y, et al. Chronic inflation of ferret lungs with CPAP reduces airway smooth muscle contractility in vivo and in vitro. J Appl Physiol (1985) 2008;104:610–5.
65. Lin CC, Lin CY. Obstructive sleep apnea syndrome and bronchial hyperreactivity. Lung 1995;173:117–26.
66. Busk M, Busk N, Puntenney P, et al. Use of continuous positive airway pressure reduces airway reactivity in adults with asthma. Eur Respir J 2013;41:317–22.
67. Martin RJ, Pak J. Nasal CPAP in nonapneic nocturnal asthma. Chest 1991;100: 1024–7.

Role of Small Airways in Asthma

Lindsay K. Finkas, MD[a],*, Richard Martin, MD[b]

KEYWORDS

- Small airways • Extrafine particle inhalers • Asthma • Nocturnal asthma

KEY POINTS

- The small airways are distal airways that measure less than 2 mm in luminal diameter.
- Inflammation and increased peripheral airway resistance have been demonstrated in the small airways of patients with asthma.
- The development of extrafine particle inhalers has improved drug delivery to the small airways.

INTRODUCTION

Asthma is a common chronic condition characterized by reversible airflow limitation. Prevalence has increased in the United States, affecting approximately 8% of the population and can be associated with high morbidity and health care costs.[1] Asthma is a heterogeneous disease affecting both small and large airways. In the past, much of the focus in asthma has been on the larger airways given the difficulty associated with measuring the small airways. The small airways, as a result, are frequently ignored, though remain an important aspect of asthma. Recently, there has been increased work in elucidating the contribution of the peripheral airways in asthma, more specifically severe asthma.[2]

The distal (small) airways are defined as those distal to the seventh or eighth division of the tracheobronchial tree and measure less than 2 mm in luminal diameter.[3] The distal airways represent most of the total surface area of the airways and play an important role in the pathophysiology of asthma.[4] The alveolar tissue area, in addition to the airways, also contributes to distal airway inflammation.[5]

Studies have been undertaken to evaluate inflammation and the physiology of the distal airway as well as develop clinical parameters that may be used to measure the small airways. New inhalers and drug formulations with improved corticosteroids

[a] Division of Allergy and Clinical Immunology, Department of Medicine, National Jewish Health, 1400 Jackson Street, Denver, CO 80206, USA; [b] Department of Medicine, National Jewish Health, 1400 Jackson Street, Denver, CO 80206, USA
* Corresponding author.
E-mail address: FinkasL@NJHealth.org

Immunol Allergy Clin N Am 36 (2016) 473–482
http://dx.doi.org/10.1016/j.iac.2016.03.009
0889-8561/16/$ – see front matter © 2016 Elsevier Inc. All rights reserved.
immunology.theclinics.com

deposition are able to reach the small airways that are an area that larger-particle corticosteroid inhalers have been unable to target in significant concentration.[6]

Nocturnal asthma (NA) can be used as a model for studying the small airways and is used in several studies. NA is common in individuals with asthma and affects approximately 30% to 75% of individuals with asthma.[7] NA is a risk factor for mortality (70% association) and respiratory arrests (80% association).[8] In asthma, the peak lung function achieved is seen at 4:00 PM with a nadir at 4:00 AM.[9] For NA, this circadian change is markedly increased. In addition, bronchial hyperreactivity increases at night as well. These changes are felt to be related to circadian changes that occur in multiple factors, including cortisol levels.[10]

INFLAMMATION

Histologic evaluation of autopsy specimens from patients with asthma has allowed airway inflammation to be evaluated in both large and small airways. Carrol and colleagues[11] demonstrated that lymphocytes and eosinophils were present in both the proximal and distal airway in patients with asthma. Further studies have demonstrated that regional variations among the small airways and large airways exist as well. Haley and colleagues[12] found that the proximal airways had a significantly greater density of CD45-positive lymphocytes in the subbasement membrane and airway smooth muscle than the same areas in small airways. The small airways were noted to have CD45-positive lymphocytes and eosinophils in the area between airway smooth muscle and alveolar attachments.

Subjects with cystic fibrosis were also studied and they showed a similar pattern of proximal airway inflammation as subjects with asthma; however, the inflammation pattern in the small airways was not present. This suggests that small airway inflammation is not a characteristic of all obstructive airway disease and may be a specific finding seen in asthma.

A study in stable patients with chronic asthma in 1996 by Kraft and colleagues[13] evaluated 21 subjects with NA and 10 subjects with non-nocturnal asthma (NNA). Subjects underwent transbronchial and endobronchial biopsy at 4:00 PM and 4:00 AM. There were significant differences in the number of eosinophils in the alveolar tissue area from the 4:00 AM sample with increased eosinophils seen in the NA group. These findings were not seen in the biopsies from the proximal airway. In comparison of the 4:00 PM and 4:00 AM samples in the NA group, there were a significantly greater number of eosinophils at 4:00 AM. Similar findings were present for macrophages as well with increased values seen at 4:00 AM in the NA group. Circadian differences were not seen in the large airways.[13] An example of the inflammation in the small airways is shown in **Fig. 1**.[14]

CD4 T lymphocytes produce inflammatory cytokines including tumor necrosis factor, interleukin (IL)-4, IL-5, and IL-13 that are important mediators in eosinophil migration. Kraft and colleagues[15] sought to evaluate whether T lymphocytes were responsible for eosinophil migration in the distal airways in patients with NA. They found the number of CD4+ T lymphocytes in alveolar tissue at 4:00 AM was greater than that seen in subjects with NNA. In addition, they found that the number of alveolar CD4+ lymphocytes in NA positively correlated with the number of EG2+ eosinophils and inversely with FEV1 at 4:00 AM. Interestingly, proximal tissue inflammation of the larger airways did not have a significant correlation.[15]

Mediator release was also studied by Schulman and colleagues.[16] Human lung parenchyma tissue mediator release was measured and compared with airway tissue in a ragweed-challenged in vitro study. The model allowed investigators to compare if bronchus or parenchyma had greater mediator release following allergen challenge.

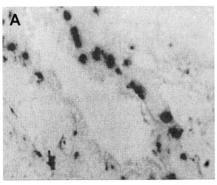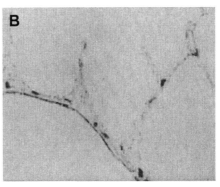

Fig. 1. Representative distal airway inflammation. (*A*) Small airway less than 2 mm in an subject with asthma with EG2-positive cells (activated eosinophils). (*B*) Major basic protein-stained lung parenchyma from a subject with asthma. (*From* Hamid Q, Song Y, Kotsimbos TC, et al. Inflammation of small airways in asthma. J Allergy Clin Immunol 1997;100(1):46; with permission.)

They found twofold to threefold greater concentrations of prostaglandins and thromboxane B2 in the lung parenchyma compared with the airway. Histamine was also measured and there was a fivefold greater concentration in the lung parenchyma than in the larger airways. These findings support differences in inflammatory responses in different airway tissue.

Conventional computed tomography (CT) and chest radiographic imaging have been unable to measure the distal airways. With the development of high-resolution CT (HRCT), there is now the ability to measure the small airway with diameter of 1.5 to 2.0 mm as well as wall thickness as small as 0.25 mm.[17] Okazawa and colleagues[18] used HRCT to evaluate airway wall thickness as well as the site and magnitude of narrowing of the airway in response to methacholine in subjects with asthma and healthy controls. In the subjects with asthma, the small airways were thickened compared with healthy controls. The small airways also showed a significantly decreased luminal area following methacholine inhalation. Goldin and colleagues[19] also used HRCT, and found that methacholine induced bronchoconstriction in up to 95% of airways with diameter between 1.6 and 2.5 mm.

PHYSIOLOGY

Wagner and colleagues[20] improved our understanding of physiology of the small airways by using a peripheral airway resistance technique. With this technique, a bronchoscope is wedged into the airway and airflow rate is progressively increased via one port and pressure change is measured in the second port. Peripheral airway resistance (Rp) is then calculated dividing the change in pressure by the change in flow (ΔPressure/Δflow). They used this method to compare healthy controls with individuals with mild asthma who had similar lung function. They found significantly increased peripheral airway resistance in the subjects with asthma (**Fig. 2**).[20]

A study by Kraft and colleagues[21] subsequently evaluated peripheral airway resistance in NA, NNA, and healthy controls. In addition, they assessed peripheral function to B-2 agonist by administering subcutaneous terbutaline in all groups. All subjects underwent bronchoscopy with Rp at 4:00 PM and 4:00 AM separated by 1 week. Peripheral airway resistance was measured via wedge bronchoscope as discussed previously. The peripheral airway resistance was highest in the NA group at both 4:00 PM and 4:00 AM compared with both NNA and control groups; however, there

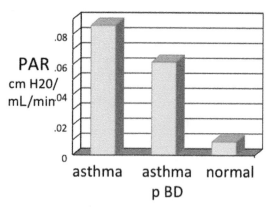

Fig. 2. Measurement of peripheral airways resistance: wedged bronchoscopic technique. pBD, post bronchodilator; PAR, peripheral airway resistance. (*Data from* Wagner EM, Liu MC, Weinmann GG, et al. Peripheral lung resistance in normal and asthmatic subjects. Am Rev Respir Dis 1990;141(3):584–8.)

was no significant difference found in Rp within the NA group at both times. Plateau pressures were noted to significantly increase from 4:00 PM to 4:00 AM in the NA group only. Closing pressures were found to be decreased in the NA group compared with NNA and control groups at both times. Following beta agonist treatment, Rp decreased in both asthma groups, although was significant only at 4:00 AM. The increase in plateau pressure in the NA group from 4:00 AM to 4:00 PM is suggestive of a loss of collateral channels and this may be due to smooth muscle contraction, inflammation, and/or edema.[21]

As direct measurement of peripheral airway resistance is invasive, surrogate markers to measure the small airways is desirable and multiple modalities and testing have been investigated. Spirometry is the most common test used to evaluate and monitor asthma. It is a simple, noninvasive method. Reproducibility on testing is important, as measurements such as the forced vital capacity (FVC) are highly effort dependent.[22] The forced expiratory volume in 1 second (FEV1) and FVC are reflective of the proximal airways, whereas the forced expiratory flow 25% to75% of the forced vital capacity (FEF25%–75%) has long been purposed as a measurement of the small airways. It is highly dependent on the validity of the FVC measurement and the level of expiratory effort.[23]

A pediatric study by Rao and colleagues[24] found a low FEF 25% to 75% in the setting of normal FEV1 was associated with increased asthma severity. The FEF 25% to 75%, however, has shown poor reproducibility and comparability if not adjusted for lung volumes. The FEF 25% to 75% is also often normal when the FEV1/FVC ratio is greater than 75.[25]

Closing volume (CV) is defined as the volume of gas remaining in the vital capacity (VC) at the intersection of phases III and IV. It is typically expressed as a percentage of the VC (CV/VC%). Higher CV has been attributed to earlier closing of the distal airways. In a pediatric study by In't Veen and colleagues,[26] CV was found to be elevated in the severe asthma group with recurrent exacerbations. This suggests that recurrent exacerbations may be related to the distal airway.

A study by Sutherland and Martin[27] looked at the relationship between physiology and distal lung inflammation by comparing transbronchial biopsy, spirometry, and plethysmography in patients with asthma. Distal lung tissue inflammation at

4:00 AM poorly correlated with previously suggested measurements of small airways FEF 25% to 75% and maximal to partial VC maneuver (M:P ratio). The distal lung tissue eosinophils at 4:00 AM, however, did correlate with both the thoracic gas volume and total lung capacity. This study suggests that FEF 25% to 75% and M:P ratio may not be reflective of distal airway inflammation and may not be the best reliable measurements of the inflammation in distal airways. Thoracic gas volume and total lung capacity may be better measurements of distal airway inflammation, as they correlate with distal airway eosinophil count.[27]

Impulse oscillometry (IOS) is another noninvasive objective measurement of lung function and particular values are associated with the small airways. IOS is a tool that is of benefit, as it is independent of effort and requires minimal patient cooperation. The R5 is a measurement that includes both small and large airways, whereas the R20 reflects the large airways only. Therefore, the difference between the R5 and R20 (R5 – R20) is reflective of the small airways only. Reactance area (AX) may also be used as a measurement of small airways and is the reactance at all frequencies between 5 Hz and the frequency at which the reactance is 0. In a study in children with asthma as well as controls, there was a significant difference in the R5 – R20, as was reactance in subjects with poorly controlled asthma versus those with controlled asthma and healthy controls.[28] Additionally, a study by Takeda and colleagues[29] used IOS in subjects to assess associations with health status, dyspnea, and asthma control. They found the R20 as well the R5 – R20 to be independently associated with lower health status as well as dyspnea. The AX was associated with loss of asthma control.[29]

OTHER MODALITIES

Exhaled nitric oxide (NO) is a newer, safe, noninvasive measurement of airway inflammation that is standardized. As NO is produced throughout the airway, it is recommended to obtain the measurement during exhalation against positive pressure to close the velum, and therefore exclude the upper airway contributions.[30] NO is produced by the reaction catalyzed by NO synthase. The inducible form of the enzyme is increased by proinflammatory mediators.[22] Fraction of exhaled nitric oxide measurements are flow dependent and require a constant expiratory flow and measurements obtained at a single flow rate are primarily reflective of the proximal airway.[31]

Two compartment models of pulmonary NO productions can be used to calculate the alveolar production of exhaled NO concentration.[32] Alveolar NO was calculated using a nonlinear model. Elevated alveolar NO can be seen in other conditions involving distal airway inflammation, such as pulmonary fibrosis and chronic obstructive pulmonary disease. A study from the United Kingdom compared subjects with refractory asthma, mild-to-moderate asthma, and healthy controls. They found that alveolar NO concentration was reproducible in subjects with refractory asthma. The study also showed there was also a positive correlation between alveolar NO concentration and bronchoalveolar lavage eosinophil count, but a similar association was not seen in bronchial wash or sputum eosinophil count. In addition, alveolar NO was found to be higher in subjects with refractory asthma as compared with mild-to-moderate asthma and healthy controls and values decreased following treatment with prednisolone. Alveolar NO, however, was not decreased following a doubling dose of inhaled steroids. This suggests that alveolar NO is a measurement of the distal lung and that refractory asthma is associated with increased distal airway inflammation.[33]

Lehtimäki and colleagues[34] found that subjects with asthma with nocturnal symptoms had higher levels of alveolar NO compared with both patients with asthma without nocturnal symptoms and healthy controls. This again suggests the role of the small airways in NA.

Nitrogen breath washout has also been proposed as a noninvasive measurement of the peripheral airways. By using a slope III analysis of multiple washout versus single washout, the ability to distinguish between the conductive airways (proximal airways) from acinar (distal airways) is achieved.[35]

THERAPEUTICS

Inhaled corticosteroids (ICS) are the mainstay of treatment for persistent asthma in both pediatric and adult populations. Inhaled drug delivery to the distal lung is dependent on numerous factors, with the most important being drug particle size. Formulation and preparation of the drug, patient technique, as well as the device in which the drug is delivered can also play a role in deposition in the distal airway. Studies have shown that the ideal particle size for drug delivery to the distal airway is a mass median aerodynamic diameter between 1 μm and 2 μm. Particle size less than 1 μm tends to be inhaled and exhaled without deposition. Particle size between 2 and 5 μm is deposited mainly in the medium-sized and large-sized airways. Particle size greater than 5 μm is associated with deposition in the oropharynx as well as in the larger, central airways.[36]

Particle size and drug efficacy have been well studied in inhaled bronchodilators. Improvements in FEF 25% to 75% have been shown with smaller particle size inhaled isoproterenol 2.5 μm compared with 5.0 μm. Studies looking at varying particle size with inhaled ipratropium bromide demonstrated peak bronchodilation was achieved with smaller particle size. This improvement is felt to be due to improved deposition into the small airways.[37]

In 1987, the Montreal Protocol mandated elimination of substances that deplete the ozone layer and included chlorofluorocarbons (CFCs) that were used as propellants in pressurized metered-dose inhalers (MDIs).[38] This led to the development of alternative forms of propellants, including hydrofluoroalkane (HFAs) that are currently used. With the development of HFAs, there were also changes in drug formulation. For beclomethasone dipropionate (BDP), this meant reformulation from a suspension to a solution. This change in formulation resulted in a change in particle size as well as a decrease in speed in which the drug leaves the MDI, both positively effecting drug delivery.[39] In addition to HFAs, breath-actuated dry powder inhalers (DPIs) have also been developed and are increasing in use. Particle sizes in DPIs are in some cases larger than previously used in MDIs with CFCs.[40] See **Table 1** for selected ICS and particle size.

Table 1
Particle size of select inhaled corticosteroids

Drug	Particle Size (MMAD), μm
Beclomethasone-HFA[a]	1.1
Beclomethasone-CFC[b]	3.5
Ciclesonide-HFA[a]	1.1
Flunisolide-HFA[a]	1.2
Flunisolide-CFC[b]	3.8
Fluticasone-DPI	5.4
Flucticasone-CFC[b]	2.4

Abbreviations: CFC, chlorofluorocarbon; DPI, dry powder inhaler; HFA, hydrofluoroalkane; MMAD, mass median aerodynamic diameter.
[a] Indicates extrafine particle inhalers.
[b] No longer available.

The smaller the particle size of the ICS, the greater the distal airway deposition and possibly, improved efficacy. CFC and DPI inhalers typically have larger particle sizes and, as a result, only approximately 5% to 30% of the drug is delivered to the lungs. The remainder of the drug is deposited in the oropharynx. The change in BDP to solution form with HFA resulted in a reduced mass median aerodynamic diameter to 1.1 μm from 3.5 μm.[41]

To evaluate drug delivery and deposition in the airway and relation to particle size, Leach and colleagues[42] used technetium-99m-radiolabled BDP. Beclomethasone was then delivered via CFC suspension or with HFA solution. There was a significant difference between airway deposition between the 2 products, with a significantly increased airway deposition associated with the BDP-HFA. In healthy subjects, BDP-HFA delivered 55% to 60% of the drug to the airways with 29% to 30% deposited in the oropharynx compared with the CFC, in which 4% to 7% of the drug was delivered to the lung with the remaining 90% to 94% having oropharyngeal deposition. Similar findings were also seen in the subjects with asthma. The pattern of delivery also differed between the 2 formulations. CFC-BDP had more central distribution as opposed to the HFA-BDP that had more diffuse delivery, in which the investigators concluded as improved delivery to the distal airways.

A randomized, placebo-controlled trial in 1999 by Gross and colleagues[43] compared HFA-BDP 400 μg/d, CFC-BDP 800 μg/d and placebo for 12 weeks. Peak expiratory flow rates were used as an outcome and HFA-BDP was shown to be equivalent to CFC-BDP. The investigators concluded that there was similar efficacy at half the dose with the HFA-BDP due to peripheral lung deposition.

Flunisolide has also been studied and compared in HFA versus CFC formulations. Corren and colleagues[44] studied varying dosing of HFA flunisolide and CFC flunisolide in asthmatic subjects. FEV1 was used as the primary endpoint and similar improvement in FEV1 was achieved in flunisolide HFA at one-third the dose compared with the CFC flunisolide–treated group.

Particle size has also been studied radiographically by following air trapping on HRCT. Goldin and colleagues[45] randomized subjects to HFA-BDP and CFC-DBP. Pre-HRCT and post-HRCT performed at residual volume before and after methacholine challenge. Following 4 weeks of treatment, subjects in the HFA-BDP group had greater improvement in regional airtrapping than those in the CFC-BDP group.

Increased dose of small-particle ICS as well as standard-size ICS as compared with the addition of long-acting beta agonists (LABA) has also been studied retrospectively by Israel and colleagues.[46] Increased dose of small and standard particle ICS was as effective as adding LABA as evaluated by asthma control and rates of severe exacerbations over 1 year.

In a retrospective matched cohort study, the cost-effectiveness of extrafine particle ICS as compared with standard-size particle ICS for both the United States and the United Kingdom in patients older than 12 demonstrated that the odds of overall control were greater in the extrafine ICS cohorts in both countries. Cost related to asthma was also significantly lower with the extrafine ICS cohorts in both countries.[47]

SUMMARY

Asthma is an obstructive airway disease that involves both large and small airways. Studies evaluating the small airways have shown increased inflammation as well as increased peripheral airway resistance in individuals with asthma. Additional studies are needed to correlate airway inflammation and resistance with surrogate markers that may readily provide information about the distal airways and assist in the evaluation of patients with asthma. With the development of new inhalers and drug formulations, there is an increased ability to deliver drugs to the distal airway that may improve asthma control and reduce exacerbations.

REFERENCES

1. Akinbami LJ, Bailey C, Zahran HS, et al. Trends in asthma prevalence, health care use, and mortality in the United States, 2001–2010. NCHS Data Brief 2012;(94):1–8.
2. van der Wiel E, ten Hacken NH, Postma DS, et al. Small-airways dysfunction associates with respiratory symptoms and clinical features of asthma: a systematic review. J Allergy Clin Immunol 2013;131(3):646–57.
3. Hogg JC, Macklem PT, Thurlbeck WM. Site and nature of airway obstruction in chronic obstructive lung disease. N Engl J Med 1968;278(25):1355–60.
4. Tulic MK, Christodoulopoulos P, Hamid Q. Small airway inflammation in asthma. Respir Res 2001;2(6):333–9.
5. Martin RJ. Exploring the distal lung: new direction in asthma. Isr Med Assoc J 2008;10(12):846–9.
6. Trikha AM, Martin RJ. Small airways in asthma. Curr Respir Care Rep 2013;2: 226–32.
7. Turner-Warwick M. Epidemiology of nocturnal asthma. Am J Med 1988;85(1B):6–8.
8. Hetzel MR, Clark TJ, Branthwaite MA. Asthma: analysis of sudden deaths and ventilatory arrests in hospital. Br Med J 1977;1(6064):808–11.
9. Hetzel MR, Clark TJ. Comparison of normal and asthmatic circadian rhythms in peak expiratory flow rate. Thorax 1980;35(10):732–8.
10. Martin RJ. Small airway and alveolar tissue changes in nocturnal asthma. Am J Respir Crit Care Med 1998;157(5 Pt 2):S188–90.
11. Carroll N, Elliot J, Morton A, et al. The structure of large and small airways in nonfatal and fatal asthma. Am Rev Respir Dis 1993;147(2):405–10.
12. Haley KJ, Sunday ME, Wiggs BR, et al. Inflammatory cell distribution within and along asthmatic airways. Am J Respir Crit Care Med 1998;158(2):565–72.
13. Kraft M, Djukanovic R, Wilson S, et al. Alveolar tissue inflammation in asthma. Am J Respir Crit Care Med 1996;154(5):1505–10.
14. Hamid Q, Song Y, Kotsimbos TC, et al. Inflammation of small airways in asthma. J Allergy Clin Immunol 1997;100(1):44–51.
15. Kraft M, Martin RJ, Wilson S, et al. Lymphocyte and eosinophil influx into alveolar tissue in nocturnal asthma. Am J Respir Crit Care Med 1999;159(1):228–34.
16. Schulman ES, Adkinson NF Jr, Newball HH. Cyclooxygenase metabolites in human lung anaphylaxis: airway vs. parenchyma. J Appl Physiol Respir Environ Exerc Physiol 1982;53(3):589–95.
17. King GG, Muller NL, Pare PD. Evaluation of airways in obstructive pulmonary disease using high-resolution computed tomography. Am J Respir Crit Care Med 1999;159(3):992–1004.
18. Okazawa M, Muller N, McNamara AE, et al. Human airway narrowing measured using high resolution computed tomography. Am J Respir Crit Care Med 1996; 154(5):1557–62.
19. Goldin JG, McNitt-Gray MF, Sorenson SM, et al. Airway hyperreactivity: assessment with helical thin-section CT. Radiology 1998;208(2):321–9.
20. Wagner EM, Liu MC, Weinmann GG, et al. Peripheral lung resistance in normal and asthmatic subjects. Am Rev Respir Dis 1990;141(3):584–8.
21. Kraft M, Pak J, Martin RJ, et al. Distal lung dysfunction at night in nocturnal asthma. Am J Respir Crit Care Med 2001;163(7):1551–6.

22. Liang BM, Lam DC, Feng YL. Clinical applications of lung function tests: a revisit. Respirology 2012;17(4):611–9.
23. Miller MR, Hankinson J, Brusasco V, et al. Standardisation of spirometry. Eur Respir J 2005;26(2):319–38.
24. Rao DR, Gaffin JM, Baxi SN, et al. The utility of forced expiratory flow between 25% and 75% of vital capacity in predicting childhood asthma morbidity and severity. J Asthma 2012;49(6):586–92.
25. van den Berge M, ten Hacken NH, Cohen J, et al. Small airway disease in asthma and COPD: clinical implications. Chest 2011;139(2):412–23.
26. in 't Veen JC, Beekman AJ, Bel EH, et al. Recurrent exacerbations in severe asthma are associated with enhanced airway closure during stable episodes. Am J Respir Crit Care Med 2000;161(6):1902–6.
27. Sutherland ER, Martin RJ. Distal lung inflammation in asthma. Ann Allergy Asthma Immunol 2002;89(2):119–24 [quiz: 124–5, 211].
28. Shi Y, Aledia AS, Tatavoosian AV, et al. Relating small airways to asthma control by using impulse oscillometry in children. J Allergy Clin Immunol 2012;129(3):671–8.
29. Takeda T, Oga T, Niimi A, et al. Relationship between small airway function and health status, dyspnea and disease control in asthma. Respiration 2010;80(2):120–6.
30. Silkoff PE, McClean PA, Slutsky AS, et al. Marked flow-dependence of exhaled nitric oxide using a new technique to exclude nasal nitric oxide. Am J Respir Crit Care Med 1997;155(1):260–7.
31. Linkosalo L, Lehtimaki L, Holm K, et al. Relation of bronchial and alveolar nitric oxide to exercise-induced bronchoconstriction in atopic children and adolescents. Pediatr Allergy Immunol 2012;23(4):360–6.
32. Tsoukias NM, George SC. A two-compartment model of pulmonary nitric oxide exchange dynamics. J Appl Physiol (1985) 1998;85(2):653–66.
33. Berry M, Hargadon B, Morgan A, et al. Alveolar nitric oxide in adults with asthma: evidence of distal lung inflammation in refractory asthma. Eur Respir J 2005; 25(6):986–91.
34. Lehtimäki L, Kankaanranta H, Saarelainen S, et al. Increased alveolar nitric oxide concentration in asthmatic patients with nocturnal symptoms. Eur Respir J 2002; 20(4):841–5.
35. Verbanck S, Schuermans D, Paiva M, et al. Nonreversible conductive airway ventilation heterogeneity in mild asthma. J Appl Physiol (1985) 2003;94(4):1380–6.
36. Sutherland ER, Martin RJ. Targeting the distal lung in asthma: do inhaled corticosteroids treat all areas of inflammation? Treat Respir Med 2005;4(4):223–9.
37. Zanen P, Go LT, Lammers JW. Optimal particle size for beta 2 agonist and anticholinergic aerosols in patients with severe airflow obstruction. Thorax 1996; 51(10):977–80.
38. UNEP Environmental Effects Panel, United Nations Environment Programme. Environmental effects of ozone depletion: 1994 assessment: pursuant to article 6 of the Montreal Protocol on substances that deplete the ozone layer. Nairobi (Kenya): UNEP; 1994.
39. Anderson PJ. Delivery options and devices for aerosolized therapeutics. Chest 2001;120(Suppl 3):89S–93S.
40. Martin RJ. Therapeutic significance of distal airway inflammation in asthma. J Allergy Clin Immunol 2002;109(Suppl 2):S447–60.
41. Vanden Burgt JA, Busse WW, Martin RJ, et al. Efficacy and safety overview of a new inhaled corticosteroid, QVAR (hydrofluoroalkane-beclomethasone extrafine inhalation aerosol), in asthma. J Allergy Clin Immunol 2000;106(6):1209–26.

42. Leach CL, Davidson PJ, Boudreau RJ. Improved airway targeting with the CFC-free HFA-beclomethasone metered-dose inhaler compared with CFC-beclomethasone. Eur Respir J 1998;12(6):1346–53.
43. Gross G, Thompson PJ, Chervinsky P, et al. Hydrofluoroalkane-134a beclomethasone dipropionate, 400 microg, is as effective as chlorofluorocarbon beclomethasone dipropionate, 800 microg, for the treatment of moderate asthma. Chest 1999;115(2):343–51.
44. Corren J, Nelson H, Greos LS, et al. Effective control of asthma with hydrofluoroalkane flunisolide delivered as an extrafine aerosol in asthma patients. Ann Allergy Asthma Immunol 2001;87(5):405–11.
45. Goldin JG, Tashkin DP, Kleerup EC, et al. Comparative effects of hydrofluoroalkane and chlorofluorocarbon beclomethasone dipropionate inhalation on small airways: assessment with functional helical thin-section computed tomography. J Allergy Clin Immunol 1999;104(6):S258–67.
46. Israel E, Roche N, Martin RJ, et al. Increased dose of inhaled corticosteroid versus add-on long-acting beta-agonist for step-up therapy in asthma. Ann Am Thorac Soc 2015;12(6):798–806.
47. Martin RJ, Price D, Roche N, et al. Cost-effectiveness of initiating extrafine- or standard size-particle inhaled corticosteroid for asthma in two health-care systems: a retrospective matched cohort study. NPJ Prim Care Respir Med 2014; 24:14081.

Chronic Infection and Severe Asthma

Tara F. Carr, MD*, Monica Kraft, MD

KEYWORDS

- Severe asthma • Chronic infection • *Mycoplasma pneumoniae*
- *Chlamydophila pneumoniae* • Macrolides • Microbiome

KEY POINTS

- *Mycoplasma pneumoniae* can induce type 2 airway inflammation, which resembles asthma.
- *Chlamydophila pneumoniae* can induce profound systemic and local inflammation.
- Both *M pneumoniae* and *C pneumoniae* have been associated with the development, chronicity, and severity of asthma in humans.
- The use of macrolides in treatment of severe asthma, although controversial, may benefit those with confirmed atypical bacterial infection.
- The effect of the airway microbiome on the development and severity of asthma is an area of active research, with potential for high impact.

INTRODUCTION

The role of lung infection in the development, persistence, severity, and exacerbation of asthma has undergone investigation for decades. This article discusses current understanding of chronic bacterial infection in asthma as it pertains to pathogens, pathobiology, severity, and treatment. Future research will likely explore the impact of the lung microbiome because it may confer protection from asthma or contribute to development of disease.

MYCOPLASMA PNEUMONIAE

Mycoplasma pneumoniae is an extracellular atypical bacterium, transmitted by contact with respiratory droplets. *M pneumoniae* colonizes mucosal surfaces, predominantly of the respiratory tract. In addition to causing infectious disease, *M pneumoniae*

Financial Disclosure Statement: Dr T.F. Carr reports no financial conflicts of interest as a result of this work. Dr M. Kraft reports no financial conflicts of interest as a result of this work.
Division of Pulmonary, Allergy, Critical Care, and Sleep Medicine, University of Arizona, 1501 North Campbell Avenue, Tucson, AZ 85724, USA
* Corresponding author. Division of Pulmonary, Allergy, Critical Care, and Sleep Medicine, University of Arizona, 1501 North Campbell Avenue, PO 24030, Tucson, AZ 85724.
E-mail address: tcarr@deptofmed.arizona.edu

exposure can induce a variety of autoimmune diseases. Importantly, *M pneumoniae* has been implicated in development of airway inflammation, development of asthma, and severity of asthma.

M pneumoniae contributes to community-acquired lower respiratory tract infection (LRTI) in children through the clinical syndromes of tracheobronchitis, pneumonia, and wheezing illnesses in both asthmatic and nonasthmatic children. Indeed, *M pneumoniae*-induced LRTI in children can cause wheezing in 40%[1] and has been identified as a pathogen in 19% of children older than 5 years with pneumonia.[2] In adults, *M pneumoniae* is a common cause of community-acquired pneumonia.[3] Although a systematic surveillance for *M pneumoniae* infection is not performed in the United States, data exist from outbreaks and were collected by the Centers for Disease Control and Prevention between 2006 and 2013,[4] through which macrolide resistance was identified in 10% of infections.

Mycoplasma pneumoniae Pathogenicity

M pneumoniae depends on a host for survival and replication. *M pneumoniae* has no cell wall and limited metabolic capacity; therefore, it depends on utilization of host cells for replication. *M pneumoniae* can have structural and functional effects through cytotoxic effects on ciliated cells. On exposure of a host cell, mainly of the respiratory epithelium, *M pneumoniae* projects a specialized attachment organelle, comprised of a filamentous core and adhesin-rich tip, which facilitates the cytadhesin necessary for the pathogen's survival.[5,6] This process is necessary for the development of lung inflammation associated with the infectious phenotype. *M pneumoniae* then synthesizes hydrogen peroxide and superoxide radicals, which induce cellular oxidative stress in the respiratory epithelium. However, the glycerol metabolic pathways, which may be responsible for cytotoxic effects and pathogenicity of oxidative stress,[7,8] have been identified and provide possible targets for development of novel therapies.[9] Interestingly, inhaled fluticasone may improve *M pneumoniae*-associated asthma through blocking adherence of *M pneumoniae* in the lung tissue, leading to prevention of subsequent inflammation-related physiologic effects.[10]

M pneumoniae can induce significant inflammation in the host. *M pneumoniae* produces a unique bacterial adenosine diphosphate (ADP)-ribosylating and vacuolating toxin, termed the community-acquired respiratory distress syndrome (CARDS) toxin, which can activate the NLRP3 inflammasome, leading to subsequent formation of interleukin (IL)-1β and resultant inflammation.[11] CARDS can also bind surfactant protein A (SP-A)[12] and interacts with a host protein annexin A2[13] which is involved in multiple cellular functions, including phagocytosis and tight junction maintenance.[14,15] *M pneumoniae* lipoproteins can initiate inflammation through toll-like receptor (TLR)-2,[16] thereby inducing IL-8 expression in airway epithelial cells.[17] Further, *M pneumoniae* causes cytadherence-induced inflammation through TLR4 and autophagy pathways.[18]

Clearance of *M pneumoniae* from the lung is primarily though macrophage activation, requiring MyD88-NF-kB signaling.[19] Polymorphisms of SP-A2 may affect binding of this protein to *M pneumoniae* and contribute to impaired clearance with disease susceptibility, as shown in a novel humanized transgenic mouse model.[20] Mast cells may play a role in protection from severe mycoplasma infection.[21]

Experimental and Mechanistic Models of Mycoplasma pneumoniae and Asthma

The association between *M pneumoniae* infection and asthma has been evaluated through in vitro and murine models. These experiments reveal a variety of mechanisms through which *M pneumoniae* and abnormal host responses to the infectious insult combine and additively contribute to the development or severity of asthma. For example, in murine models, airway hyperresponsiveness (AHR) can be induced by *M pneumoniae* infection by inducing increased mast cell burden.[22] The *M pneumoniae* CARDS toxin can induce and exacerbate experimental asthma.[23,24] Particularly in the setting of allergic airway sensitization, *M pneumoniae* infection can cause AHR,[25] airway inflammation,[26] wheeze,[27] airway mucin expression,[28,29] and remodeling through collagen deposition.[30]

The existing literature also provides strong evidence that, indeed, *M pneumoniae* infection induces type-2 inflammation in humans, particularly in the setting of allergic disease or asthma. For example, in subjects with *M pneumoniae* pneumonia, bronchoalveolar lavage (BAL) sampling has revealed induction of type-2 inflammatory cytokines,[31] eosinophilia,[32] and abnormal cellular responses.[33] In those with atopic disease or asthma, *M pneumoniae* infection markedly induced eosinophils[34] and eosinophil-associated cytokines.[35–37] Asthmatics seem disproportionately affected by severe disease,[38] perhaps related to defective SHP-1 in airway epithelial cells of asthmatics, resulting in enhanced inflammatory response to *M pneumoniae* infection.[39] The importance of TLRs as a receptor for *M pneumoniae* infection and severity is illustrated by increased expression of TLR2 and TLR4 on peripheral blood dendritic cells from children with asthma compared with those without asthma or *M pneumoniae* infection.[40] Notably, and perhaps related, airway tissue analyses reveal increased expression of TLR2, 3, and 4 and TSLP in fatal asthma.[41]

Mycoplasma pneumoniae and Asthma in Humans

With data supporting the contribution of *M pneumoniae* to airway inflammation and type-2 inflammation, the relationship between asthma and *M pneumoniae* infection cannot be discounted. Indeed, the contribution of airway *M pneumoniae* infection to development, chronicity, and severity of asthma has been long studied and previously reviewed.[42–45] However, despite the breadth of published literature, guidelines for the evaluation and treatment of *M pneumoniae* in asthma have not been established, due in large part to heterogeneity among studies and challenges due to diagnostic techniques. This article presents relevant studies in human subjects, which attempt to elucidate the relationship between asthma development, severity, and *M pneumoniae* infection.

Onset of wheeze or asthma

Although direct causation has not been established, atypical infection is correlated with asthma development[46] or the onset of wheezing. Indeed, in pediatric cohorts, *M pneumoniae* infection is diagnosed in higher frequencies among those with acute wheezing associated with febrile upper respiratory tract infection[47] and can be related to structural changes seen on cross-sectional imaging of the lung.[48] Those with *M pneumoniae* lower respiratory infections without preexisting asthma may have persistently impaired lung function years later.[1] In light of the high frequency of *M pneumoniae* exposure and variability of infection, a nonselected longitudinal cohort study may be a more powerful tool to study the contribution of *M pneumoniae* to development of asthma and wheeze.

Chronic asthma, exacerbations, and severity

Acute or prior *M pneumoniae* infection is frequently detected in children and adults with diagnosed asthma, seemingly more frequently than in those without asthma. Further, *M pneumoniae* may be implicated in refractory disease or asthma exacerbations, thereby conferring significant disease morbidity and severity. Studies assessing the presence of *M pneumoniae* infection in the pediatric and adult populations are listed in **Table 1**.

Table 1
Studies evaluating *Mycoplasma pneumoniae* role in chronic asthma, exacerbations, and/or severity

Reference	Population	Type of Study, Number (N) of Subjects	Testing Method	Outcome
Pediatric Studies				
Smith-Norowitz et al,[121] 2013	Stable asthmatics	Cohort, N = 36	Serologic	Higher concentrations of anti–*M pneumoniae* IgM in asthmatics compared with nonasthmatic controls
Bebear et al,[122] 2014	Chronic asthma, exacerbations	Cohort, N = 168, N = 88	Serologic and blood PCR	*M pneumoniae* detected in 13.6% with chronic asthma, 7% of asthma exacerbations
Fonseca-Aten et al,[123] 2006	Exacerbations of wheeze or asthma seen in the emergency room	Cohort, N = 43	Nasopharyngeal PCR	*M pneumoniae* infection in 48% by PCR-based methods, and coinfection with *C pneumoniae* in 9 by PCR and/or serology
Wood et al,[124] 2013	Acute or refractory asthma	Cohort, N = 143	Serologic	*M pneumoniae* detected in 64% of subjects with acute asthma, 65% with refractory asthma, and 56% of healthy controls
Biscardi et al,[81] 2004	Hospitalization for acute severe asthma or wheeze	Cohort, N = 352	Serologic	*M pneumoniae* detected in 20% of those with preexisting asthma, 50% of those for whom the hospitalization represented the initial asthma presentation, 5% in stable asthmatic controls

Adult Studies

Study	Population	Study Type	Method	Findings
Bebear et al,[122] 2014	Chronic asthma, exacerbations	Cohort, N = 68	Serologic and blood PCR	M pneumoniae detected in 6.3% with chronic asthma, 10% of asthma exacerbations
Kraft et al,[125] 1998	Chronic stable asthma	Cohort, N = 29	Blood and respiratory tract culture, PCR	Half of the asthmatic group had M pneumoniae detected from the lower airway by PCR, compared with 1 in the nonasthmatic group
Martin et al,[126] 2001	Chronic stable asthma	Cohort, N = 55	Blood and respiratory tract culture, PCR	M pneumoniae identified in 45% of asthmatics
Lieberman et al,[127] 2003	Hospitalization for acute asthma	Cohort, N = 100	Serology	18% had evidence of acute M pneumoniae infection; clinical parameters suggested that these subjects had more severe exacerbations
Peters et al,[128] 2011	Refractory asthmatics	Cohort, N = 64	Respiratory and blood serology, antigens	52% had evidence of M pneumoniae: M pneumoniae antigens, antibodies against CARDS toxin and P1 adhesin

Abbreviations: Ig, immunoglobulin; PCR, polymerase chain reaction.

CHLAMYDOPHILA PNEUMONIAE

Chlamydophila pneumoniae, formerly known as Chlamydia pneumoniae, is a common human respiratory pathogen. This ubiquitous, obligate intracellular microorganism is transmitted via the respiratory route and widely distributed, with seropositivity noted in well more than half of adults. Most C pneumoniae infections are asymptomatic or mildly symptomatic; however, a significant proportion of individuals suffer more severe illnesses such as upper respiratory tract infection, community-acquired pneumonia, and bronchitis. The clinical course of C pneumoniae infections can be expected to follow a biphasic timeline, with chronic cough for several weeks after resolution of the initial infectious syndrome. C pneumoniae infection has also been linked to coronary atherosclerosis, bronchiectasis, chronic obstructive pulmonary disease, Alzheimer disease, and multiple sclerosis. Despite the evidence of widespread infection from C pneumoniae in the general population, genetic susceptibility and/or differences in immune responsiveness may be responsible for the spectrum of disease severity and sequelae.[49]

Chlamydophila pneumoniae Pathogenicity

Chlamydial organisms have a unique biphasic developmental cycle wherein the transmissible agent, the dense and metabolically inactive elementary body, transforms on host-cellular endocytosis to become the metabolically active reticulate body. After the acute infection, C pneumoniae can achieve a latent, metabolically inert state in which it does not multiply but remains viable. However, during this state of chronic infection or colonization, the C pneumoniae can continue to produce its heat shock protein 60 (HSP60), a highly immunogenic protein that can induce a pronounced inflammatory response through TLR2, TLR4,[50–52] and cytosolic pathogen recognition receptors,[53] effectively inducing the transcription factor NF-κB[54] and subsequent downstream proinflammatory events. HSP60 has also been shown to directly stimulate peripheral blood lymphocyte proliferation and interferon (IFN)-γ secretion, and induce T helper (Th)1 polarization through dendritic cell-expressed signals.[55,56] Furthermore, C pneumoniae can induce inflammatory activity through host NLRP3 signaling, leading to IL-1β upregulation.[57–60] Finally, C pneumoniae can inhibit proliferation of activated human T cells through apoptotic and pyroptotic pathways.[61] Chronic C pneumoniae infection in a murine model[62] induced bronchus-associated lymphoid tissue, classically and alternatively activated macrophages, and pulmonary fibrosis.

Experimental and Mechanistic Models of Chlamydophila pneumoniae and Asthma

Similar to M pneumoniae, there is a relationship between C pneumoniae infection and the induction of an asthmatic phenotype and type-2 inflammation. In particular, early-life C pneumoniae respiratory infections in mice have been shown to irreversibly modify immunity, confer risk for asthma, and impair lung physiology.[63–66] C pneumoniae infection in mice can induce immunoglobulin (Ig)E production,[67] lung eosinophilia, IL-5 production, mucus cell hyperplasia, and AHR.[68] Interestingly, neutrophilic inflammation[68,69] is often induced in these models and identified in human BAL,[70] similar to that seen in neutrophilic asthma. C pneumoniae can further contribute to airway inflammation through the production of MUC5AC mucin[71] and to airway remodeling through the matrix metalloproteinases[72,73] and vascular endothelial growth factor.[73,74] However, the degree of infection of C pneumoniae[75,76] or mast cell burden[77] may be related to risk of antigen sensitization and airway inflammation.

Chlamydophila pneumoniae and Asthma in Humans

Onset of wheeze or asthma

C pneumoniae has been repeatedly identified in and associated with initial asthma presentation. Diagnosis of acute C pneumoniae infection in pediatric cohorts, followed longitudinally, is associated with wheezing[78] and incident diagnosis of asthma.[78,79] Data support a role of repeated or chronic C pneumoniae infection in children with recurrent respiratory symptoms.[80] Diagnosis of asthma is also associated with C pneumoniae in both children[81] and adults.[82,83]

Chronic asthma, exacerbations, and severity

Literature suggests C pneumoniae infection is detected more frequently among asthmatics than nonasthmatics, further supporting theories implicating C pneumoniae in asthma pathogenesis. Further, C pneumoniae infection has been implicated in severity of asthma through contribution to exacerbations. C pneumoniae is also implicated in poor asthma control, worse quality of life, and lung function decline, which all contribute to severity of asthma. Studies measuring these effects are shown in **Table 2**.

MACROLIDES FOR ASTHMA

The effect of macrolide therapy on asthma may be due to a direct antibacterial effect, particularly against the atypical bacteria M pneumoniae and C pneumoniae; however, the impact of these drugs on corticosteroid pharmacokinetics or as direct immunomodulatory therapy is potentially significant. This article discusses the evidence supporting use of macrolides to treat asthma irrespective of infection status, the use of macrolides in asthmatics with evidence of atypical infection, and the impact of macrolide therapy as steroid-sparing therapy.

Use of Macrolides in Asthma, Irrespective of Atypical Infection

In clinical trials of macrolide therapy for asthma irrespective of atypical infection status, benefit is not clear. Although trials have showed some improvement in AHR[84,85] or quality of life[86,87] in adult persistent asthmatics, these benefits were inconsistent. Macrolide therapy has been shown to affect airway inflammation in asthmatics, in both noneosinophilic[88] and aspirin-exacerbated respiratory disease phenotypes.[89]

Bacterial infection can induce asthma exacerbation, suggesting antibacterial therapy may reduce exacerbation rates. The Azithromycin for prevention of exacerbations in severe asthma (AZISAST) trial[90] was a randomized, double-blinded, placebo-controlled study of low-dose, long-term azithromycin as add-on therapy to inhaled corticosteroids and long-acting beta-2 agonists in adult subjects with exacerbation-prone severe asthma. Although the primary outcome, rate of exacerbations, and/or LRTI requiring antibiotics, was not different between the treatment groups, a predefined subgroup analysis according to blood cellular phenotype identified relative benefit of azithromycin in the noneosinophilic severe asthma phenotype. M pneumoniae or C pneumoniae status was not assessed in these participants.

Macrolides as Steroid-Sparing Agents for Asthma

Interest in the use of macrolides as steroid-sparing therapy in severe asthma has been ongoing for decades. The macrolide troleandomycin was shown in several studies[91–93] to improve clinical and laboratory markers of asthma, as well as aid in steroid dose reduction; other studies found little benefit.[94,95] Clarithromycin was used in a small cohort to reduce steroid requirements and improve quality of life.[96]

Table 2
Studies evaluating *Chlamydophila pneumoniae* role in chronic asthma, exacerbations, and/or severity

Reference	Population	Type of Study, Number (N) of Subjects	Testing Method	Outcome
Pediatric Studies				
Fonseca-Aten et al,[123] 2006	Exacerbations of wheeze or asthma seen in the emergency room	Cohort, N = 43	Nasopharyngeal PCR	*C pneumoniae* identified in 12 (28%) of acute exacerbations
Awasthi et al,[129] 2012	Hospitalization for asthma exacerbation, or uncontrolled asthma in clinic	Cohort, N = 89	Serologic	25% of asthmatic children presenting with exacerbations in the hospital had evidence of *C pneumoniae*, compared with 7% of those with uncontrolled asthma presenting to clinic
Adult Studies				
Lieberman et al,[127] 2003	Hospitalization for acute asthma	Cohort, N = 100	Serologic	8 subjects had evidence of acute *C pneumoniae* infection
Kraft et al,[125] 1998	Chronic stable asthma	Cohort, N = 29	Blood and respiratory tract culture, PCR	Half of the asthmatics were seropositive for *C pneumoniae*
Martin et al,[126] 2001	Chronic stable asthma	Cohort, N = 55	Blood and respiratory tract culture, PCR	*C pneumoniae* identified in 13% of asthmatics using PCR, compared with no *C pneumoniae* in the upper airways of controls
Bebear et al,[122] 2014	Chronic asthma, exacerbations	Cohort, N = 68	Serologic and blood PCR	*C pneumoniae* was present in 10% of children and 6% of adults with chronic asthma
Biscione et al,[130] 2004	Spouse pairs of 1 atopic asthmatic, 1 nonatopic nonasthmatic	Cohort, N = 148	Nasopharyngeal	*C pneumoniae* was detected in 6.4% of asthmatics, 2.3% of the nonasthmatic spouses

Miyashita et al,[131] 1998	Acute exacerbation	Cohort, N = 276	Serologic	Evidence of C pneumoniae by IgG and/or IgA in 9% of asthmatics compared with 3% of controls
Allegra et al,[132] 1994	Outpatient asthma exacerbations	Cohort, N = 74	Serologic	9% were found to be infected by C pneumoniae
Black et al,[133] 2000	Asthmatics	Cohort, N = 619	Serologic	Higher antibody titers were associated with more severe asthma
Huittinen et al,[134] 2001	Asthmatics	Cohort, N = 619	Serologic	Antibodies against C pneumoniae HSP60 were associated with asthma, levels of IgA antibodies were inversely associated with lung function
Hahn et al,[135] 2001	Asthmatics	Cohort, N = 138	Serologic	27% of asthmatic subjects were C pneumoniae HSP60 seropositive vs 8% of controls, C pneumoniae HSP60 seropositivity correlated with lower FEV1
Pasternack et al,[136] 2005	New diagnosis of asthma	Longitudinal cohort, N = 245	Serologic	Neither baseline C pneumoniae status nor seroconversion was related to incident asthma; however, nonatopic asthmatics with positive C pneumoniae serology had a faster rate of lung function decline than noninfected subjects with or without asthma

Abbreviation: FEV1, forced expiratory volume in 1 second.

However, in none of these studies was *M pneumoniae* or *C pneumoniae* status reported. The mechanism by which troleandomycin may improve corticosteroid effectiveness was elucidated by Szefler and colleagues,[97] wherein pharmacokinetic studies demonstrate reduced elimination of methylprednisolone in the presence of troleandomycin. Finally, Strunk and colleagues,[98] with the Childhood Asthma Research and Education Network, sought to determine whether azithromycin or montelukast could be used as inhaled steroid-sparing therapy in children ages 6 to 18 years old with moderate to severe asthma. This study was discontinued early after futility analysis demonstrated no difference among the treatment groups.

Use of Macrolides in Asthma, with Respect to Atypical Infection

For those asthmatics with evidence of *C pneumoniae* or *M pneumoniae* infection, however, treatment with an appropriate macrolide may lead to symptom improvement or reduction of inflammation. Similarly, for those with asthma exacerbations and evidence of *C pneumoniae* or *M pneumoniae* infection, macrolide therapy may be beneficial. Studies assessing the impact of antibiotic therapy on *C pneumoniae* or *M pneumoniae* infection in asthma are described in **Table 3**.

A Cochrane Database systematic review was performed to determine whether macrolides are effective in the management of patients with chronic asthma.[99] Twenty-three studies met inclusion criteria of randomized, placebo-controlled clinical trials involving both children and adult subjects with chronic asthma treated with macrolides for more than 4 weeks. The investigators concluded that, although existing evidence does not show macrolides to be better than placebo for most clinical outcomes, they may affect some measures of lung function, and the possible benefit of macrolides in subjects with noneosinophilic asthma based on subgroup analyses in 2 of the included studies may require further investigation. Further recommendations were not given because the evidence was determined to be of very low quality due to heterogeneity among subjects and interventions, imprecision, and reporting biases. Clearly, additional clinical trials are needed in this area to address impact of atypical infection evaluation and treatment among the severe asthmatic, frequent exacerbator, or noneosinophilic asthmatic phenotype.

MICROBIOME OF THE ASTHMATIC LUNG

The respiratory mucosa, once thought to be sterile, is known to host a large variety of commensal bacteria, which are proposed to contribute to the maintenance of immune homeostasis and protection from disease.[100–103] It is estimated that more than 10,000 different microbial species live in and on humans, representing 100 trillion organisms existing in a symbiotic relationship, most of which are bacterial. The airway microbiome likely develops in early life, may be altered by diet or antibiotic exposure, and is related to the gut microbiome. Similarly, the gut microbiome develops in early life, with a rapid increase in diversity that seems necessary for health[104] and is susceptible to alterations through diet and antibiotic therapy.

The hygiene hypothesis proposes that reduction in the diversity and quantity of microbial exposure confers risk for the development of atopic disease and inflammation.[105–107] Indeed, in individuals with asthma, abnormal microbiological characteristics have been identified in the gut,[108–110] upper airway,[111] and lower airway.

The degree and nature of the contribution of lung microbiome to severity of asthma is not yet clear. Marri and colleagues[112] reported alterations in the microbial composition of induced sputum of asthmatics that were similar among asthmatics suffering from mild or severe disease but distinguished asthmatics from normal controls. Huang

Table 3
Clinical trials of macrolide therapy for asthma, with respect to *Mycoplasma pneumoniae* or *Chlamydophila pneumoniae* infection status

Reference	Population	*M pneumoniae* or *C pneumoniae* Assessment	N	Intervention	Outcomes
Kraft et al,[137] 2002	Stable adult asthma	*M pneumoniae* or *C pneumoniae* on PCR	N = 55	Clarithromycin or placebo for 6 wk	Improvement in FEV_1 in those with infection, with reduction in BAL cytokine expression, particularly TNF-α, IL-5, and IL-12
Black et al,[138] 2001	Adult asthma	Elevated *C pneumoniae* antibody titers	N = 232	Roxithromycin or placebo for 6 wk	Those receiving treatment had greater improvement in morning and evening peak expiratory flow rates
Hahn et al,[139] 1995	Adult asthma, moderate to severe	*C pneumoniae* antibodies	N = 46	Doxycycline, azithromycin, or erythromycin for 4 wk	Half of subjects had clinical improvement, measured by pulmonary function or symptom scores
Sutherland et al,[140] 2010	Adult asthma, mild to moderate uncontrolled	*M pneumoniae* or *C pneumoniae* on PCR	N = 92	Clarithromycin or placebo for 16 wk	PCR-negative subjects had no benefit by asthma control questionnaire, PCR-positive group was underpowered
Emre et al,[141] 1994	Children with acute wheezing	*C pneumoniae* antibodies	N = 159	Erythromycin or clarithromycin for standard course	For wheezing with *C pneumoniae* antibodies, treatment led to eradication of infection and improvement in clinical outcomes
Fonseca-Aten et al,[123] 2006	Children with acute wheezing	*M pneumoniae* or *C pneumoniae* on PCR	N = 43	Clarithromycin or placebo for standard course	No differences were noted between the treatment groups, even among those with infection; however, nasal aspirate concentrations of TNF-α, IL-1β, and IL-10 decreased after treatment
Johnston et al,[142] 2006	Adults with acute asthma exacerbation	*M pneumoniae* or *C pneumoniae* on PCR, culture or antibodies	N = 278	Telithromycin or placebo for 10 d	The treatment group had improvement in symptoms and lung function, not restricted to the 61% of participants positive for *C pneumoniae* or *M pneumoniae*

Abbreviation: TNF, tumor necrosis factor.

and colleagues[113] identified differences in the bronchial airway microbiota to be associated with suboptimally controlled asthma and bronchial hyperresponsiveness.

However, literature supports a significant association between asthma severity and changes in microbiota profiles. Huang and colleagues[114] studied severe asthma, identifying specific microbiota of the bronchial brushings to be associated with inflammatory processes such as the relationship of Proteobacteria and Th17 gene expression. Green and colleagues[115] identified dominant bacterial profiles, particularly Moraxella, hemophilus, or streptococcal species, in the airway associated with severe airway obstruction and airway neutrophilia. Goleva and colleagues[116] identified an impact of gram-negative bacteria on corticosteroid resistance in asthma.

As anticipated, antibiotic therapy affects the airway microbiome in asthma. Slater and colleagues[117] treated 5 adult subjects with moderate to severe persistent asthma with 6 weeks of daily azithromycin therapy. Microbiome samples were obtained from the lung via BAL before and after therapy. In this pilot study, the investigators reported decreased bacterial richness after treatment, with reduction in *Pseudomonas*, *Haemophilus*, and *Staphylococcus* spp.

Therefore, aberrations of the microbiome in asthmatics not only contribute to the development and perpetuation of abnormal inflammation in asthma[118,119] but, theoretically, could confer susceptibility to infections such as *M pneumoniae* and *C pneumoniae*. Further, knowledge of the abnormal microbiome patterns and manipulation thereof will likely lead to novel therapies.[120]

SUMMARY

Understanding of the impact of atypical bacterial infection on the development of asthma and contribution to severity is based on mostly associative evidence, supported by translational and mechanistic experiments. Future clinical trials examining the impact of atypical infection, or treatment of that infection, on asthma severity will require careful phenotyping of participants. Longitudinal cohort studies seeking to understand the contribution of these atypical bacteria to the development or severity of asthma will be challenged to study these infections in the setting of the host's microbiota.

REFERENCES

1. Sabato AR, Martin AJ, Marmion BP, et al. *Mycoplasma pneumoniae*: acute illness, antibiotics, and subsequent pulmonary function. Arch Dis Child 1984; 59(11):1034–7.
2. Jain S, Williams DJ, Arnold SR, et al. Community-acquired pneumonia requiring hospitalization among U.S. children. N Engl J Med 2015;372(9):835–45.
3. Saraya T, Kurai D, Nakagaki K, et al. Novel aspects on the pathogenesis of *Mycoplasma pneumoniae* pneumonia and therapeutic implications. Front Microbiol 2014;5:410.
4. Diaz MH, Benitez AJ, Winchell JM. Investigations of *Mycoplasma pneumoniae* infections in the United States: trends in molecular typing and macrolide resistance from 2006 to 2013. J Clin Microbiol 2015;53(1):124–30.
5. Waites KB, Talkington DF. *Mycoplasma pneumoniae* and its role as a human pathogen. Clin Microbiol Rev 2004;17(4):697–728.
6. Waites KB, Balish MF, Atkinson TP. New insights into the pathogenesis and detection of *Mycoplasma pneumoniae* infections. Future Microbiol 2008;3(6):635–48.
7. Pilo P, Vilei EM, Peterhans E, et al. A metabolic enzyme as a primary virulence factor of *Mycoplasma mycoides* subsp. *mycoides* small colony. J Bacteriol 2005;187(19):6824–31.

8. Hames C, Halbedel S, Hoppert M, et al. Glycerol metabolism is important for cytotoxicity of *Mycoplasma pneumoniae*. J Bacteriol 2009; 191(3):747–53.

9. Elkhal CK, Kean KM, Parsonage D, et al. Structure and proposed mechanism of l-alpha-glycerophosphate oxidase from *Mycoplasma pneumoniae*. FEBS J 2015;282(16):3030–42.

10. Chu HW, Campbell JA, Harbeck RJ, et al. Effects of inhaled fluticasone on bronchial hyperresponsiveness and airway inflammation in *Mycoplasma pneumoniae*-infected mice. Chest 2003;123(Suppl 3):427s.

11. Bose S, Segovia JA, Somarajan SR, et al. ADP-ribosylation of NLRP3 by *Mycoplasma pneumoniae* CARDS toxin regulates inflammasome activity. MBio 2014;5(6).

12. Kannan TR, Baseman JB. ADP-ribosylating and vacuolating cytotoxin of *Mycoplasma pneumoniae* represents unique virulence determinant among bacterial pathogens. Proc Natl Acad Sci U S A 2006;103(17):6724–9.

13. Somarajan SR, Al-Asadi F, Ramasamy K, et al. Annexin A2 mediates *Mycoplasma pneumoniae* community-acquired respiratory distress syndrome toxin binding to eukaryotic cells. MBio 2014;5(4).

14. Becker A, Kannan TR, Taylor AB, et al. Structure of CARDS toxin, a unique ADP-ribosylating and vacuolating cytotoxin from *Mycoplasma pneumoniae*. Proc Natl Acad Sci U S A 2015;112(16):5165–70.

15. Fang YT, Lin CF, Wang CY, et al. Interferon-gamma stimulates p11-dependent surface expression of annexin A2 in lung epithelial cells to enhance phagocytosis. J Cell Physiol 2012;227(6):2775–87.

16. Shimizu T, Kida Y, Kuwano K. Triacylated lipoproteins derived from *Mycoplasma pneumoniae* activate nuclear factor-kappaB through toll-like receptors 1 and 2. Immunology 2007;121(4):473–83.

17. Lee KE, Kim KW, Hong JY, et al. Modulation of IL-8 boosted by *Mycoplasma pneumoniae* lysate in human airway epithelial cells. J Clin Immunol 2013; 33(6):1117–25.

18. Shimizu T, Kimura Y, Kida Y, et al. Cytadherence of *Mycoplasma pneumoniae* induces inflammatory responses through autophagy and toll-like receptor 4. Infect Immun 2014;82(7):3076–86.

19. Lai JF, Zindl CL, Duffy LB, et al. Critical Role of Macrophages and Their Activation via MyD88-NFκB Signaling in Lung Innate Immunity to *Mycoplasma pneumoniae*. PLoS One 2010;5(12):e14417.

20. Ledford JG, Voelker DR, Addison KJ, et al. Genetic variation in SP-A2 leads to differential binding to *Mycoplasma pneumoniae* membranes and regulation of host responses. J Immunol 2015;194(12):6123–32.

21. Xu X, Zhang D, Lyubynska N, et al. Mast cells protect mice from *Mycoplasma pneumonia*. Am J Respir Crit Care Med 2006;173(2):219–25.

22. Hsia BJ, Ledford JG, Potts-Kant EN, et al. Mast cell TNF receptors regulate responses to *Mycoplasma pneumoniae* in surfactant protein A (SP-A)-/- mice. J Allergy Clin Immunol 2012;130(1):205–14.e202.

23. Medina JL, Coalson JJ, Brooks EG, et al. *Mycoplasma pneumoniae* CARDS toxin induces pulmonary eosinophilic and lymphocytic inflammation. Am J Respir Cell Mol Biol 2012;46(6):815–22.

24. Medina JL, Coalson JJ, Brooks EG, et al. *Mycoplasma pneumoniae* CARDS toxin exacerbates ovalbumin-induced asthma-like inflammation in BALB/c mice. PLoS One 2014;9(7):e102613.

25. Chu HW, Honour JM, Rawlinson CA, et al. Effects of respiratory *Mycoplasma pneumoniae* infection on allergen-induced bronchial hyperresponsiveness and lung inflammation in mice. Infect Immun 2003;71(3):1520–6.

26. Martin RJ, Chu HW, Honour JM, et al. Airway inflammation and bronchial hyperresponsiveness after *Mycoplasma pneumoniae* infection in a murine model. Am J Respir Cell Mol Biol 2001;24(5):577–82.

27. Zhang H, Wei B, Shang YX, et al. Effects of *Mycoplasma pneumoniae* infection on airway neurokinin-1 receptor expression in BALB/c mice. Genet Mol Res 2014;13(4):8320–8.

28. Hao Y, Kuang Z, Jing J, et al. *Mycoplasma pneumoniae* modulates STAT3-STAT6/EGFR-FOXA2 signaling to induce overexpression of airway mucins. Infect Immun 2014;82(12):5246–55.

29. Wu Q, Case SR, Minor MN, et al. A novel function of MUC18: amplification of lung inflammation during bacterial infection. Am J Pathol 2013;182(3):819–27.

30. Chu HW, Rino JG, Wexler RB, et al. *Mycoplasma pneumoniae* infection increases airway collagen deposition in a murine model of allergic airway inflammation. Am J Physiol Lung Cell Mol Physiol 2005;289(1):L125–33.

31. Koh YY, Park Y, Lee HJ, et al. Levels of interleukin-2, interferon-gamma, and interleukin-4 in bronchoalveolar lavage fluid from patients with Mycoplasma pneumonia: implication of tendency toward increased immunoglobulin E production. Pediatrics 2001;107(3):E39.

32. Wu SH, Chen XQ, Kong X, et al. Characteristics of respiratory syncytial virus-induced bronchiolitis co-infection with *Mycoplasma pneumoniae* and add-on therapy with montelukast. World J Pediatr 2016;12(1):88–95.

33. Guo L, Liu F, Lu MP, et al. Increased T cell activation in BALF from children with *Mycoplasma pneumoniae* pneumonia. Pediatr Pulmonol 2015;50(8):814–9.

34. Kim JH, Cho TS, Moon JH, et al. Serial Changes in Serum Eosinophil-associated Mediators between Atopic and Non-atopic Children after *Mycoplasma pneumoniae* pneumonia. Allergy Asthma Immunol Res 2014;6(5):428–33.

35. Ye Q, Xu XJ, Shao WX, et al. *Mycoplasma pneumoniae* infection in children is a risk factor for developing allergic diseases. ScientificWorldJournal 2014;2014: 986527.

36. Wang L, Chen Q, Shi C, et al. Changes of serum TNF-alpha, IL-5 and IgE levels in the patients of mycoplasma pneumonia infection with or without bronchial asthma. Int J Clin Exp Med 2015;8(3):3901–6.

37. Jeong YC, Yeo MS, Kim JH, et al. *Mycoplasma pneumoniae* infection affects the serum levels of vascular endothelial growth factor and interleukin-5 in atopic children. Allergy Asthma Immunol Res 2012;4(2):92–7.

38. Shin JE, Cheon BR, Shim JW, et al. Increased risk of refractory *Mycoplasma pneumoniae* pneumonia in children with atopic sensitization and asthma. Korean J Pediatr 2014;57(6):271–7.

39. Wang Y, Zhu Z, Church TD, et al. SHP-1 as a critical regulator of *Mycoplasma pneumoniae*-induced inflammation in human asthmatic airway epithelial cells. J Immunol 2012;188(7):3371–81.

40. Shao L, Cong Z, Li X, et al. Changes in levels of IL-9, IL-17, IFN-gamma, dendritic cell numbers and TLR expression in peripheral blood in asthmatic children with *Mycoplasma pneumoniae* infection. Int J Clin Exp Pathol 2015;8(5): 5263–72.

41. Ferreira DS, Annoni R, Silva LF, et al. Toll-like receptors 2, 3 and 4 and thymic stromal lymphopoietin expression in fatal asthma. Clin Exp Allergy 2012; 42(10):1459–71.

42. Sutherland ER, Martin RJ. Asthma and atypical bacterial infection. Chest 2007; 132(6):1962–6.
43. Hong SJ. The role of *Mycoplasma pneumoniae* infection in asthma. Allergy Asthma Immunol Res 2012;4(2):59–61.
44. Darveaux JI, Lemanske RF Jr. Infection-related asthma. J Allergy Clin Immunol Pract 2014;2(6):658–63.
45. Friedlander AL, Albert RK. Chronic macrolide therapy in inflammatory airways diseases. Chest 2010;138(5):1202–12.
46. Yano T, Ichikawa Y, Komatu S, et al. Association of *Mycoplasma pneumoniae* antigen with initial onset of bronchial asthma. Am J Respir Crit Care Med 1994;149(5):1348–53.
47. Esposito S, Blasi F, Arosio C, et al. Importance of acute *Mycoplasma pneumoniae* and *Chlamydia pneumoniae* infections in children with wheezing. Eur Respir J 2000;16(6):1142–6.
48. Kim CK, Chung CY, Kim JS, et al. Late abnormal findings on high-resolution computed tomography after *Mycoplasma pneumonia*. Pediatrics 2000;105(2): 372–8.
49. Puolakkainen M. Innate immunity and vaccines in chlamydial infection with special emphasis on *Chlamydia pneumoniae*. FEMS Immunol Med Microbiol 2009;55(2):167–77.
50. Costa CP, Kirschning CJ, Busch D, et al. Role of chlamydial heat shock protein 60 in the stimulation of innate immune cells by *Chlamydia pneumoniae*. Eur J Immunol 2002;32(9):2460–70.
51. Da Costa CU, Wantia N, Kirschning CJ, et al. Heat shock protein 60 from *Chlamydia pneumoniae* elicits an unusual set of inflammatory responses via Toll-like receptor 2 and 4 in vivo. Eur J Immunol 2004;34(10):2874–84.
52. Zhou Z, Wu Y, Chen L, et al. Heat shock protein 10 of *Chlamydophila pneumoniae* induces proinflammatory cytokines through Toll-like receptor (TLR) 2 and TLR4 in human monocytes THP-1. In Vitro Cell Dev Biol Anim 2011;47(8):541–9.
53. Ishii KJ, Koyama S, Nakagawa A, et al. Host innate immune receptors and beyond: making sense of microbial infections. Cell Host Microbe 2008;3(6): 352–63.
54. Kang Y, Wang F, Lu Z, et al. MAPK kinase 3 potentiates *Chlamydia* HSP60-induced inflammatory response through distinct activation of NF-kappaB. J Immunol 2013;191(1):386–94.
55. Ausiello CM, Palazzo R, Spensieri F, et al. 60-kDa heat shock protein of *Chlamydia pneumoniae* is a target of T-cell immune response. J Biol Regul Homeost Agents 2005;19(3–4):136–40.
56. Ausiello CM, Fedele G, Palazzo R, et al. 60-kDa heat shock protein of *Chlamydia pneumoniae* promotes a T helper type 1 immune response through IL-12/IL-23 production in monocyte-derived dendritic cells. Microbes Infect 2006;8(3):714–20.
57. Itoh R, Murakami I, Chou B, et al. *Chlamydia pneumoniae* harness host NLRP3 inflammasome-mediated caspase-1 activation for optimal intracellular growth in murine macrophages. Biochem Biophys Res Commun 2014;452(3):689–94.
58. Matsuo J, Nakamura S, Takeda S, et al. Synergistic costimulatory effect of *Chlamydia pneumoniae* with carbon nanoparticles on NLRP3 inflammasome-mediated interleukin-1beta secretion in macrophages. Infect Immun 2015; 83(7):2917–25.
59. Shimada K, Crother TR, Karlin J, et al. Caspase-1 dependent IL-1beta secretion is critical for host defense in a mouse model of *Chlamydia pneumoniae* lung infection. PLoS One 2011;6(6):e21477.

60. He X, Mekasha S, Mavrogiorgos N, et al. Inflammation and fibrosis during *Chlamydia pneumoniae* infection is regulated by IL-1 and the NLRP3/ASC inflammasome. J Immunol 2010;184(10):5743–54.

61. Olivares-Zavaleta N, Carmody A, Messer R, et al. *Chlamydia pneumoniae* inhibits activated human T lymphocyte proliferation by the induction of apoptotic and pyroptotic pathways. J Immunol 2011;186(12):7120–6.

62. Jupelli M, Shimada K, Chiba N, et al. *Chlamydia pneumoniae* infection in mice induces chronic lung inflammation, iBALT formation, and fibrosis. PLoS One 2013;8(10):e77447.

63. Horvat JC, Starkey MR, Kim RY, et al. Early-life chlamydial lung infection enhances allergic airways disease through age-dependent differences in immunopathology. J Allergy Clin Immunol 2010;125(3):617–25, 625.e1–6.

64. Asquith KL, Horvat JC, Kaiko GE, et al. Interleukin-13 promotes susceptibility to chlamydial infection of the respiratory and genital tracts. PLoS Pathog 2011; 7(5):e1001339.

65. Starkey MR, Essilfie AT, Horvat JC, et al. Constitutive production of IL-13 promotes early-life Chlamydia respiratory infection and allergic airway disease. Mucosal Immunol 2013;6(3):569–79.

66. Starkey MR, Nguyen DH, Brown AC, et al. PD-L1 Promotes Early-life Chlamydia Respiratory Infection-induced Severe Allergic Airway Disease. Am J Respir Cell Mol Biol 2016;54(4):493–503.

67. Dzhindzhikhashvili MS, Joks R, Smith-Norowitz T, et al. Doxycycline suppresses *Chlamydia pneumoniae*-mediated increases in ongoing immunoglobulin E and interleukin-4 responses by peripheral blood mononuclear cells of patients with allergic asthma. J Antimicrob Chemother 2013;68(10):2363–8.

68. Horvat JC, Starkey MR, Kim RY, et al. Chlamydial respiratory infection during allergen sensitization drives neutrophilic allergic airways disease. J Immunol 2010;184(8):4159–69.

69. Essilfie AT, Horvat JC, Kim RY, et al. Macrolide therapy suppresses key features of experimental steroid-sensitive and steroid-insensitive asthma. Thorax 2015; 70(5):458–67.

70. Patel KK, Vicencio AG, Du Z, et al. Infectious *Chlamydia pneumoniae* is associated with elevated interleukin-8 and airway neutrophilia in children with refractory asthma. Pediatr Infect Dis J 2010;29(12):1093–8.

71. Morinaga Y, Yanagihara K, Miyashita N, et al. Azithromycin, clarithromycin and telithromycin inhibit MUC5AC induction by *Chlamydophila pneumoniae* in airway epithelial cells. Pulm Pharmacol Ther 2009;22(6):580–6.

72. Park CS, Lee YS, Kwon HS, et al. *Chlamydophila pneumoniae* inhibits corticosteroid-induced suppression of metalloproteinase-9 and tissue inhibitor metalloproteinase-1 secretion by human peripheral blood mononuclear cells. J Med Microbiol 2012;61(Pt 5):705–11.

73. Park CS, Kim TB, Moon KA, et al. *Chlamydophila pneumoniae* enhances secretion of VEGF, TGF-beta and TIMP-1 from human bronchial epithelial cells under Th2 dominant microenvironment. Allergy Asthma Immunol Res 2010;2(1):41–7.

74. Kim TB, Moon KA, Lee KY, et al. *Chlamydophila pneumoniae* triggers release of CCL20 and vascular endothelial growth factor from human bronchial epithelial cells through enhanced intracellular oxidative stress and MAPK activation. J Clin Immunol 2009;29(5):629–36.

75. Dutow P, Lingner S, Laudeley R, et al. Severity of allergic airway disease due to house dust mite allergen is not increased after clinical recovery of lung infection with *Chlamydia pneumoniae* in mice. Infect Immun 2013;81(9):3366–74.

76. Crother TR, Schroder NW, Karlin J, et al. *Chlamydia pneumoniae* infection induced allergic airway sensitization is controlled by regulatory T-cells and plasmacytoid dendritic cells. PLoS One 2011;6(6):e20784.
77. Chiba N, Shimada K, Chen S, et al. Mast cells play an important role in *Chlamydia pneumoniae* lung infection by facilitating immune cell recruitment into the airway. J Immunol 2015;194(8):3840–51.
78. Zaitsu M. The development of asthma in wheezing infants with *Chlamydia pneumoniae* infection. J Asthma 2007;44(7):565–8.
79. Hahn DL, Dodge RW, Golubjatnikov R. Association of *Chlamydia pneumoniae* (strain TWAR) infection with wheezing, asthmatic bronchitis, and adult-onset asthma. JAMA 1991;266(2):225–30.
80. Cunningham AF, Johnston SL, Julious SA, et al. Chronic *Chlamydia pneumoniae* infection and asthma exacerbations in children. Eur Respir J 1998;11(2):345–9.
81. Biscardi S, Lorrot M, Marc E, et al. *Mycoplasma pneumoniae* and asthma in children. Clin Infect Dis 2004;38(10):1341–6.
82. Hahn DL, Anttila T, Saikku P. Association of *Chlamydia pneumoniae* IgA antibodies with recently symptomatic asthma. Epidemiol Infect 1996;117(3):513–7.
83. Hahn DL. *Chlamydia pneumoniae* antibodies and adult-onset asthma. J Allergy Clin Immunol 2000;106:404.
84. Miyatake H, Taki F, Taniguchi H, et al. Erythromycin reduces the severity of bronchial hyperresponsiveness in asthma. Chest 1991;99(3):670–3.
85. Kostadima E, Tsiodras S, Alexopoulos EI, et al. Clarithromycin reduces the severity of bronchial hyperresponsiveness in patients with asthma. Eur Respir J 2004;23(5):714–7.
86. Hahn DL, Grasmick M, Hetzel S, et al. Azithromycin for bronchial asthma in adults: an effectiveness trial. J Am Board Fam Med 2012;25(4):442–59.
87. Hahn DL, Plane MB, Mahdi OS, et al. Secondary outcomes of a pilot randomized trial of azithromycin treatment for asthma. PLoS Clin Trials 2006;1(2):e11.
88. Simpson JL, Powell H, Boyle MJ, et al. Clarithromycin targets neutrophilic airway inflammation in refractory asthma. Am J Respir Crit Care Med 2008;177(2):148–55.
89. Shoji T, Yoshida S, Sakamoto H, et al. Anti-inflammatory effect of roxithromycin in patients with aspirin-intolerant asthma. Clin Exp Allergy 1999;29(7):950–6.
90. Brusselle GG, Vanderstichele C, Jordens P, et al. Azithromycin for prevention of exacerbations in severe asthma (AZISAST): a multicentre randomised double-blind placebo-controlled trial. Thorax 2013;68(4):322–9.
91. Itkin IH, Menzel ML. The use of macrolide antibiotic substances in the treatment of asthma. J Allergy 1970;45(3):146–62.
92. Zeiger RS, Schatz M, Sperling W, et al. Efficacy of troleandomycin in outpatients with severe, corticosteroid-dependent asthma. J Allergy Clin Immunol 1980;66(6):438–46.
93. Siracusa A, Brugnami G, Fiordi T, et al. Troleandomycin in the treatment of difficult asthma. J Allergy Clin Immunol 1993;92(5):677–82.
94. Kamada AK, Hill MR, Iklé DN, et al. Efficacy and safety of low-dose troleandomycin therapy in children with severe, steroid-requiring asthma. J Allergy Clin Immunol 1993;91(4):873–82.
95. Nelson HS, Hamilos DL, Corsello PR, et al. A double-blind study of troleandomycin and methylprednisolone in asthmatic subjects who require daily corticosteroids. Am Rev Respir Dis 1993;147(2):398–404.

96. Garey KW, Rubinstein I, Gotfried MH, et al. Long-term clarithromycin decreases prednisone requirements in elderly patients with prednisone-dependent asthma. Chest 2000;118(6):1826–7.

97. Szefler SJ, Rose JQ, Ellis EF, et al. The effect of troleandomycin on methylpred-nisolone elimination. J Allergy Clin Immunol 1980;66(6):447–51.

98. Strunk RC, Bacharier LB, Phillips BR, et al. Azithromycin or montelukast as inhaled corticosteroid-sparing agents in moderate-to-severe childhood asthma study. J Allergy Clin Immunol 2008;122(6):1138–44.e4.

99. Kew KM, Undela K, Kotortsi I, et al. Macrolides for chronic asthma. Cochrane Database Syst Rev 2015;(9):CD002997.

100. Hansel TT, Johnston SL, Openshaw PJ. Microbes and mucosal immune responses in asthma. Lancet 2013;381(9869):861–73.

101. Huang YJ. The respiratory microbiome and innate immunity in asthma. Curr Opin Pulm Med 2015;21(1):27–32.

102. Gollwitzer ES, Saglani S, Trompette A, et al. Lung microbiota promotes tolerance to allergens in neonates via PD-L1. Nat Med 2014;20(6):642–7.

103. Marsland BJ, Gollwitzer ES. Host-microorganism interactions in lung diseases. Nat Rev Immunol 2014;14(12):827–35.

104. Fujimura KE, Slusher NA, Cabana MD, et al. Role of the gut microbiota in defining human health. Expert Rev Anti Infect Ther 2010;8(4):435–54.

105. Brooks C, Pearce N, Douwes J. The hygiene hypothesis in allergy and asthma: an update. Curr Opin Allergy Clin Immunol 2013;13(1):70–7.

106. Lynch SV, Wood RA, Boushey H, et al. Effects of early-life exposure to allergens and bacteria on recurrent wheeze and atopy in urban children. J Allergy Clin Immunol 2014;134(3):593–601.e12.

107. McCoy KD, Koller Y. New developments providing mechanistic insight into the impact of the microbiota on allergic disease. Clin Immunol 2015;159(2):170–6.

108. Bisgaard H, Li N, Bonnelykke K, et al. Reduced diversity of the intestinal microbiota during infancy is associated with increased risk of allergic disease at school age. J Allergy Clin Immunol 2011;128(3):646–52.e1-5.

109. Fujimura KE, Lynch SV. Microbiota in allergy and asthma and the emerging relationship with the gut microbiome. Cell Host Microbe 2015;17(5):592–602.

110. Trompette A, Gollwitzer ES, Yadava K, et al. Gut microbiota metabolism of dietary fiber influences allergic airway disease and hematopoiesis. Nat Med 2014; 20(2):159–66.

111. Park H, Shin JW, Park SG, et al. Microbial communities in the upper respiratory tract of patients with asthma and chronic obstructive pulmonary disease. PLoS One 2014;9(10):e109710.

112. Marri PR, Stern DA, Wright AL, et al. Asthma-associated differences in microbial composition of induced sputum. J Allergy Clin Immunol 2013;131(2): 346–52.e1-3.

113. Huang YJ, Nelson CE, Brodie EL, et al. Airway microbiota and bronchial hyper-responsiveness in patients with suboptimally controlled asthma. J Allergy Clin Immunol 2011;127(2):372–81.e1-3.

114. Huang YJ, Nariya S, Harris JM, et al. The airway microbiome in patients with severe asthma: associations with disease features and severity. J Allergy Clin Immunol 2015;136(4):874–84.

115. Green BJ, Wiriyachaiporn S, Grainge C, et al. Potentially pathogenic airway bacteria and neutrophilic inflammation in treatment resistant severe asthma. PLoS One 2014;9(6):e100645.

116. Goleva E, Jackson LP, Harris JK, et al. The effects of airway microbiome on corticosteroid responsiveness in asthma. Am J Respir Crit Care Med 2013;188(10): 1193–201.
117. Slater M, Rivett DW, Williams L, et al. The impact of azithromycin therapy on the airway microbiota in asthma. Thorax 2014;69:673–4.
118. Huang YJ, Lynch SV. The emerging relationship between the airway microbiota and chronic respiratory disease: clinical implications. Expert Rev Respir Med 2011;5(6):809–21.
119. Huang YJ, Boushey HA. The microbiome and asthma. Ann Am Thorac Soc 2014;11(Suppl 1):S48–51.
120. Huang YJ. Asthma microbiome studies and the potential for new therapeutic strategies. Curr Allergy Asthma Rep 2013;13(5):453–61.
121. Smith-Norowitz TA, Silverberg JI, Kusonruksa M, et al. Asthmatic children have increased specific anti-*Mycoplasma pneumoniae* IgM but not IgG or IgE-values independent of history of respiratory tract infection. Pediatr Infect Dis J 2013; 32(6):599–603.
122. Bebear C, Raherison C, Nacka F, et al. Comparison of *Mycoplasma pneumoniae* Infections in asthmatic children versus asthmatic adults. Pediatr Infect Dis J 2014;33(3):e71–5.
123. Fonseca-Aten M, Okada PJ, Bowlware KL, et al. Effect of clarithromycin on cytokines and chemokines in children with an acute exacerbation of recurrent wheezing: a double-blind, randomized, placebo-controlled trial. Ann Allergy Asthma Immunol 2006;97(4):457–63.
124. Wood PR, Hill VL, Burks ML, et al. *Mycoplasma pneumoniae* in children with acute and refractory asthma. Ann Allergy Asthma Immunol 2013;110(5):328–34.e1.
125. Kraft M, Cassell GH, Henson JE, et al. Detection of *Mycoplasma pneumoniae* in the airways of adults with chronic asthma. Am J Respir Crit Care Med 1998; 158(3):998–1001.
126. Martin RJ, Kraft M, Chu HW, et al. A link between chronic asthma and chronic infection. J Allergy Clin Immunol 2001;107(4):595–601.
127. Lieberman D, Lieberman D, Printz S, et al. Atypical Pathogen Infection in Adults with Acute Exacerbation of Bronchial Asthma. Am J Respir Crit Care Med 2003; 167(3):406–10.
128. Peters J, Singh H, Brooks EG, et al. Persistence of community-acquired respiratory distress syndrome toxin-producing *Mycoplasma pneumoniae* in refractory asthma. Chest 2011;140(2):401–7.
129. Awasthi S, Yadav KK, Agarwal J. *Chlamydia pneumoniae* infection associated with uncontrolled asthma: a hospital based cross sectional study. Indian J Pediatr 2012;79(10):1318–22.
130. Biscione GL, Corne J, Chauhan AJ, et al. Increased frequency of detection of *Chlamydophila pneumoniae* in asthma. Eur Respir J 2004;24(5):745–9.
131. Miyashita N, Kubota Y, Nakajima M, et al. *Chlamydia pneumoniae* and exacerbations of asthma in adults. Ann Allergy Asthma Immunol 1998;80(5):405–9.
132. Allegra L, Blasi F, Centanni S, et al. Acute exacerbations of asthma in adults: role of *Chlamydia pneumoniae* infection. Eur Respir J 1994;7(12):2165–8.
133. Black PN, Scicchitano R, Jenkins CR, et al. Serological evidence of infection with *Chlamydia pneumoniae* is related to the severity of asthma. Eur Respir J 2000;15(2):254–9.
134. Huittinen T, Hahn D, Anttila T, et al. Host immune response to *Chlamydia pneumoniae* heat shock protein 60 is associated with asthma. Eur Respir J 2001; 17(6):1078–82.

135. Hahn DL, Peeling RW. Airflow limitation, asthma, and *Chlamydia pneumoniae*-specific heat shock protein 60. Ann Allergy Asthma Immunol 2008;101(6):614–8.
136. Pasternack R, Huhtala H, Karjalainen J. *Chlamydophila (Chlamydia) pneumoniae* serology and asthma in adults: a longitudinal analysis. J Allergy Clin Immunol 2005;116(5):1123–8.
137. Kraft M, Cassell GH, Pak J, et al. *Mycoplasma pneumoniae* and *Chlamydia pneumoniae* in asthma: effect of clarithromycin. Chest 2002;121(6):1782–8.
138. Black PN, Blasi F, Jenkins CR, et al. Trial of roxithromycin in subjects with asthma and serological evidence of infection with *Chlamydia pneumoniae*. Am J Respir Crit Care Med 2001;164(4):536–41.
139. Hahn DL. Treatment of *Chlamydia pneumoniae* infection in adult asthma: a before-after trial. J Fam Pract 1995;41(4):345–51.
140. Sutherland ER, King TS, Icitovic N, et al. A trial of clarithromycin for the treatment of suboptimally controlled asthma. J Allergy Clin Immunol 2010;126(4):747–53.
141. Emre U, Roblin PM, Gelling M, et al. The association of *Chlamydia pneumoniae* infection and reactive airway disease in children. Arch Pediatr Adolesc Med 1994;148(7):727–32.
142. Johnston SL, Blasi F, Black PN, et al. The effect of telithromycin in acute exacerbations of asthma. N Engl J Med 2006;354(15):1589–600.

Chronic Rhinosinusitis and Aspirin-Exacerbated Respiratory Disease

Neha M. Dunn, MD, Rohit K. Katial, MD*

KEYWORDS

- Aspirin-exacerbated respiratory disease • Asthma • Chronic rhinosinusitis
- Chronic sinusitis • Nasal polyps

KEY POINTS

- Patients with concomitant chronic rhinosinusitis and asthma often have more severe disease that is difficult to control with standard pharmacotherapy.
- Treatment must focus on treating both the upper and lower airway inflammation because an insult in one area often leads to subsequent inflammation in the other.
- A subset of patients have aspirin-exacerbated respiratory disease (AERD) characterized by asthma, chronic rhinosinusitis with nasal polyposis, and intolerance of COX-1 inhibitors.
- In addition to standard anti-inflammatory therapy, patients with AERD often require an aspirin desensitization followed by long-term aspirin therapy to manage their disease.
- Recognizing the presence of chronic rhinosinusitis in patients with severe asthma allows for management of the upper and lower respiratory tracts and improved disease control.

INTRODUCTION

A large percentage of patients with severe asthma have concomitant chronic rhinosinusitis (CRS), which represents a distinct group of patients with severe, often refractory upper and lower airway inflammation.[1,2] Such patients frequently have similar inflammatory mediators throughout the upper and lower airways as described by the unified airway concept. CRS is a broad clinical syndrome defined by persistent mucosal inflammation of the nasal and paranasal cavities and can impact asthma control.[3] This article discusses definitions, phenotypes, evaluation, and treatment of CRS.

DEFINITIONS

The terminology for rhinosinusitis is variable and often classified by duration (**Table 1**).[4,5] CRS is a heterogeneous disease with complex pathophysiology and is

Department of Allergy and Immunology, National Jewish Health, 1400 Jackson Street, Denver, CO 80206, USA
* Corresponding author.
E-mail address: katialr@njhealth.org

Immunol Allergy Clin N Am 36 (2016) 503–514
http://dx.doi.org/10.1016/j.iac.2016.03.011   immunology.theclinics.com
0889-8561/16/$ – see front matter © 2016 Elsevier Inc. All rights reserved.

Table 1	
Rhinosinusitis classifications	
Classification	**Duration**
Acute rhinosinusitis	Rhinosinusitis symptoms lasting <4 wk
Subacute rhinosinusitis	Rhinosinusitis symptoms lasting 4–12 wk
Chronic rhinosinusitis	Rhinosinusitis symptoms lasting >12 wk
Acute bacterial rhinosinusitis	Acute sinusitis with bacterial etiology
Viral rhinosinusitis	Acute sinusitis with viral etiology
Recurrent acute rhinosinusitis	4 or more annual episodes of rhinosinusitis without persistent inflammation in between

often simplified into patients with or without nasal polyps (CRSwNP; CRSsNP). CRSwNP is further subdivided into those who do not tolerate aspirin or other cyclooxygenase (COX)-1 inhibitors, termed aspirin-exacerbated respiratory disease (AERD). AERD was previously termed Samter triad and is often referred to as aspirin-sensitive rather than aspirin-tolerant asthma.

UNIFIED AIRWAY HYPOTHESIS

The unified airway hypothesis is a concept that closely links the upper airways, including the middle ear, nose, paranasal sinuses, and the entire lower airway as one functional, interconnected group with shared inflammatory features.[6,7] Prior studies have shown that 78% of patients with asthma have nasal symptoms[8] and up to greater than 84% of sinus computed tomography (CT) scans were abnormal in patients with severe asthma.[2] The prevalence of asthma in CRS ranges from 45% to 65% in patients with CRSwNP and 18% in CRSsNP. One study found that 94% of patients with CRS had asthma with 88% having severe persistent disease.[9–11]

Patients with CRS and asthma often have severe respiratory disease requiring more aggressive management.[12] Such patients have been found to have lower quality of life measures, higher rhinosinusitis severity scores, and poor outcomes after functional endoscopic sinus surgery compared with the nonasthmatic group.[13,14] Moreover, when CRS is treated (medically or surgically), asthma symptoms improve and the need for asthma-related medications decreases.[12,15,16]

CRS had been found to have similar airway remodeling as the bronchial mucosa in patients with asthma with nearly indistinguishable microscopic findings including mucosal edema, submucosal gland and bronchial smooth muscle hypertrophy, collagen deposition, basement membrane thickening, and subepithelial fibrosis in the lamina reticularis.[17] However, Chanez and colleagues[18] showed that the extent of eosinophilic inflammation, reticular basement membrane thickness, and percent of the epithelium shedding is greater in bronchial than nasal mucosa of patients with asthma with perennial rhinitis. Several studies have shown that antigens placed in the nose up-regulate inflammatory cells, primarily eosinophils, and their mediators in the distal bronchi. Similarly, antigen placement into the bronchi with a bronchoscope results in upregulation of inflammatory mediators in the nose, suggesting that stimulation can occur anywhere within the unified airway.[19,20] Corren and colleagues[21] found that nasal provocation with allergen delivery to the nose led to a significant increase in bronchial hyperresponsiveness compared with placebo, but there were no changes in forced expiratory volume in 1 second (FEV_1). Generally, it seems that either challenging or treating the upper airway effects bronchial hyperactivity but does not truly impact lung function as measured by FEV_1.

PATHOPHYSIOLOGY

CRS is no longer considered primarily an infectious disease but rather a disease of endogenously driven inflammation.[22] CSwNP is a distinct phenotype with a Th2 cytokine signature similar to eosinophilic/allergic asthma with robust expression of interleukin (IL)-4, IL-5, and IL-13. White patients with nasal polyps usually have high levels of tissue eosinophils, neutrophils, mast cells, and B cells. Epithelial cytokines TSLP[23] and IL-33[24] have been implicated in driving Th2 inflammation by directly activating innate lymphocyte cells-2, which release substantial amounts of IL-5 and IL-13. Conversely, Asian patients with nasal polyps have a more variable pattern of tissue infiltration and cytokine expression with more neutrophils, fewer eosinophils, and a Th1/Th17 pattern with elevated interferon (IFN)-γ, IL-6, IL-1β, and IL-17.[25,26] The pathophysiology of CRSsNP is thought to be driven by a breakdown of innate immunity leading to frequent recurrent episodes of acute sinusitis, bacterial colonization, and biofilm formation.[27]

ALLERGIC FUNGAL RHINOSINUSITIS

It was previously believed that nearly all cases of CRS were driven by response to common airborne fungal elements.[28] Fungal elements, specifically *Alternaria*, were thought to stimulate peripheral blood mononuclear cells and lead to the release of Th1 and Th2 cytokines, including IFN-g, IL-4, IL-5, and IL-13. It was thought that these sensitized T cells activated eosinophils and led to degranulation with subsequent tissue damage causing the symptoms of CRS.[29] Since then, this hypothesis has become more controversial. First, eosinophils are not generally important cells types in host defense against fungi. Second, attempts at replicating the sensitization of peripheral blood mononuclear cells to fungal antigens have failed.[30,31] Most importantly, although smaller studies have shown some improvement in nasal polyps with topical antifungals,[32] double-blind placebo-controlled trials have failed to show efficacy of antifungal therapy modifying the disease process.[33,34] Now, fungi are no longer viewed as the primary cause of the development of all CRS, but some investigators suspect fungi play a role in a subgroup of patients with CRS.

BACTERIA IN CHRONIC RHINOSINUSITIS

Although the microbiome of the sinonasal tract remains poorly characterized, there are several theories regarding the proposed role of bacteria in CRS.[3] The superantigen hypothesis suggests exotoxins from *Staphylococcus* bacteria behave as superantigens amplifying local inflammatory responses fostering polyp formation.[35,36] Patients with CRSwNP have been shown to carry *Staphylococcus aureus* in a high percent of patients.[37] It is not clear whether superantigens from these bacteria are causative but they may accentuate the pre-existing inflammatory response in these tissues.[3] The biofilm hypothesis describes bacterial biofilms that have been found in 42% to 75% of patients with CRS with or without nasal polyps.[38,39] Biofilms form a highly organized protective extracellular matrix that allows bacteria to evade host defenses and conventional antibiotics. However, there is no direct evidence to suggest that biofilms play a role in the initial establishment of CRS.[40] Although Tatar and colleagues[41] found regression of biofilms in patients treatment with oral macrolides for 2 weeks, Videler and colleagues[42] found a lack of efficacy of low-dose azithromycin in patients with

CRS treated for 3 months with regards to symptom scores, nasal endoscopic findings, peak nasal inspiratory flow, and microbiology.

ATOPY

Allergic rhinitis often precedes the development of asthma and has been shown to worsen asthma control.[8,43,44] However, severity of CRS by clinical and radiographic parameters has not been found to demonstrate significant correlations with atopic status.[45] AR is thought to be a superimposed factor rather than a causative factor in CRS that contributes to the overall inflammatory burden seen in CRS.[46] There are limited data with poor evidence to support that allergen avoidance or immunotherapy improves CRS, but rather treatment of AR along with aggressive therapy for the underlying eosinophilic inflammation is necessary.[46–48] Allergy testing via skin prick testing or allergen-specific immunoassays to detect IgE-specific antibody may be helpful in patients with seasonal exacerbations of rhinitis or asthma, but is not routinely necessary in all patients with CRS.

ASPIRIN-EXACERBATED RESPIRATORY DISEASE

Patients with AERD (**Box 1**) have greater morbidity than patients with aspirin-tolerant asthma with more emergency department visits, hospitalizations, and corticosteroid bursts.[54] Patients often suffer hyposmia or anosmia, which correlates strongly with the diagnosis.[55] The authors have previously reported that CRSwNP patients with AERD had more severe sinus CT scores, more sinus surgeries, and prednisone use than aspirin-tolerant individuals.[10] Berges-Gimeno and colleagues[51] studied 300 patients with AERD and showed that nearly all (94%) had either complete sinus opacification or mucoperiosteal thickening on radiography. Patients with asthma often have an increased dependency on systemic corticosteroids and a higher frequency of severe exacerbations and reduced lung function.[54]

The exact mechanism of AERD is uncertain but is characterized by eosinophilic infiltration with abnormal arachidonic acid metabolism.[56] Most patients with AERD are not atopic suggesting that the pathogenesis is independent of atopy.[50] Both the respiratory tract and polypoid tissue from patients with AERD have shown eosinophilic infiltration and activation with the presence of eosinophilic granule contents, cysteinyl leukotrienes (cysLTs), IL-5, eotaxin, RANTES, and IFN-γ.[56,57] In addition to these

---

Box 1
AERD Facts

- AERD is manifested by adult-onset asthma, CRSwNP, and intolerance of COX-1 inhibitors.

- Patients usually present in the third or fourth decade of life.

- Estimate of AERD prevalence from 2014 meta-analysis: 7% of patients with asthma have AERD and twice as many patients with severe asthma have it.

- COX-inhibitor sensitivity can develop in any stage of the disease as AERD evolves over time. Commonly begins with rhinitis initially. One study showed asthma appeared 2 years after onset of rhinitis on average, with intolerance to COX-1 inhibitors and nasal polyposis 4 years after.

- Ingestion of COX-1 inhibitors is usually dose-dependent and leads to an exacerbation of underlying rhinosinusitis and asthma with nasal congestion, conjunctivitis, rhinorrhea, laryngospasm, and/or bronchoconstriction within 30 minutes to 3 hours.

Data from Refs.[49–53]

cytokines the authors have shown that aspirin desensitization in this cohort decreases sputum IL-4 levels, which in part regulates the cysteinyl leukotriene expression.[57] Therefore, the increase in proinflammatory cysLTs, such as LTC4, LTD4, and LTE4 and their receptors, may be a consequence of the rich TH2 environment consisting of IL-4, IL-5, and IL-13. Additionally, there is a decrease in regulatory prostaglandins, such as prostaglandin E_2 and its receptors, in sinonasal passages of patients with AERD.[58,59]

In patients with AERD, CRS and asthma are severe and relatively refractory to pharmacotherapy.[60] Nasal polyps in patients with AERD tend to require surgical treatment and have high rates of recurrence after surgery compared with patients with CRSwNP who tolerate aspirin.[60,61] Inflammation progresses despite avoidance of COX-1 inhibitors and often aspirin desensitization is warranted for added therapeutic benefit. Patients with AERD should be managed with topical therapies, such as nasal saline rinses and off-label use of topical steroids. For patients who fail medical therapy, surgical intervention may be indicated. Unfortunately, patients with AERD respond less well to surgery than aspirin-tolerant patients and often require multiple procedures.[62] McMains and Kountakis[63] reported that up to 80% of patients with AERD who had not undergone aspirin desensitization required an additional sinus surgery within 24 months of their last surgery. Despite surgical intervention, medical treatment with topical nasal steroids is necessary following surgery. Moreover, aspirin desensitization followed by continuous aspirin therapy has been shown to improve quality of life, nasal, and asthma symptoms scores. It also reduces the frequency of polyp formation, sinus infections, and need for systemic corticosteroids 6 and 12 months after therapy.[64–66]

EVALUATION AND TREATMENT

Accurate diagnosis of CRS not only requires a thorough history, but also confirmation of sinonasal mucosal inflammation, such as polyps, mucosal edema, or purulent mucus.[67,68] Symptoms of CRS most commonly include nasal obstruction (81%–95%), facial congestion, pressure or fullness (70%–85%), discolored nasal discharge (51%–83%), and hyposmia (61%–69%). Two or more of these symptoms is highly sensitive for diagnosing CRS but symptoms alone are fairly nonspecific.[67,69,70] Several studies have shown that greater olfactory dysfunction indicates greater sinonasal disease, correlates with the degree of inflammation in patients with polyps, and is predictive of radiographic sinus scores.[67,71] Loss of smell was found to be the sole predictor of persistent mucosal inflammation after sinus surgery.[72]

Imaging

CT and MRI can be used to confirm the diagnosis of CRS, but based on the increased cost and possible overdiagnosis, CT scan without contrast is preferred.[5] CT scanning allows for the ability to quantify the extent of disease based on opacification of paranasal sinuses,[73] monitor disease progression, and provide anatomic detail necessary to guide potential surgery,[74] but it does not necessarily correlate with symptom severity.[75] Ten Brinke and colleagues[2] found that patients with more extensive sinus disease on CT scans were more likely to have evidence of airway inflammation based on peripheral and sputum eosinophilia and elevated exhaled nitric oxide. Patients had more severe CT sinus scores were more likely to have aspirin sensitivity but CT scores did not correlate with nasal symptoms, asthma control, or FEV_1. CT scanning is also helpful in excluding aggressive infection or neoplastic disease that could mimic CRS. If such findings are noted, follow-up MRI should be performed.[74]

Corticosteroids

Topical corticosteroids are widely recommended in the treatment of CRS,[76] and their efficacy at reducing nasal symptoms has been supported by multiple systematic reviews but some subgroup analyses have shown more benefit in patients with polyps rather than those without.[77–80] Ragab and colleagues[12] found that treating with an oral macrolide, nasal irrigation, and topical steroids resulted in significant improvement in asthma symptom scores, increased FEV_1, reduced need for bronchodilators, and systemic steroids with decreased hospitalizations. However, when evaluating nasal steroids alone, a meta-analysis by Lohia and colleagues[81] showed nasal steroids improved FEV_1, asthma symptom scores, and rescue medication use compared with placebo, but in patients already on orally inhaled corticosteroids, the addition of intranasal steroids did not lead to any specific changes in clinical asthma outcomes.

A short course of oral corticosteroids has been shown to shrink polyp size and improve nasal symptoms and nasal flow.[82,83] Oral corticosteroids can be used as a bridge to surgery or in severe cases of CRSwNP that are refractory to topical therapy. However, the latter is preferred because of less adverse systemic effects. Aukema and colleagues[84] found that fluticasone nasal drops reduced the need for surgery in patients with CRS compared with placebo and hypothesized that nasal drops allow for better delivery into the middle meatus than nasal sprays. Long-term treatment with budesonide saline irrigation for at least 12 weeks has been reported to maintain improvement in nasal symptoms, polyp size, and nasal flow in those first treated with oral corticosteroids.[85] Jang and colleagues[86] evaluated postoperative patients who used budesonide saline irrigation versus those who did not and found lower CRS symptom scores and improved endoscopy findings in the treatment group.

Antibiotics

There is no clear evidence that oral antibiotics are beneficial in CRS. Unnecessary prescription of antibiotics can lead to unwanted side effects, increased health care costs, and induce antimicrobial resistance. Patients with CRS may have occasional episodes of acute bacterial sinusitis, which may require oral antibiotics. Acute bacterial rhinosinusitis must be recognized and treated because it can lead to serious complications including meningitis, brain abscess, orbital cellulitis, and orbital abscess.[87,88] For CRSwNP, chronic topical or intravenous antibiotics are not recommended but select oral antibiotics, especially macrolides, have shown some benefit based on their anti-inflammatory effects.[46,89]

Leukotriene Modifiers

Elevated cysLT concentrations in patients with CRSwNP suggest that leukotriene modifiers would have clinical benefit.[90] Leukotriene modifiers have shown benefit in upper airway disease with improvement in nasal congestion and hyposmia.[91] Furthermore, in a systematic review, Rix and colleagues[11] found that montelukast significantly improved nasal symptoms, nasal endoscopy and CT imaging, pulmonary symptoms, and asthma medication intake, whereas no effect was seen on pulmonary function tests.

Surgery

Various authors have studied the effect of surgical treatment of CRS on asthma outcomes with variable findings. Ragab and colleagues[12] found surgical intervention led to a decrease in asthma medication use, hospitalization, exhaled nitric oxide and improved FEV_1 but no significant change in asthma symptom scores. The overall conclusion was that medical therapy was superior to surgical therapy. In another systematic review, Vashishta and colleagues[92] found that endoscopic sinus surgery improves asthma control with decreased exacerbations, hospitalizations, and use of systemic and inhaled corticosteroids. However, pulmonary function was unchanged. Chen and colleagues[93] found functional endoscopic sinus surgery improved asthma control as measured by symptom scores but asthma medication use and pulmonary function testing remained stable. In a systematic review, Rix and colleagues[11] reported that two studies found significant improvement in FEV_1, whereas one did not. These variable results emphasize the need for high-quality research to answer such questions.

BIOLOGIC THERAPY

There is a large unmet need for newer therapies for CRS, because of the poor therapeutic response to current treatments with a high rate of recurrence or persistence of disease, Recent studies with biologic agents have shown promising results. A small study of CRSwNP and asthma patients treated with omalizumab, a human monoclonal antibody against IgE, resulted in improved rhinitis and asthma symptom scores and improved sinus CT scores but no improvement in FEV_1.[94] A larger study showed that omalizumab reduced nasal endoscopic polyp scores, improved CT scans, decreased nasal and asthma symptoms, and improved quality of life scores in patients with nasal polyps and asthma regardless of atopic status.[95] Mepolizumab, a humanized IgG1 monoclonal antibody against IL-5, was used to treat 20 subjects with nasal polyps with prominent eosinophilia. Twelve subjects showed improvement in symptom scores and sinus CT score.[96] A recent phase II multinational, randomized, double-blind, placebo-controlled study evaluated dupilumab, a human monoclonal antibody against IL-4Rα, which inhibits IL-4 and IL-13 activity, in patients with bilateral nasal polyposis but the results have not yet been released.[97]

SUMMARY

CRS and concomitant asthma often lead to a severe, persistent clinical course that is often difficult to treat and refractory to therapy. Patients with CRSwNP are often more difficult to treat than those without nasal polyps and have a Th2 cytokine pattern. A subset of patients have AERD with CRSwNP, asthma, and intolerance to COX-1 inhibitors. Such patients often have an even more severe clinical course with recurrent nasal polyps often requiring multiple surgeries and asthma that does not respond to traditional therapies. Diagnostic measures include a thorough history, direct visualization, imaging with CT, and an aspirin challenge when indicated. Successful treatment requires addressing inflammation in the upper and lower airways and focuses on the use of topical anti-inflammatory therapies, nasal irrigation, and leukotriene modifiers. In select cases, the use of aspirin desensitization, endoscopic sinus surgery, and occasionally oral corticosteroids or antibiotics are indicated. Novel monoclonal antibody therapies have shown some promising results, but more studies need to be performed.

REFERENCES

1. Pfister R, Lutolf M, Schapowal A, et al. Screening for sinus disease in patients with asthma: a computed tomography-controlled comparison of A-mode ultrasonography and standard radiography. J Allergy Clin Immunol 1994;94(5): 804–9.

2. ten Brinke A, Grootendorst DC, Schmidt JT, et al. Chronic sinusitis in severe asthma is related to sputum eosinophilia. J Allergy Clin Immunol 2002;109(4): 621–6.

3. Lam K, Schleimer R, Kern RC. The etiology and pathogenesis of chronic rhinosinusitis: a review of current hypotheses. Curr Allergy Asthma Rep 2015;15(7):41.

4. Scadding GK, Durham SR, Mirakian R, et al. BSACI guidelines for the management of rhinosinusitis and nasal polyposis. Clin Exp Allergy 2008;38(2):260–75.

5. Rosenfeld RM, Piccirillo JF, Chandrasekhar SS, et al. Clinical practice guideline (update): adult sinusitis. Otolaryngol Head Neck Surg 2015;152(Suppl 2):S1–39.

6. Krouse JH, Brown RW, Fineman SM, et al. Asthma and the unified airway. Otolaryngol Head Neck Surg 2007;136(Suppl 5):S75–106.

7. Stachler RJ. Comorbidities of asthma and the unified airway. Int Forum Allergy Rhinol 2015;5(Suppl 1):S17–22.

8. Corren J. Allergic rhinitis and asthma: how important is the link? J Allergy Clin Immunol 1997;99(2):S781–6.

9. Jarvis D, Newson R, Lotvall J, et al. Asthma in adults and its association with chronic rhinosinusitis: the GA2LEN survey in Europe. Allergy 2012;67(1):91–8.

10. Fountain CR, Mudd PA, Ramakrishnan VR, et al. Characterization and treatment of patients with chronic rhinosinusitis and nasal polyps. Ann Allergy Asthma Immunol 2013;111(5):337–41.

11. Rix I, Hakansson K, Larsen CG, et al. Management of chronic rhinosinusitis with nasal polyps and coexisting asthma: a systematic review. Am J Rhinol Allergy 2015;29(3):193–201.

12. Ragab S, Scadding GK, Lund VJ, et al. Treatment of chronic rhinosinusitis and its effects on asthma. Eur Respir J 2006;28(1):68–74.

13. Alobid I, Benitez P, Bernal-Sprekelsen M, et al. Nasal polyposis and its impact on quality of life: comparison between the effects of medical and surgical treatments. Allergy 2005;60(4):452–8.

14. Al Badaai Y, Samaha M. Outcome of endoscopic sinus surgery for chronic rhinosinusitis patients: a Canadian experience. J Laryngol Otol 2010;124(10):1095–9.

15. Palmer JN, Conley DB, Dong RG, et al. Efficacy of endoscopic sinus surgery in the management of patients with asthma and chronic sinusitis. Am J Rhinol 2001;15(1):49–53.

16. Ikeda K, Tanno N, Tamura G, et al. Endoscopic sinus surgery improves pulmonary function in patients with asthma associated with chronic sinusitis. Ann Otol Rhinol Laryngol 1999;108(4):355–9.

17. Ponikau JU, Sherris DA, Kephart GM, et al. Features of airway remodeling and eosinophilic inflammation in chronic rhinosinusitis: is the histopathology similar to asthma? J Allergy Clin Immunol 2003;112(5):877–82.

18. Chanez P, Vignola AM, Vic P, et al. Comparison between nasal and bronchial inflammation in asthmatic and control subjects. Am J Respir Crit Care Med 1999;159(2):588–95.

19. Braunstahl GJ, Overbeek SE, Kleinjan A, et al. Nasal allergen provocation induces adhesion molecule expression and tissue eosinophilia in upper and lower airways. J Allergy Clin Immunol 2001;107(3):469–76.

20. Braunstahl GJ, Overbeek SE, Fokkens WJ, et al. Segmental bronchoprovocation in allergic rhinitis patients affects mast cell and basophil numbers in nasal and bronchial mucosa. Am J Respir Crit Care Med 2001;164(5):858–65.

21. Corren J, Adinoff AD, Irvin CG. Changes in bronchial responsiveness following nasal provocation with allergen. J Allergy Clin Immunol 1992;89(2):611–8.

22. Borish L. Chronic rhinosinusitis: more than just "asthma of the upper airway". Am J Respir Crit Care Med 2015;192(6):647–8.

23. Nagarkar DR, Poposki JA, Tan BK, et al. Thymic stromal lymphopoietin activity is increased in nasal polyps of patients with chronic rhinosinusitis. J Allergy Clin Immunol 2013;132(3):593–600.e12.

24. Shaw JL, Fakhri S, Citardi MJ, et al. IL-33-responsive innate lymphoid cells are an important source of IL-13 in chronic rhinosinusitis with nasal polyps. Am J Respir Crit Care Med 2013;188(4):432–9.

25. Busse WW, Holgate S, Kerwin E, et al. Randomized, double-blind, placebo-controlled study of brodalumab, a human anti-IL-17 receptor monoclonal antibody, in moderate to severe asthma. Am J Respir Crit Care Med 2013;188(11): 1294–302.

26. Zhang N, Van Zele T, Perez-Novo C, et al. Different types of T-effector cells orchestrate mucosal inflammation in chronic sinus disease. J Allergy Clin Immunol 2008;122(5):961–8.

27. Lee RJ, Kofonow JM, Rosen PL, et al. Bitter and sweet taste receptors regulate human upper respiratory innate immunity. J Clin Invest 2014;124(3):1393–405.

28. Davis LJ, Kita H. Pathogenesis of chronic rhinosinusitis: role of airborne fungi and bacteria. Immunol Allergy Clin North Am 2004;24(1):59–73.

29. Shin SH, Ponikau JU, Sherris DA, et al. Chronic rhinosinusitis: an enhanced immune response to ubiquitous airborne fungi. J Allergy Clin Immunol 2004; 114(6):1369–75.

30. Douglas R, Bruhn M, Tan LW, et al. Response of peripheral blood lymphocytes to fungal extracts and staphylococcal superantigen B in chronic rhinosinusitis. Laryngoscope 2007;117(3):411–4.

31. Orlandi RR, Marple BF, Georgelas A, et al. Immunologic response to fungus is not universally associated with rhinosinusitis. Otolaryngol Head Neck Surg 2009; 141(6):750–6.e1-e2.

32. Ponikau JU, Sherris DA, Kita H, et al. Intranasal antifungal treatment in 51 patients with chronic rhinosinusitis. J Allergy Clin Immunol 2002;110(6):862–6.

33. Ebbens FA, Scadding GK, Badia L, et al. Amphotericin B nasal lavages: not a solution for patients with chronic rhinosinusitis. J Allergy Clin Immunol 2006;118(5): 1149–56.

34. Ebbens FA, Fokkens WJ. The mold conundrum in chronic rhinosinusitis: where do we stand today? Curr Allergy Asthma Rep 2008;8(2):93–101.

35. Bachert C, Gevaert P, Holtappels G, et al. Total and specific IgE in nasal polyps is related to local eosinophilic inflammation. J Allergy Clin Immunol 2001;107(4): 607–14.

36. Bachert C, Zhang N, Patou J, et al. Role of staphylococcal superantigens in upper airway disease. Curr Opin Allergy Clin Immunol 2008;8(1):34–8.

37. Van Zele T, Gevaert P, Watelet JB, et al. Staphylococcus aureus colonization and IgE antibody formation to enterotoxins is increased in nasal polyposis. J Allergy Clin Immunol 2004;114(4):981–3.

38. Suh JD, Ramakrishnan V, Palmer JN. Biofilms. Otolaryngol Clin North Am 2010; 43(3):521–30, viii.

39. Calo L, Passali GC, Galli J, et al. Role of biofilms in chronic inflammatory diseases of the upper airways. Adv Otorhinolaryngol 2011;72:93–6.

40. Foreman A, Jervis-Bardy J, Wormald PJ. Do biofilms contribute to the initiation and recalcitrance of chronic rhinosinusitis? Laryngoscope 2011;121(5):1085–91.

41. Tatar EC, Tatar I, Ocal B, et al. Prevalence of biofilms and their response to medical treatment in chronic rhinosinusitis without polyps. Otolaryngol Head Neck Surg 2012;146(4):669–75.
42. Videler WJ, Badia L, Harvey RJ, et al. Lack of efficacy of long-term, low-dose azithromycin in chronic rhinosinusitis: a randomized controlled trial. Allergy 2011; 66(11):1457–68.
43. Corren J, Manning BE, Thompson SF, et al. Rhinitis therapy and the prevention of hospital care for asthma: a case-control study. J Allergy Clin Immunol 2004; 113(3):415–9.
44. Brozek JL, Bousquet J, Baena-Cagnani CE, et al. Allergic Rhinitis and its Impact on Asthma (ARIA) guidelines: 2010 revision. J Allergy Clin Immunol 2010;126(3): 466–76.
45. Pearlman AN, Chandra RK, Chang D, et al. Relationships between severity of chronic rhinosinusitis and nasal polyposis, asthma, and atopy. Am J Rhinol Allergy 2009;23(2):145–8.
46. Fokkens WJ, Lund VJ, Mullol J, et al. European position paper on rhinosinusitis and nasal polyps 2012. Rhinol Suppl 2012;(23):3.
47. Slavin RG, Spector SL, Bernstein IL, et al. The diagnosis and management of sinusitis: a practice parameter update. J Allergy Clin Immunol 2005;116(Suppl 6):S13–47.
48. Bernstein IL, Storms WW. Practice parameters for allergy diagnostic testing. Joint Task Force on Practice Parameters for the Diagnosis and Treatment of Asthma. The American Academy of Allergy, Asthma and Immunology and the American College of Allergy, Asthma and Immunology. Ann Allergy Asthma Immunol 1995;75(6 Pt 2):543–625.
49. Rajan JP, Wineinger NE, Stevenson DD, et al. Prevalence of aspirin-exacerbated respiratory disease among asthmatic patients: a meta-analysis of the literature. J Allergy Clin Immunol 2015;135(3):676–81.e1.
50. Szczeklik A, Nizankowska E, Duplaga M. Natural history of aspirin-induced asthma. AIANE Investigators. European Network on Aspirin-Induced Asthma. Eur Respir J 2000;16(3):432–6.
51. Berges-Gimeno MP, Simon RA, Stevenson DD. The natural history and clinical characteristics of aspirin-exacerbated respiratory disease. Ann Allergy Asthma Immunol 2002;89(5):474–8.
52. Fahrenholz JM. Natural history and clinical features of aspirin-exacerbated respiratory disease. Clin Rev Allergy Immunol 2003;24(2):113–24.
53. Stevenson DD. Aspirin and NSAID sensitivity. Immunol Allergy Clin North Am 2004;24(3):491–505, vii.
54. Mascia K, Haselkorn T, Deniz YM, et al. Aspirin sensitivity and severity of asthma: evidence for irreversible airway obstruction in patients with severe or difficult-to-treat asthma. J Allergy Clin Immunol 2005;116(5):970–5.
55. Young J, Frenkiel S, Tewfik MA, et al. Long-term outcome analysis of endoscopic sinus surgery for chronic sinusitis. Am J Rhinol 2007;21(6):743–7.
56. Payne SC, Early SB, Huyett P, et al. Evidence for distinct histologic profile of nasal polyps with and without eosinophilia. Laryngoscope 2011;121(10):2262–7.
57. Steinke JW, Liu L, Huyett P, et al. Prominent role of IFN-gamma in patients with aspirin-exacerbated respiratory disease. J Allergy Clin Immunol 2013;132(4): 856–65.e1-e3.
58. Roca-Ferrer J, Garcia-Garcia FJ, Pereda J, et al. Reduced expression of COXs and production of prostaglandin E(2) in patients with nasal polyps with or without aspirin-intolerant asthma. J Allergy Clin Immunol 2011;128(1):66–72.e1.

59. Perez-Novo CA, Watelet JB, Claeys C, et al. Prostaglandin, leukotriene, and lipoxin balance in chronic rhinosinusitis with and without nasal polyposis. J Allergy Clin Immunol 2005;115(6):1189–96.
60. Kim JE, Kountakis SE. The prevalence of Samter's triad in patients undergoing functional endoscopic sinus surgery. Ear Nose Throat J 2007;86(7):396–9.
61. Batra PS, Kern RC, Tripathi A, et al. Outcome analysis of endoscopic sinus surgery in patients with nasal polyps and asthma. Laryngoscope 2003;113(10): 1703–6.
62. Awad OG, Lee JH, Fasano MB, et al. Sinonasal outcomes after endoscopic sinus surgery in asthmatic patients with nasal polyps: a difference between aspirin-tolerant and aspirin-induced asthma? Laryngoscope 2008;118(7):1282–6.
63. McMains KC, Kountakis SE. Medical and surgical considerations in patients with Samter's triad. Am J Rhinol 2006;20(6):573–6.
64. Berges-Gimeno MP, Simon RA, Stevenson DD. Long-term treatment with aspirin desensitization in asthmatic patients with aspirin-exacerbated respiratory disease. J Allergy Clin Immunol 2003;111(1):180–6.
65. Stevenson DD, Hankammer MA, Mathison DA, et al. Aspirin desensitization treatment of aspirin-sensitive patients with rhinosinusitis-asthma: long-term outcomes. J Allergy Clin Immunol 1996;98(4):751–8.
66. Klimek L, Pfaar O. Aspirin intolerance: does desensitization alter the course of the disease? Immunol Allergy Clin North Am 2009;29(4):669–75.
67. Bhattacharyya N. Clinical and symptom criteria for the accurate diagnosis of chronic rhinosinusitis. Laryngoscope 2006;116(7 Pt 2 Suppl 110):1–22.
68. Arango P, Kountakis SE. Significance of computed tomography pathology in chronic rhinosinusitis. Laryngoscope 2001;111(10):1779–82.
69. Younis RT, Anand VK, Davidson B. The role of computed tomography and magnetic resonance imaging in patients with sinusitis with complications. Laryngoscope 2002;112(2):224–9.
70. Stankiewicz JA, Chow JM. Nasal endoscopy and the definition and diagnosis of chronic rhinosinusitis. Otolaryngol Head Neck Surg 2002;126(6):623–7.
71. Konstantinidis I, Witt M, Kaidoglou K, et al. Olfactory mucosa in nasal polyposis: implications for FESS outcome. Rhinology 2010;48(1):47–53.
72. Downey LL, Jacobs JB, Lebowitz RA. Anosmia and chronic sinus disease. Otolaryngol Head Neck Surg 1996;115(1):24–8.
73. Meltzer EO, Hamilos DL, Hadley JA, et al. Rhinosinusitis: developing guidance for clinical trials. J Allergy Clin Immunol 2006;118(Suppl 5):S17–61.
74. Mafee MF, Tran BH, Chapa AR. Imaging of rhinosinusitis and its complications: plain film, CT, and MRI. Clin Rev Allergy Immunol 2006;30(3):165–86.
75. Kenny TJ, Duncavage J, Bracikowski J, et al. Prospective analysis of sinus symptoms and correlation with paranasal computed tomography scan. Otolaryngol Head Neck Surg 2001;125(1):40–3.
76. Fokkens W, Lund V, Mullol J. European position paper on rhinosinusitis and nasal polyps 2007. Rhinol Suppl 2007;(20):1–136.
77. Joe SA, Thambi R, Huang J. A systematic review of the use of intranasal steroids in the treatment of chronic rhinosinusitis. Otolaryngol Head Neck Surg 2008; 139(3):340–7.
78. Wei CC, Adappa ND, Cohen NA. Use of topical nasal therapies in the management of chronic rhinosinusitis. Laryngoscope 2013;123(10):2347–59.
79. Rudmik L, Hoy M, Schlosser RJ, et al. Topical therapies in the management of chronic rhinosinusitis: an evidence-based review with recommendations. Int Forum Allergy Rhinol 2013;3(4):281–98.

80. Kalish L, Snidvongs K, Sivasubramaniam R, et al. Topical steroids for nasal polyps. Cochrane Database Syst Rev 2012;(12):CD006549.
81. Lohia S, Schlosser RJ, Soler ZM. Impact of intranasal corticosteroids on asthma outcomes in allergic rhinitis: a meta-analysis. Allergy 2013;68(5):569–79.
82. Meltzer EO, Hamilos DL. Rhinosinusitis diagnosis and management for the clinician: a synopsis of recent consensus guidelines. Mayo Clin Proc 2011;86(5): 427–43.
83. Hissaria P, Smith W, Wormald PJ, et al. Short course of systemic corticosteroids in sinonasal polyposis: a double-blind, randomized, placebo-controlled trial with evaluation of outcome measures. J Allergy Clin Immunol 2006;118(1):128–33.
84. Aukema AA, Mulder PG, Fokkens WJ. Treatment of nasal polyposis and chronic rhinosinusitis with fluticasone propionate nasal drops reduces need for sinus surgery. J Allergy Clin Immunol 2005;115(5):1017–23.
85. Benitez P, Alobid I, de Haro J, et al. A short course of oral prednisone followed by intranasal budesonide is an effective treatment of severe nasal polyps. Laryngoscope 2006;116(5):770–5.
86. Jang DW, Lachanas VA, Segel J, et al. Budesonide nasal irrigations in the postoperative management of chronic rhinosinusitis. Int Forum Allergy Rhinol 2013; 3(9):708–11.
87. Clayman GL, Adams GL, Paugh DR, et al. Intracranial complications of paranasal sinusitis: a combined institutional review. Laryngoscope 1991;101(3):234–9.
88. Hytonen M, Atula T, Pitkaranta A. Complications of acute sinusitis in children. Acta Otolaryngol Suppl 2000;543:154–7.
89. Soler ZM, Oyer SL, Kern RC, et al. Antimicrobials and chronic rhinosinusitis with or without polyposis in adults: an evidenced-based review with recommendations. Int Forum Allergy Rhinol 2013;3(1):31–47.
90. Steinke JW, Bradley D, Arango P, et al. Cysteinyl leukotriene expression in chronic hyperplastic sinusitis-nasal polyposis: importance to eosinophilia and asthma. J Allergy Clin Immunol 2003;111(2):342–9.
91. Borish L. The role of leukotrienes in upper and lower airway inflammation and the implications for treatment. Ann Allergy Asthma Immunol 2002;88(4 Suppl 1): 16–22.
92. Vashishta R, Soler ZM, Nguyen SA, et al. A systematic review and meta-analysis of asthma outcomes following endoscopic sinus surgery for chronic rhinosinusitis. Int Forum Allergy Rhinol 2013;3(10):788–94.
93. Chen FH, Zuo KJ, Guo YB, et al. Long-term results of endoscopic sinus surgery-oriented treatment for chronic rhinosinusitis with asthma. Laryngoscope 2014; 124(1):24–8.
94. Tajiri T, Matsumoto H, Hiraumi H, et al. Efficacy of omalizumab in eosinophilic chronic rhinosinusitis patients with asthma. Ann Allergy Asthma Immunol 2013; 110(5):387–8.
95. Gevaert P, Calus L, Van Zele T, et al. Omalizumab is effective in allergic and nonallergic patients with nasal polyps and asthma. J Allergy Clin Immunol 2013;131(1):110–6.e1.
96. Gevaert P, Van Bruaene N, Cattaert T, et al. Mepolizumab, a humanized anti-IL-5 mAb, as a treatment option for severe nasal polyposis. J Allergy Clin Immunol 2011;128(5):989–95.e1-e8.
97. Pauwels B, Jonstam K, Bachert C. Emerging biologics for the treatment of chronic rhinosinusitis. Expert Rev Clin Immunol 2015;11(3):349–61.

Asthma–Chronic Obstructive Pulmonary Disease Overlap Syndrome
Nothing New Under the Sun

Nirupama Putcha, MD, MHS*, Robert A. Wise, MD

KEYWORDS

- Asthma • COPD • Overlap • Subtypes • ACOS

KEY POINTS

- It is increasingly recognized that there is a group of individuals having characteristics of both chronic obstructive pulmonary disease (COPD) and asthma.
- This group is thought to have characteristics of both diseases and might be at higher risk for respiratory events, exacerbations, and heightened symptoms.
- Understanding this subgroup is important in understanding the mechanisms for adverse outcomes and determining if specialized treatments have utility.
- Patients with asthma–COPD overlap syndrome include patients with COPD and eosinophilia, smoking asthmatics, long-standing asthmatics with airway remodeling, and steroid-resistant asthmatics with neutrophilic inflammation.

INTRODUCTION

The debate about the relationship between asthma and chronic obstructive pulmonary disease (COPD) on the spectrum of obstructive lung disease is far from new. The earliest and most famous example of such a debate can be found in the juxtaposition of the "Dutch" and the "British" hypotheses. Orie and colleagues from the Netherlands first described their hypothesis in 1961 that one disease termed "Chronic Nonspecific Lung Disease (CNSLD)" existed, which described all individuals with asthma, chronic bronchitis, and emphysema. They hypothesized that all of these individuals had shared endogenous and exogenous factors (now called gene–environment interaction) that contributed to the development of the disease. Host factors included allergic disease and bronchial hyperresponsiveness, and environmental factors included

Division of Pulmonary and Critical Care Medicine, Johns Hopkins University School of Medicine, 5501 Hopkins Bayview Circle, JHAAC 4B.74, Baltimore, MD 21224, USA
* Corresponding author.
E-mail address: Nputcha1@jhmi.edu

Immunol Allergy Clin N Am 36 (2016) 515–528
http://dx.doi.org/10.1016/j.iac.2016.03.003   immunology.theclinics.com
0889-8561/16/$ – see front matter © 2016 Elsevier Inc. All rights reserved.

cigarette smoke and pollution.[1,2] Conflicting with this position was the "British" hypothesis, which distinguished a syndrome of chronic, irreversible airflow obstruction resulting from, most notably, exposure to smoking in susceptible individuals.[3] This was thought to be separate from asthma, which was related to allergic disease and airways hyperreactivity. Patients with chronic airflow obstruction were considered to differ from those with asthma based on clinical course and pathogenesis.

Studies such as those reported by Burrows and colleagues[4] in 1987, which demonstrated in a large, longitudinal epidemiologic study that nonsmoking individuals with a more asthmatic, atopic phenotype had significantly less decline in forced expiratory volume in 1 second (FEV_1) over time as well as much lower mortality rate than the group of nonatopic former and current smokers, seemed to lend substantial weight to the British hypothesis of 2 distinct clinical syndromes. Beyond outcome measures, other important evidence pointing to 2 distinct clinical syndromes drew from work that describes asthma and COPD as having distinct physiologic, inflammatory, and radiologic patterns. Asthma has been described to involve more eosinophilic inflammation[5] as opposed to the neutrophilic inflammation thought to be more dominant in individuals with COPD. Fabbri and colleagues[5] also showed that, in individuals with a history of asthma with a similar degree of fixed airflow obstruction and airway hyperreactivity as a group of individuals with COPD, those with asthma had less emphysema on computed tomography scans, lower residual volume, and higher diffusing capacity on pulmonary function testing. Patients with a history of asthma also showed more eosinophilic inflammation in blood, sputum, airway histology, and higher levels of expired nitric oxide. With regard to describing a distinct COPD diagnosis, in an early paper on the subject, Vermeire and Pride[6] proposed a COPD phenotype comprising individuals with airflow obstruction, bronchial hypersecretion, and alveolar destruction. In contrast with asthma patients, this group of patients with smoking-related airflow obstruction has neutrophil-predominant airways inflammation.[7]

Research endeavors, drug development, and clinical guidelines about COPD and asthma in the past few decades have focused on the diseases as distinct entities. However, it has always been recognized by clinicians, as evidenced by the Dutch versus British hypothesis debate, that the distinctions between COPD and asthma are less clear, with a spectrum of disease. In recent years, there has been a resurgence of thought about the presence of a significant group of individuals that have attributes of both asthma and COPD, recently termed the asthma–COPD overlap syndrome (ACOS). Understanding this historical context of the Dutch versus British debate is a reminder that the idea of asthma and COPD as potentially overlapping entities is not an entirely novel perspective, but also highlights the importance of this topic given its implications for our understanding of obstructive airways disease and treatment strategies. The resurgent interest in ACOS has been kindled by the recognition by both the Global Initiative for Asthma (GINA; in asthma) and Global Initiative of Chronic Obstructive Lung Disease (GOLD; in COPD) expert panels that many patients were not adequately addressed by either group, and the acronym ACOS was put forth.

PREVALENCE AND EPIDEMIOLOGY OF ASTHMA–CHRONIC OBSTRUCTIVE PULMONARY DISEASE OVERLAP SYNDROME

Recent studies have focused on understanding the scope, characteristics and epidemiology of individuals with ACOS.[8] The estimated prevalence of the syndrome seems to vary based on the population studied and the definitions used to describe the syndrome, but has been estimated between 13% and 38% of the population with obstructive lung disease.[9–21] Most estimates of prevalence of ACOS among a population of individuals with asthma seems to be slightly higher, with estimates ranging from 27.1% to 38%,[13,16,18] whereas estimates of ACOS within a population of individuals with COPD seem to be slightly lower, ranging mostly from 13% to 28.6%.[9–11,14,17,19–21] Other than the differences in population characteristics, which may account for the variation in prevalence estimates, the definitions used to identify individuals with ACOS also differ greatly. Several studies, particularly those in which the population studied is primarily composed of individuals with COPD, have defined ACOS as an individual with a spirometric diagnosis of COPD, most commonly using the GOLD criteria,[22] American Thoracic Society/European Respiratory Society criteria,[23] or some slight variation of these criteria, and also reporting a diagnosis of asthma earlier in life, such as before the age of 40.[9,14,20] Others use functional characteristics such as bronchial hyperresponsiveness or bronchodilator reversibility in their diagnostic criteria,[11,18,19,21,24] and still others use formal criteria for asthma (eg, Global Initiative for Asthma [GINA][25] or British Asthma guidelines) and COPD (eg, American Thoracic Society/European Respiratory Society[23] or GOLD criteria[22]) and define overlap as meeting both sets of criteria.[15,17,21]

Regardless of the heterogeneity of the populations studied and the inconsistencies of the definitions of ACOS applied, the group having ACOS seem to have differing characteristics from populations having COPD or asthma alone. For the most part, individuals with ACOS are younger[14,15] and have less cumulative smoking burden[9,14,15,20] than individuals with COPD alone. Additionally, the group with ACOS have a higher body mass index[14,20] than counterparts with COPD or asthma alone. Inconsistent findings were a higher prevalence of women[9,14,17] and better lung function (as measured by FEV_1)[9,15] in the ACOS group than in those with COPD alone.

Most studies show that individuals with ACOS have worse clinical outcomes than individuals with COPD alone or asthma alone. Compared with individuals with COPD alone, those with COPD and asthma have a greater risk of exacerbations, respiratory adverse events, and hospitalizations.[9,10,14,17,19,20,26] These patients have more dyspnea,[20] respiratory symptoms,[20,26] physical impairment,[26] worse quality of life,[14,15,19,20] and poorer disease control[19,21] compared with those with COPD or asthma alone.

Paradoxically, several studies have demonstrated that, despite having more exacerbations and respiratory symptoms, the ACOS group has less disease severity than the group with COPD alone. One study of a large Spanish COPD cohort showed that individuals with ACOS had lower 1-year mortality than those with COPD alone.[11] Findings on lung function have been less consistent, with some observing that the group with ACOS have better lung function[9,15] and slower decline in lung function[12] than the group with COPD alone, whereas others observed that lung function was lower[17,20] in the group with ACOS. In addition to lower mortality and slower lung function decline, Fu and colleagues[24] found that the group with ACOS had slower age-related decline in exercise capacity assessed by the 6-minute walk test than the group with COPD alone.

Despite the inconsistent findings about differences in severity of disease, there is a consistent message from the many studies performed on this subject that the group with ACOS seems to have different characteristics than those with COPD alone. For example, Hardin and colleagues[14] found in the large COPDGene study that the group with ACOS had less emphysema but more airways wall thickness on computed tomography scans. The finding of higher wall thickness was later also demonstrated by Suzuki and colleagues[21] when studying a smaller clinical cohort.

CONSENSUS STATEMENTS

Ultimately, because of the recent interest in characterizing the group with asthma and COPD overlap in the setting of many different working definitions, there have been 2 recent consensus statements that aimed to better define the ACOS group.

Spanish Statement

The first of these statements to be published was a consensus statement of Spanish Pulmonologists.[27] After performing a literature review, this group of experts used a step-wise approach to reach consensus about the following topics: (1) determining a name for the syndrome, (2) agreeing on major and minor criteria for diagnosis, (3) suggesting treatment strategies, and (4) addressing gaps in understanding for future research attention. The group agreed that there was a subtype of COPD that included patients having both COPD and asthma-type characteristics, and they chose to describe this subtype as the "mixed COPD–asthma phenotype." Then, among several proposed criteria, they agreed on 3 major and 3 minor criteria for identifying an individual with this subtype of disease (**Table 1**), agreeing that 2 major criteria or 1 major and 2 minor criteria would need to be present for an individual to qualify as having this disease subtype. These criteria include lung function measures and historical elements as well as laboratory testing. Other criteria that were considered but did not gain enough consensus among the experts to be included were peripheral eosinophilia, symptom variability, positive skin prick testing, increased exhaled nitric oxide, positive methacholine testing, peak flow variability, family history of asthma or atopy, rhinitis, bronchodilator reversibility, and a positive oral corticosteroid test.

This statement also addressed treatment considerations and future research targets. Notably, 100% of the experts agreed that individuals classified as mixed COPD–asthma phenotype should have early use of inhaled corticosteroids (ICS), citing positive drug trials of ICS in individuals with COPD as well as eosinophilic airways inflammation measured by sputum eosinophilia.[28,29] A majority of the group also agreed that ICS should be used as part of a "triple therapy" strategy (ICS, long-acting beta-agonist and long-acting anticholinergic agents) in the most severe cases of asthma–COPD overlap, titrating the ICS component to symptom burden as is done with asthma, paying careful attention to the high risks associated with withdrawing the ICS component leading to higher exacerbation risk.[27]

Table 1
Major and minor criteria for "mixed chronic obstructive pulmonary disease/asthma phenotype"

Major Criteria	Minor Criteria
Positive bronchodilator testing (FEV$_1$ increases by ≥15% and ≥400 mL)	Elevated total IgE level
Sputum eosinophilia	Personal history of atopy
Personal history of asthma (diagnosed before the age of 40)	Positive bronchodilator testing (FEV$_1$ increases by ≥12% and ≥200 mL) on ≥2 occasions

To be considered as having this phenotype, the authors suggest 2 major criteria are met. Alternatively, 1 major and 2 minor criteria can be met as well.

Abbreviations: FEV$_1$, forced expiratory volume in 1 second; IgE, immunoglobulin E.

Adapted from Soler-Cataluna JJ, Cosio B, Izquierdo JL, et al. Consensus document on the overlap phenotype COPD-asthma in COPD. Arch Bronconeumol 2012;48:331–7.

Combined Global Initiative for Asthma/Global Initiative of Chronic Obstructive Lung Disease Statement

The other consensus document published was the combined GINA/GOLD statement,[30] first published in 2014 and updated recently. This statement, acknowledging the difficulty of defining ACOS with the limited available research to date, was less precise about defining the syndrome, but has clearly outlined the methodology of characterizing ACOS clinically and considerations for initiation of therapy. This group defines ACOS as "characterized by persistent airflow limitation with several features usually associated with asthma and several features usually associated with COPD." Further, 5 important steps are outlined to aid in assessing individuals with respiratory symptoms to better characterize them as having asthma, COPD, or ACOS. The first step includes taking a thorough history and examination to determine if the patient has chronic airways disease. Next, it is suggested that the provider review a list of characteristics more typical of asthma or COPD, and count the number of these characteristics that the patient exhibits (**Table 2**). If the preponderance of characteristics points to asthma or COPD, then a diagnosis of one or the other is made; otherwise, a diagnosis of ACOS is considered. The characteristics include age of onset of disease, variability vs persistence of symptoms, spirometric characteristics, medical history, family and past exposure history, progression of symptoms over time, and radiographic characteristics. The third step is to perform spirometry, and spirometric characteristics of asthma, COPD, or ACOS are outlined. This information is suggested to be used to revise the diagnosis if needed. In step 4, therapy is commenced based on the diagnosis. If asthma, the GINA guidelines[25] are used, if COPD, the GOLD guidelines are used,[22] and if ACOS, the group advocates starting treatment for asthma, given that ICS is an important aspect of control, and to add long acting bronchodilators if they are not already being used. Finally, in step 5, the document recommends referral for further investigation if there is continued uncertainly, the patient is unresponsive to treatment, if atypical symptoms or signs are present, or if there are further issues with tolerating or prescribing treatment, such as interfering comorbidities or other issues.

PROPOSED PATHWAYS TO ASTHMA CHRONIC OBSTRUCTIVE PULMONARY DISEASE OVERLAP SYNDROME, PRESENTED AS 4 PHENOTYPES

To date, studies have attempted to describe the ACOS subgroup with differing definitions as if it were a single entity. We propose that ACOS, as it is now recognized, comprises several different entities that have different clinical presentations and different pathophysiologic mechanisms. Attempts at reaching consensus have been informative but more work is needed if operational definitions of ACOS can be established and validated. We describe 4 operational definitions of ACOS that correspond to clinically recognizable patterns: (1) the smoker with airflow limitation and an eosinophilic inflammatory pattern, (2) the asthmatic who is resistant to steroid treatment and has a more neutrophilic pattern of inflammation, (3) the elderly asthmatic who has had remodeling of their airways and developed irreversible airflow obstruction, and (4) the childhood asthmatic who takes up smoking and develops irreversible airflow obstruction (**Fig. 1**).

Smokers with Eosinophilic Inflammation

There have been several studies that have attempted to describe the subgroup of individuals with COPD having a higher burden of eosinophilic inflammation. Bafadhel and colleagues[31] investigated biomarkers during COPD exacerbations and detected

Table 2
Characteristics that support a diagnosis of asthma or COPD, grouped by category

	Characteristics Favoring Diagnosis of Asthma	Characteristics Favoring Diagnosis of COPD
Age	Onset <20 y	Onset >40 y
Respiratory symptoms	Variation of symptoms with time	Symptoms persist regardless of treatment
	Worsening of symptoms at night or in morning	Usually have daily symptoms and dyspnea with good and bad days
	Triggers for symptoms noted including exercise, emotion, dust or allergen exposure	Chronic bronchitis symptoms precede onset of dyspnea and not necessarily related to triggers
Lung function	Variability in airflow obstruction using peak flows or spirometry	Airflow obstruction often persistent or fixed
Lung function between symptoms	Lung function normal between symptoms	Lung function abnormal between symptoms
History	Previously diagnosed by doctor with asthma	Previously diagnosed by doctor with COPD, emphysema, chronic bronchitis
	Family history of asthma, allergic disease	Heavy exposure history common: tobacco smoke, biomass fuels
Time course	Symptoms do not worsen over time, but vary seasonally or from year to year	Symptoms progress slowly over time
	Can improve quickly and respond quickly to therapies such as ICS or bronchodilators	Symptoms often have limited response to short acting inhalers
Imaging	Chest radiograph usually normal	Chest radiograph reveals severe hyperinflation

The Global Initiative for Asthma/Global Initiative of Chronic Obstructive Lung Disease statement notes that if ≥3 characteristics are present for one either asthma or COPD, it is suggested that the patient likely has that disease; however, if there are a similar number of boxes checked for both, then a diagnosis of asthma–COPD overlap syndrome is considered.

Abbreviations: COPD, chronic obstructive pulmonary disease; ICS, inhaled corticosteroids.

Adapted from Global Initiative of Chronic Obstructive Lung Disease (GOLD). Diagnosis of diseases of chronic airflow limitation: asthma, COPD, and asthma-COPD overlap syndrome (ACOS). 2015.

3 clusters or phenotypes of exacerbations including exacerbations driven by bacteria, viruses, and eosinophilic airway inflammation (as detected by sputum and serum eosinophil counts). They found that 28% of exacerbations in their series were attributed to eosinophilic inflammation. In addition, around 37.4% of the ECLIPSE cohort was shown to have persistent blood and sputum eosinophilia (defined as ≥2%). This subgroup was shown to have better lung function, fewer symptoms (lower St George's Respiratory Questionnaire score and Modified Medical Research Council scores) and less progression of emphysema than the group with persistently low eosinophil counts.[32] Both of these studies are highly suggestive of a subgroup of individuals with COPD having a higher burden of eosinophilic inflammation, but also that this subgroup likely has a different pattern of disease progression and severity.

There have been other attempts to distinguish a subgroup of COPD with eosinophilic inflammation, particularly with regard to understanding whether this group has enhanced response to inhaled or oral corticosteroid treatment. Brightling and

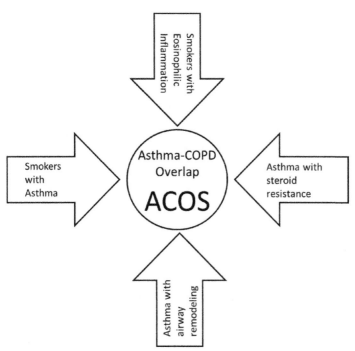

Fig. 1. Four distinct pathways to asthma–chronic obstructive pulmonary disease (COPD) overlap syndrome. ACOS, asthma–chronic obstructive pulmonary disease overlap syndrome.

colleagues[33] showed that individuals with more baseline sputum eosinophilia, treated with systemic corticosteroids, showed a greater increase in FEV_1 and improvement in respiratory symptoms than those with little or no eosinophilia before treatment. Similar findings were noted for outcomes of dyspnea, quality of life, and lung function in a small study of patients with severe COPD and bronchitis, of whom 40% had sputum eosinophilia before treatment.[34] A few studies have shown that ICS have more benefit for improvement in lung function and respiratory symptoms in individuals with more sputum eosinophilia than those without.[29,35] Going further, Siva and colleagues[28] tested the value of targeting eosinophilia with treatment strategies by randomizing patients to standard treatment versus standard treatment with the additional aim of reducing sputum eosinophilia. They found a modest reduction in the number of severe exacerbations experienced in the group where eosinophilia was targeted with the use of corticosteroids.

Further support for this phenotype of individuals can be found in the recent work of Christenson and colleagues,[36] who studied airway epithelial gene expressions in asthma and COPD. They found overlap in around 100 genes altered in the airway epithelium in asthma with those upregulated in COPD, noting that the gene expression changes present in this overlap were found in large and small airways. Additionally, they went on to develop at 100-gene signature of gene expression related to T helper (Th)2-related inflammation, termed the T2S score. They showed that this specific Th2 signature was upregulated in a subgroup of COPD having eosinophilic inflammation (airways and systemic eosinophilia), as well as clinical characteristics thought to be associated with ACOS including bronchial hyperresponsiveness and treatment response to ICS.

Related to this phenotype, there have been several studies that have attempted to understand the prevalence of atopy among those with COPD and how this relates to outcomes. Jamieson and colleagues[37] found the prevalence of atopy was around 30% (measured by sensitization to a panel of common indoor and outdoor allergens) in individuals with COPD, and noted that these people had a higher risk for respiratory symptoms, exacerbations, and adverse outcomes. Within the European Respiratory Society Study on Chronic Obstructive Pulmonary Disease (EUROSCOP) study, Fattahi and colleagues[38] showed a prevalence of 18.3% of atopy in those with COPD, and noted a higher risk for respiratory symptoms in this group. They went further to show that ICS was more effective to reduce symptoms in atopic COPD patients than those without atopy, echoing the results described above for individuals with COPD and sputum and serum eosinophilia, suggesting a common Th2, allergy-mediated pathway for this group of patients.

Resistant Asthmatic

Another subgroup of patients that has been described is a group of asthmatics who clinically seem very resistant to treatment with steroids and often have irreversible airflow obstruction. These individuals often have elements of both asthma and COPD. Additionally, it is thought that asthmatics resistant to steroids have more neutrophil-predominant airway inflammation, which, as noted, is traditionally thought to be the predominant type of inflammation found in individuals with COPD.[7,39]

Periostin, a marker of severe steroid-resistant asthma and CD8-driven eosinophilic inflammation, has been associated with airway remodeling and a greater decline in lung function in patients with asthma.[40]

Interestingly, there have been at least a few studies that have suggested that latent infection in asthmatics is associated with the phenotype of steroid resistance. Green and colleagues[41] used non–culture-based techniques to detect colonization with Streptococcus, Moraxella, or Haemophilus species in the sputum of more than 60% of resistant asthmatics in a small cohort. They went on to show that these individuals had more sputum neutrophils than those without colonization. Others have demonstrated supportive findings using mouse models of allergic airways disease and Haemophilus infection.[42] It has also been suggested that latent adenoviral infection is associated with heightened cigarette smoke–induced inflammation and a pattern of steroid resistance in asthma.[43] Additionally, some animal models of latent adenovirus infection have shown more rapid progression of emphysema in the setting of cigarette smoke exposure.[44] The mechanism for the link between indolent infection and steroid resistant asthma is the activation of the innate immune system through latent bacterial or viral infections, which lead to neutrophilic inflammation that is less responsive to steroid therapy.[43]

Elderly Asthmatic with Irreversible Airflow Obstruction

Older asthmatics, particularly those with long-standing asthma, do demonstrate irreversible airflow obstruction and a shift to more neutrophilic inflammation.[45] One of the earliest documented references to this group of asthmatics with only partial reversibility of airflow obstruction is found in the work of Woolcock and Read[46] from 1968. In this work, pressure–volume curves of the lungs were estimated during an acute exacerbation and then after resolution for 10 patients with asthma from differing age categories, the youngest being 9 years old and the oldest 52. The authors found that, in one-half of the sample, the pressure–volume curves did not normalize after exacerbations and were indicative of loss of elastic recoil and hyperinflation of the lungs, consistent with possible emphysema.[46] McCarthy and colleagues[47] noted similarly when studying a cohort of 16 stable asthmatics that nearly one-half had findings indicative of loss of lung elastic recoil concerning for early emphysema. Another study of 18 adults with chronic persistent asthma documented loss of lung elastic recoil in a majority of these participants, which seemed to be more pronounced in the older participants compared with younger.[48] In a separate study, this group went on to study adult asthmatics based on the severity of asthma and noted that loss of lung elastic recoil was present in all participants with moderate persistent and severe persistent asthma, but less prevalent in the group with mild persistent asthma, suggesting that not only is duration, but also severity of illness is a factor in the long-term impacts on lung structure and function.[49] One large longitudinal study in Europe followed individuals aged 20 to 44 years for 9 years, and attempted to characterize a group of individuals with airflow obstruction as asthma, COPD, or ACOS. Clinically, they noted a similar profile of symptoms and history of those with asthma and those with ACOS, having similar prevalence of allergic disease, eczema, and airway hyperresponsiveness. They found that those individuals with ACOS had more decline in lung function over time than those with asthma alone but less than those with COPD alone. They went on to note that those with ACOS had earlier onset, longer duration of asthma with more exposure history to cigarettes, thus leading them to the conclusion that likely those individuals with ACOS may largely constitute a group with longstanding poorly controlled asthma that have "progressed to fixed airflow obstruction,"[12] and may constitute one of the subtypes of working definitions of ACOS.

Childhood Asthmatic Who Smokes and Develops Chronic Obstructive Pulmonary Disease

The final proposed subtype includes individuals who have asthma from childhood or early adulthood, then later develop fixed airflow obstruction and COPD-type features owing to long-term primary smoking exposure. In 1 study of a Finnish primary care cohort, among 190 current and former smokers with a history of asthma but without a previous diagnosis of COPD, 27.4% had fixed airflow obstruction, consistent with a possible ACOS picture. Age greater than 60 years and higher burden of smoking history (>20 pack-years) were associated with being part of the overlap group in this study.[16] A similar study of 256 Korean patients with asthma (defined by bronchodilator reversibility or positive methacholine challenge) found that 38% had incompletely reversible airflow obstruction on 2 separate occasions at least 3 months apart. This group was noted to be older, higher proportion male, and have more current and former smokers than the group with asthma alone. Interestingly, the overlap group in this study had lower peripheral eosinophil count but a higher total immunoglobulin E level.[18]

This subtype is not only described in the context of studies of adult asthmatics, but is also captured in studies of adults with a primary diagnosis of COPD who self-report a diagnosis of asthma from childhood or early adulthood. In the COPDGene study, Hardin and colleagues[14] defined ACOS as a report of doctor diagnosis of asthma before the age 40. Studies that describe ACOS in the framework of populations with asthma show the ACOS group to be older, with a higher proportion of males and a higher burden of smoke exposure than the group with asthma alone. In contrast, ACOS patients derived from a group of COPD patients as described by Hardin and associates[14] tend to be younger, with a higher proportion of females, and a significantly lower burden of smoking history than those with COPD alone. The ACOS group was also noted to have less emphysema and significantly higher FEV_1/forced vital capacity ratio than the group with COPD alone, despite having more respiratory symptoms and exacerbation events. Taking this and other similar studies into account, it seems that the smoking asthmatic ACOS group is a hybrid of both asthma and

COPD with clinical features and inflammatory pathways of both diseases. These patients seem to have a much higher burden of respiratory symptoms and health care use than the group with either disease alone.

OTHER CONSIDERATIONS
Genetic Overlap

Another topic that has been studied with regard to asthma and COPD overlap is understanding shared genetic loci of both diseases to help better elucidate the overlap phenotype. Hardin and colleagues[14] performed an adjusted genome-wide analysis comparing ACOS cases with COPD controls in non-Hispanic whites and African Americans. They found that no single nucleotide polymorphisms reached the predetermined significance threshold but there were several loci that were close, including the CSMD1 gene on chromosome 8 and a variant on the SOX5 gene on chromosome 12, both among non-Hispanic whites. Although they tested several known asthma and COPD single nucleotide polymorphisms for associations with overlap syndrome, no single nucleotide polymorphisms that were significant in their associations after applying multiple testing thresholds. The CSMD1 gene was found to be associated with emphysema findings radiographically, whereas the SOX5 gene has thought to be involved in lung development. It was postulated from the associations with SOX5 in ACOS that participants with ACOS might have started with asthma and then developed fixed airways obstruction owing to abnormalities in lung development.[14] Related to this, Christenson and colleagues[36] studied airway epithelial gene expression in asthma and COPD and found around 100 common genes that are upregulated in both asthma and COPD. They additionally noted a specific gene expression signature in a subgroup of individuals with COPD having eosinophilic inflammation, thought to have a clinical picture consistent with ACOS. These individuals interestingly had higher treatment response to ICS. Smolonska and colleagues[50] conducted a genome-wide association study for both asthma and COPD that suggested the common presence of 2 single nucleotide polymorphisms in genes DDX1 and COMMD10 that both participate in the nuclear factor-$\kappa\beta$ inflammatory pathway, but the findings could not be replicated in other cohorts.

Therapeutic Options and Targets

As noted, there have been several studies that have attempted to understand whether the ACOS group is more responsive to corticosteroids, either inhaled or systemic. These studies have mostly targeted individuals with COPD having serum or sputum eosinophilia.[28,33–35] For the most part, it has been strongly suggested that individuals with ACOS, particularly those in the category of COPD with eosinophilic inflammation, have an accentuated treatment response to ICS compared with COPD in general.[29,35] For this reason, the GINA/GOLD combined statement on ACOS has suggested considering ICS therapy early in the group with ACOS,[30] although stronger evidence based on randomized clinical trials is still needed.

Given the studies that have shown a higher degree of eosinophilia and allergic, Th2-type inflammation in individuals with ACOS compared with those with COPD alone,[31,32] there has also been some interest in whether this subgroup of individuals would be responsive to monoclonal antibody therapy such as mepolizumab or benralizumab. Brightling and colleagues[51] recently reported the results of a phase IIa trial of benralizumab versus placebo therapy in individuals with moderate to severe COPD with history of exacerbation having sputum eosinophil count of 3% or higher. Benralizumab is an anti–interlekin-5 receptor alpha antibody, which has previously been shown to reduce sputum eosinophils in asthmatics.[52] The authors found that although overall exacerbation rate was not different between the placebo and treatment group, subgroup analyses among individuals with serum eosinophils higher than 200 or 300 cells per microliter showed a numerical but not statistically significant decrease in exacerbations, lung function (FEV_1), and disease status in the treatment group compared with placebo.[51] Mepolizumab, an anti–interlekin-5 monoclonal antibody, has been studied in severe eosinophilic asthma and found to reduce exacerbations and improve asthma control.[53] This drug has also been considered for the treatment of COPD and is currently under investigation in individuals with COPD having peripheral blood eosinophilia and eosinophilic bronchitis (NCT02105961, NCT01463644). Omalizumab, a monoclonal anti–immunoglobulin E therapy shown to improve outcomes in severe allergic asthma,[54] has not yet been studied in individuals with COPD having increased immunoglobulin E and allergic features; however, as more becomes known about ACOS and the phenotypes of individuals included in this group, it is possible this therapy could also be studied in this context.

Asthmatics who smoke, or who have a substantial smoking history, are typically excluded from studies of asthma. Thus, there is a paucity of data on this ACOS subgroup. However, 1 well-designed trial of 39 smoking asthmatics suggested that they had a blunted response to corticosteroids, but a better response to the leukotriene modifier montelukast than nonsmoking asthmatics.[55] Thus, this ACOS subgroup may have a different therapeutic response than those with COPD and eosinophilia. It has been suggested that the steroid resistance in smokers with asthma and COPD is the consequence of impaired histone deacetylase activity, which can be restored by low-dose theophylline.[56] Accordingly, pending evidence from trials in this subgroup, theophylline may be a useful adjunct to ICS.

FUTURE CONSIDERATIONS/SUMMARY

The concept of asthma and COPD belonging to a single continuum of airways disease is far from new; however, the debate over this subject has evolved over the past decades. In the past several years, there is an emerging base of literature that has strongly suggested that a group of individuals exists with a clinical syndrome intermediate between asthma and COPD, and that such individuals have features of both diseases. Importantly, this group seems in some studies to have worse symptom outcomes as well as a higher risk for respiratory events and exacerbations. There have been attempts to better characterize this population with regards to biomarkers, genetic signature, and clinical as well as phenotypes on computed tomography scans with the ultimate goal of being able to better prescribe and tailor therapy to this group; however, the evidence is still emerging to better reach these goals. Based on the available evidence, however, we do not think that ACOS can be defined as a single entity, but rather a cluster of different subtypes that likely have different mechanisms of disease and require somewhat different approaches to treatment. We have outlined 4 proposed subgroups of patients who can be considered for inclusion in the ACOS. These subgroups seem to have distinct natural histories, clinical features, and inflammatory mechanisms. Additionally, we hope that such a characterization will lend itself to a better understanding of possible treatments that can be rigorously tested as subpopulations of the ACOS.

REFERENCES

1. Orie NG, Sluiter HJ, De Vries K, et al. The host factor in bronchitis. In: Orie NGM, Sluiter HJ, editors. Bronchitis. Netherlands: Royal Vangorcum; 1961. p. 43–59.

2. Sluiter HJ, Koeter GH, de Monchy JG, et al. The Dutch hypothesis (chronic non-specific lung disease) revisited. Eur Respir J 1991;4:479–89.
3. Fletcher C, Peto R. The natural history of chronic airflow obstruction. Br Med J 1977;1:1645–8.
4. Burrows B, Bloom JW, Traver GA, et al. The course and prognosis of different forms of chronic airways obstruction in a sample from the general population. N Engl J Med 1987;317:1309–14.
5. Fabbri LM, Romagnoli M, Corbetta L, et al. Differences in airway inflammation in patients with fixed airflow obstruction due to asthma or chronic obstructive pulmonary disease. Am J Respir Crit Care Med 2003;167:418–24.
6. Vermeire PA, Pride NB. A "splitting" look at chronic nonspecific lung disease (CNSLD): common features but diverse pathogenesis. Eur Respir J 1991;4: 490–6.
7. Keatings VM, Barnes PJ. Granulocyte activation markers in induced sputum: comparison between chronic obstructive pulmonary disease, asthma, and normal subjects. Am J Respir Crit Care Med 1997;155:449–53.
8. Alshabanat A, Zafari Z, Albanyan O, et al. Asthma and COPD overlap syndrome (ACOS): a systematic review and meta analysis. PLoS One 2015;10:e0136065.
9. Barrecheguren M, Roman-Rodriguez M, Miravitlles M. Is a previous diagnosis of asthma a reliable criterion for asthma-COPD overlap syndrome in a patient with COPD? Int J Chron Obstruct Pulmon Dis 2015;10:1745–52.
10. Chung WS, Lin CL, Kao CH. Comparison of acute respiratory events between asthma-COPD overlap syndrome and COPD patients: a population-based cohort study. Medicine 2015;94:e755.
11. Cosio BG, Soriano JB, Lopez-Campos JL, et al. Defining the asthma-COPD overlap syndrome in a COPD cohort. Chest 2015;149(1):45–52.
12. de Marco R, Marcon A, Rossi A, et al. Asthma, COPD and overlap syndrome: a longitudinal study in young European adults. Eur Respir J 2015;46(3):671–9.
13. Harada T, Yamasaki A, Fukushima T, et al. Causes of death in patients with asthma and asthma-chronic obstructive pulmonary disease overlap syndrome. Int J Chron Obstruct Pulmon Dis 2015;10:595–602.
14. Hardin M, Cho M, McDonald ML, et al. The clinical and genetic features of COPD-asthma overlap syndrome. Eur Respir J 2014;44:341–50.
15. Kauppi P, Kupiainen H, Lindqvist A, et al. Overlap syndrome of asthma and COPD predicts low quality of life. J Asthma 2011;48:279–85.
16. Kiljander T, Helin T, Venho K, et al. Prevalence of asthma-COPD overlap syndrome among primary care asthmatics with a smoking history: a cross-sectional study. NPJ Prim Care Respir Med 2015;25:15047.
17. Kim MA, Noh CS, Chang YJ, et al. Asthma and COPD overlap syndrome is associated with increased risk of hospitalisation. Int J Tuberc Lung Dis 2015;19:864–9.
18. Lee HY, Kang JY, Yoon HK, et al. Clinical characteristics of asthma combined with COPD feature. Yonsei Med J 2014;55:980–6.
19. Menezes AM, Montes de Oca M, Perez-Padilla R, et al. Increased risk of exacerbation and hospitalization in subjects with an overlap phenotype: COPD-asthma. Chest 2014;145:297–304.
20. Miravitlles M, Soriano JB, Ancochea J, et al. Characterisation of the overlap COPD-asthma phenotype. Focus on physical activity and health status. Respir Med 2013;107:1053–60.
21. Suzuki T, Tada Y, Kawata N, et al. Clinical, physiological, and radiological features of asthma-chronic obstructive pulmonary disease overlap syndrome. Int J Chron Obstruct Pulmon Dis 2015;10:947–54.

22. Global Initiative of Chronic Obstructive Lung Disease (GOLD). Global strategy for diagnosis, management, and prevention of COPD. 2014. Available at: http://www.goldcopd.org/. Accessed October 2, 2015.
23. Qaseem A, Wilt TJ, Weinberger SE, et al. Diagnosis and management of stable chronic obstructive pulmonary disease: a clinical practice guideline update from the American College of Physicians, American College of Chest Physicians, American Thoracic Society, and European Respiratory Society. Ann Intern Med 2011;155:179–91.
24. Fu JJ, Gibson PG, Simpson JL, et al. Longitudinal changes in clinical outcomes in older patients with asthma, COPD and asthma-COPD overlap syndrome. Respiration 2014;87:63–74.
25. From the global strategy for asthma management and prevention; 2015.
26. de Marco R, Pesce G, Marcon A, et al. The coexistence of asthma and chronic obstructive pulmonary disease (COPD): prevalence and risk factors in young, middle-aged and elderly people from the general population. PLoS One 2013; 8:e62985.
27. Soler-Cataluna JJ, Cosio B, Izquierdo JL, et al. Consensus document on the overlap phenotype COPD-asthma in COPD. Arch Bronconeumol 2012;48:331–7.
28. Siva R, Green RH, Brightling CE, et al. Eosinophilic airway inflammation and exacerbations of COPD: a randomised controlled trial. Eur Respir J 2007;29: 906–13.
29. Leigh R, Pizzichini MM, Morris MM, et al. predicting benefit from high-dose inhaled corticosteroid treatment. Eur Respir J 2006;27:964–71.
30. Global Initiative of Chronic Obstructive Lung Disease (GOLD). Diagnosis of diseases of chronic airflow limitation: asthma, COPD, and asthma-COPD overlap syndrome (ACOS). 2015.
31. Bafadhel M, McKenna S, Terry S, et al. Acute exacerbations of chronic obstructive pulmonary disease: identification of biologic clusters and their biomarkers. Am J Respir Crit Care Med 2011;184:662–71.
32. Singh D, Kolsum U, Brightling CE, et al. Eosinophilic inflammation in COPD: prevalence and clinical characteristics. Eur Respir J 2014;44:1697–700.
33. Brightling CE, Monteiro W, Ward R, et al. Sputum eosinophilia and short-term response to prednisolone in chronic obstructive pulmonary disease: a randomised controlled trial. Lancet 2000;356:1480–5.
34. Pizzichini E, Pizzichini MM, Gibson P, et al. Sputum eosinophilia predicts benefit from prednisone in smokers with chronic obstructive bronchitis. Am J Respir Crit Care Med 1998;158:1511–7.
35. Brightling CE, McKenna S, Hargadon B, et al. Sputum eosinophilia and the short term response to inhaled mometasone in chronic obstructive pulmonary disease. Thorax 2005;60:193–8.
36. Christenson SA, Steiling K, van den Berge M, et al. Asthma-COPD overlap. Clinical relevance of genomic signatures of type 2 inflammation in chronic obstructive pulmonary disease. Am J Respir Crit Care Med 2015;191:758–66.
37. Jamieson DB, Matsui EC, Belli A, et al. Effects of allergic phenotype on respiratory symptoms and exacerbations in patients with chronic obstructive pulmonary disease. Am J Respir Crit Care Med 2013;188:187–92.
38. Fattahi F, ten Hacken NH, Lofdahl CG, et al. Atopy is a risk factor for respiratory symptoms in COPD patients: results from the EUROSCOP study. Respir Res 2013;14:10.

39. Tsoumakidou M, Tzanakis N, Kyriakou D, et al. Inflammatory cell profiles and T-lymphocyte subsets in chronic obstructive pulmonary disease and severe persistent asthma. Clin Exp Allergy 2004;34:234–40.
40. Kanemitsu Y, Ito I, Niimi A, et al. Osteopontin and periostin are associated with a 20-year decline of pulmonary function in patients with asthma. Am J Respir Crit Care Med 2014;190:472–4.
41. Green BJ, Wiriyachaiporn S, Grainge C, et al. Potentially pathogenic airway bacteria and neutrophilic inflammation in treatment resistant severe asthma. PLoS One 2014;9:e100645.
42. Essilfie AT, Simpson JL, Dunkley ML, et al. Combined Haemophilus influenzae respiratory infection and allergic airways disease drives chronic infection and features of neutrophilic asthma. Thorax 2012;67:588–99.
43. Hogg JC. Role of latent viral infections in chronic obstructive pulmonary disease and asthma. Am J Respir Crit Care Med 2001;164:S71–5.
44. Vitalis TZ, Kern I, Croome A, et al. The effect of latent adenovirus 5 infection on cigarette smoke-induced lung inflammation. Eur Respir J 1998;11:664–9.
45. Hanania NA, King MJ, Braman SS, et al. Asthma in the elderly: current understanding and future research needs–a report of a National Institute on Aging (NIA) workshop. J Allergy Clin Immunol 2011;128:S4–24.
46. Woolcock AJ, Read J. The static elastic properties of the lungs in asthma. Am Rev Respir Dis 1968;98:788–94.
47. McCarthy DS, Sigurdson M. Lung elastic recoil and reduced airflow in clinically stable asthma. Thorax 1980;35:298–302.
48. Gelb AF, Zamel N. Unsuspected pseudophysiologic emphysema in chronic persistent asthma. Am J Respir Crit Care Med 2000;162:1778–82.
49. Gelb AF, Licuanan J, Shinar CM, et al. Unsuspected loss of lung elastic recoil in chronic persistent asthma. Chest 2002;121:715–21.
50. Smolonska J, Koppelman GH, Wijmenga C, et al. Common genes underlying asthma and COPD? Genome-wide analysis on the Dutch hypothesis. Eur Respir J 2014;44:860–72.
51. Brightling CE, Bleecker ER, Panettieri RA Jr, et al. Benralizumab for chronic obstructive pulmonary disease and sputum eosinophilia: a randomised, double-blind, placebo-controlled, phase 2a study. Lancet Respir Med 2014;2:891–901.
52. Laviolette M, Gossage DL, Gauvreau G, et al. Effects of benralizumab on airway eosinophils in asthmatic patients with sputum eosinophilia. J Allergy Clin Immunol 2013;132:1086–96.e5.
53. Ortega HG, Liu MC, Pavord ID, et al. Mepolizumab treatment in patients with severe eosinophilic asthma. N Engl J Med 2014;371:1198–207.
54. Busse W, Corren J, Lanier BQ, et al. Omalizumab, anti-IgE recombinant humanized monoclonal antibody, for the treatment of severe allergic asthma. J Allergy Clin Immunol 2001;108:184–90.
55. Lazarus SC, Chinchilli VM, Rollings NJ, et al. Smoking affects response to inhaled corticosteroids or leukotriene receptor antagonists in asthma. Am J Respir Crit Care Med 2007;175:783–90.
56. Barnes PJ. Corticosteroid resistance in patients with asthma and chronic obstructive pulmonary disease. J Allergy Clin Immunol 2013;131:636–45.

Imaging of Asthma

John Caleb Richards, MD*, David Lynch, MD,
Tilman Koelsch, MD, Debra Dyer, MD

KEYWORDS

- Asthma • Radiography • High-resolution computed tomography • Bronchiectasis
- Allergic-bronchopulmonary aspergillosis

KEY POINTS

- Bronchial thickening and hyperinflation are the most common radiographic findings in asthma, although they are nonspecific.
- High-resolution computed tomography (HRCT) findings of asthma include bronchial thickening, air trapping, and bronchial dilation.
- An important role of HRCT performed in the asthmatic patient is to evaluate for complications or mimics.

INTRODUCTION

Asthma is one of the most common diseases of the lung. Asthma manifests with common, although often subjective and nonspecific, imaging features at radiography and HRCT. Perhaps of utmost importance in imaging asthma is identifying complications or mimics. This article reviews the imaging features of asthma as well as common complications and mimics.

CHEST RADIOGRAPHY

Chest radiographic findings in asthmatic patients are not entirely specific but, when present, include bronchial wall thickening and lung hyperinflation. Bronchial wall thickening is most common, identified in 48% and 71% of patients in 2 separate studies, respectively.[1,2] This degree of variability between the 2 studies emphasizes the subjectivity of the finding. The radiographic appearance of bronchial wall thickening manifests as a ring shadows when viewed in profile and tram track shadows when viewed en face (**Fig. 1**A). Other conditions, such as acute bronchitis and chronic bronchitis, may also cause bronchial wall thickening.

Lung hyperinflation is the second most common radiographic abnormality,[3] albeit less reliable. Suggestive imaging features include flattening of the hemidiaphragms, rib splaying, and increased retrosternal clear space (**Fig. 1**B). Although radiographs

Department of Radiology, National Jewish Health, 1400 Jackson Street, Room K012f, Denver, CO 80206-2761, USA
* Corresponding author.
E-mail address: richardsj@njhealth.org

Immunol Allergy Clin N Am 36 (2016) 529–545
http://dx.doi.org/10.1016/j.iac.2016.03.005
0889-8561/16/$ – see front matter © 2016 Elsevier Inc. All rights reserved.

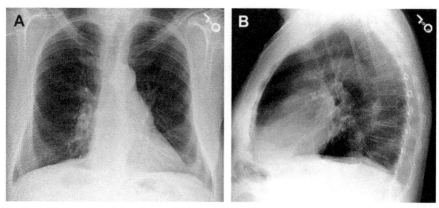

Fig. 1. (*A*) Posteroanterior radiograph in an asthmatic patient showing subtle central airway thickening. (*B*) Lateral radiograph in the same patient showing increased lucency in the retrosternal clear space and flattening of the hemidiaphragms, indicative of hyperinflation.

in asthmatic patients may show lung hyperinflation, with one study identifying this abnormality in 24%,[2] it is rare to see marked hyperinflation in an asthmatic patient who does not also have emphysema. Many patients with asthma have normal or reduced lung volumes even during an acute exacerbation of their condition.[4]

The utility of routine chest radiography in a patient admitted for severe asthma, particularly as it pertains to alteration in management, is an interesting topic. White and colleagues[5] evaluated the impact of admission chest radiography in 54 adult patients with acute asthma, who were refractory in intensive bronchodilator therapy in the emergency ward. They found that major radiographic abnormalities (focal parenchymal opacities, increased interstitial markings, enlarged cardiac silhouette, pulmonary vascular congestion, new pulmonary nodule, and/or pneumothorax) were present in 34% of patients. Instituting antibiotic therapy was more common in patients with focal parenchymal opacities or increased interstitial markings than when these findings were absent. Because of this immediate change in management, the investigators concluded that admission chest radiography is appropriate in asthmatic patients refractory to emergency room therapy.

Tsai and colleagues[6] have suggested guidelines for the selected performance of chest radiographs in patients admitted with acute exacerbations of obstructive airway disease, proposing that patients who are otherwise uncomplicated do not benefit from routine admission chest radiography. According to this proposition, patients with one or more of the following criteria are classified as "complicated" and should receive an admission chest radiograph: a clinical diagnosis of chronic obstructive pulmonary disease (as defined by the American Thoracic Society); a history of fever or temperature more than 37.8°C; clinical or ECG evidence of heart disease; history of intravenous drug abuse; seizures; immunosuppression; evidence of other lung disease; or prior thoracic surgery.[6] In a prospective study, the investigators showed that management was more likely to be changed on the basis of chest radiography in patients who met these criteria.[6] An important potential implication from this study is the reduction in unnecessary admission chest radiographs in uncomplicated patients, which in turn decreases ionizing radiation and health care costs.

Thus, although bronchial wall thickening and lung hyperinflation are the most common radiographic findings in asthmatic patients, they are ultimately nonspecific. Although admission radiographs may alter management in complicated asthma, radiographs in uncomplicated patients are likely unnecessary and may lead to increased health care costs and ionizing radiation. In addition to the aforementioned study by Tsai and colleagues, further studies have shown the utility of the implementation of guidelines and educational programs in reducing unnecessary radiographs.[7,8]

COMPUTED TOMOGRAPHY

HRCT is not recommended in the routine evaluation of suspected asthma without a specific indication based on history, symptoms, and/or results of prior investigations.[9] Chest HRCT, however, can potentially provide value if the presentation is atypical and may help identify complications from asthma or imaging features to suggest an alternative diagnosis or mimic. The most common findings related to asthma at HRCT include bronchial wall thickening, expiratory air trapping, and cylindrical bronchial dilation and have been studied regarding their implications toward severity of clinical disease.

Bronchial wall thickening is the most common finding at HRCT and several studies have shown the degree of bronchial thickening to correlate with disease severity[10–12] (Fig. 2). The variable frequency of identifying this abnormality in previous studies again

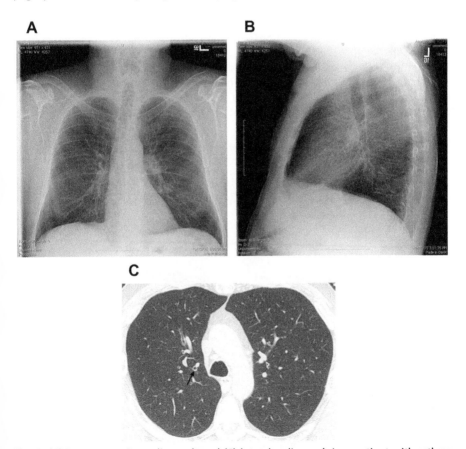

Fig. 2. (A) Posteroanterior radiograph and (B) lateral radiograph in a patient with asthma shows no abnormality. (C) Airway thickening, however, is apparent on the CT in the same patient (arrow).

highlights the subjectivity of this finding. For example, Lynch and colleagues[2] found bronchial wall thickening in 96% of patients in their study of 48 adults with uncomplicated asthma, whereas Paginin and colleagues[1] identified bronchial wall thickening in 16% of 57 adult patients with asthma of varying severity and etiology. A more recent study by Khadadah and colleagues[13] found bronchial thickening in 57% of patients. Additionally, bronchial thickening can be seen in normal patients, as identified in 19% of normal controls in 1 study.[2]

A pivotal goal in caring for patients with asthma and performing longitudinal research is developing noninvasive, reproducible means to measure airway thickening, which would allow providers to identify patients more likely to develop severe disease as well as effectively gauge response to therapy. In a study by Niimi and colleagues,[11] a method of measuring bronchial wall thickening was modified from techniques described in previous studies by McNamara and colleagues.[14,15] In this study, a region of interest was drawn around the outer and inner diameter of the apical bronchus of the right upper lobe to calculate the luminal area and total area of the airway. Wall area (Wa) was calculated by subtracting luminal area from total area and additionally corrected for body surface area (BSA). These 2 indices (Wa and Wa/BSA) were found to correlate with severity and duration of disease and degree of airflow obstruction.[11] Using a similar method of measuring airway wall thickness, Hoshino and colleagues[16] found a correlation of airway wall thickening, particularly in the third-order through fifth-order bronchi, with the degree of airflow limitation.

To further improve objectivity, reproducibility, and efficiency, automated airway segmentation methods have been implemented (**Fig. 3**). Aysola and colleagues[10] used an automated, quantitative software program to measure wall thickness and found that airway walls were thicker in patients with severe asthma than in those

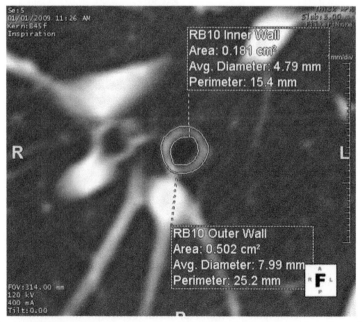

Fig. 3. An example of quantitative assessment of airway thickening, with regions of interest tracing the inner and outer wall.

with mild disease or healthy subjects, which also correlated with pathologic measures of airway remodeling and the degree of airflow obstruction.

Physiologic air trapping is defined as an increase in residual volume or as an increased ratio of residual volume to total lung capacity. Air trapping can be assessed qualitatively using HRCT at end expiration, manifesting as regions of lung with persistent low attenuation (**Fig. 4**). As with bronchial wall thickening, however, quantitative techniques have been developed to more objectively characterize air trapping and have been shown to correlate with abnormalities on pulmonary function tests (PFTs) in asthmatic patients.[17,18] Lee and colleagues,[17] using quantitative CT, showed that the percentage of lungs occupied by low attenuation areas ($\leq$950 Hounsfield units [HUs]) at end-expiratory CT was higher in asthmatic patients and was associated with airflow limitation and hyper-responsiveness.

An interesting study by Busacker and colleagues[19] showed that quantitative CT can determine air trapping in asthmatic subjects and can identify a group of individuals with a high risk of severe disease. Individuals who had greater than 9.66% of lung with less than -850 HUs were defined as having the air-trapping asthma phenotype. Because the specific volume of normal lung at total capacity, 6.0 mL/g, corresponds to a CT attenuation of -856 HUs, this threshold of -850 HUs at end expiration seems reasonable to define persistently inflated lung.[20,21] Statistical analysis showed patients with the air-trapping phenotype were significantly more likely to have a history of asthma-related hospitalizations, intensive care unit visits, and/or mechanical ventilation. History of pneumonia, duration of asthma, high levels of airway neutrophils, airflow obstruction (forced expiratory volume in the first second of expiration [FEV_1]/forced vital capacity), and atopy were identified as independent risk factors associated with the air trapping phenotype.

Bronchial dilation, or bronchiectasis (defined as a bronchus with a diameter larger than the internal diameter of the adjacent pulmonary artery), has been well documented on CT in patients with asthma[2,22,23] (**Fig. 5**). Lynch and colleagues[2] found bronchial dilation involving at least 1 airway in 37 of 48 (77%) subjects with asthma compared with 16 of 27 (59%) control subjects. Park and colleagues[24] reported a lower prevalence of this finding, however, with bronchial dilation present in 31% of asthmatic patients compared with 7% of healthy controls. As with bronchial wall thickening, there is some subjectivity in the visual assessment of this abnormality, which may account for the variability among the aforementioned studies. Some disparity between bronchial and arterial size may be related to hypoxic vasoconstriction in regions of localized air trapping.[4] Additionally, 1 study suggested that the bronchoarterial ratio

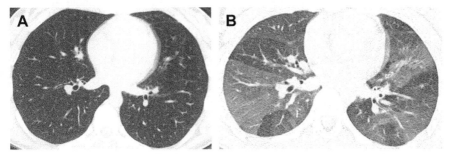

Fig. 4. (*A*) Inspiratory CT in an asthmatic patient showing homogenous lung attenuation. (*B*) Expiratory CT performed at a similar level, however, shows persistent regions of low attenuation (increased lucency), indicative of air trapping. Normal lung becomes more dense on expiratory CT.

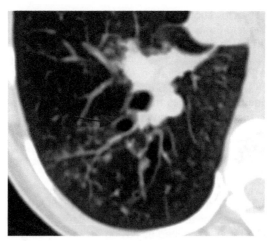

Fig. 5. Note the dilated airway in the right lower lobe (*arrow*), which is greater in diameter than the adjacent artery. A bronchoarterial ratio greater than 1 is definition of bronchiectasis.

is greater in patients who are scanned at higher altitude because of hypoxic vasocon-striction.[25] Although the studies by Park and colleagues and Takemura and colleagues did not find a correlation between bronchial dilation and airflow obstruction by PFTs, Harmanci and colleagues did find that bronchial dilation, among other abnormal HRCT findings, inversely correlated with FEV1.

Perhaps of utmost clinical importance is whether or not the bronchial dilation observed in an asthmatic patient is associated with allergic bronchopulmonary asper-gillosis (ABPA). Bronchiectasis, although an important finding, should not automati-cally decree a diagnosis of ABPA, because previous studies have indicated bronchiectasis can be present in asthmatic patients without concomitant ABPA.[26,27] For example, Neeld and colleagues[26] performed HRCT in 16 asthmatic patients, 8 of whom had clinical and immunologic evidence of ABPA, and found bronchial dilation present in 41% of lobes in the ABPA group compared with 15% of lobes in the non-ABPA asthma control group. Mitchell and colleagues performed a study to quantify distribution and severity of CT and radiographic findings in 19 patients with docu-mented ABPA, 10 with probable ABPA and 18 asthmatic controls. On CT examination, 89% of the patients with documented ABPA had cylindrical or varicoid bronchiectasis involving at least 1 lobe compared with 100% of patients with probable ABPA and 17% of asthmatic controls. Ward and colleagues[28] found bronchiectasis in 95% of pa-tients with ABPA compared with 29% of an asthmatic control group. Presence of bronchiectasis in 3 or more lobes, along with centrilobular nodules and mucoid impac-tion, were concluded to be highly suggestive of ABPA. Further findings of ABPA are discussed later.

ASSOCIATED CONDITIONS

Gastroesophageal reflux (GER) is prevalent among patients with asthma, estimated to be found in 33% to 89% of asthmatics, and has been identified as a potential trigger.[29,30] Previous studies have shown that treatment of GER may reduce symp-toms and physiologic impairment due to asthma, highlighting the importance of iden-tifying this condition. A critical review of the literature by Field and Sutherland[31] revealed that patients on medical antireflux therapy experienced reduced asthma symptoms in approximately 69% of patients and that antireflux treatment may reduce asthma medication use but has little to no effect on lung function. Thus, radiologic identification of signs suggesting GER, such as esophageal thickening or hiatal hernia, may be helpful to the clinician in the treatment of asthmatic patients. Ambulatory 24-hour pH monitoring is the gold standard for detecting GER, with sensitivity and specificity greater than 95%.[32,33] Barium studies are limited in the detection of GER, with overall sensitivity approximately 35%, in part because lower esophageal sphincter tone may intermittently be normal in subjects with reflux.[34,35] CT should not be the primary modality for assessing reflux esophagitis, because CT findings of esophagitis are not well validated. The subjective finding of esophageal wall thickening on CT often indicates underlying GER. Using a threshold of 5 mm to indicate esophageal wall thickening, Berkovich and colleagues[36] found that 55% of patients with a diagnosis of esophagitis demonstrated esophageal wall thickening on thoracic CT compared with only 4% of normal controls.

Sinusitis and asthma have been shown to coexist in 47% to 76% of asthma cases.[37] Sinus CT is commonly performed to accurately image the anatomy and extent of mucosal inflammation[38] (**Fig. 6**). In an observational study of 201 patients with asthma who underwent sinus CT, 68% revealed abnormalities at CT, with 30% having severe mucosal thickening (as scored by the Lund-Mackay staging scale) and 9% showing osteitis.[39] Furthermore, there was a positive correlation between CT scores and the eosinophil levels in the peripheral blood and induced sputum, supporting the hypothesis that asthma and chronic rhinosinusitis are mediated by similar inflammatory processes.[39] Imaging findings, however, require clinical correlation before a diagnosis of chronic rhinosinusitis is made, because symptoms do not necessarily correlate with CT findings, and mucosal thickening and opacification can be seen in up to 30% to 40% of asymptomatic individuals.[40–43]

COMPLICATIONS

Imaging plays an important role in identifying the complications of asthma. Acute complications of asthma include spontaneous pneumothorax, pneumomediastinum, subcutaneous emphysema, mucus plugging with or without atelectasis, and pneumonia.[44] Although rare, pneumopericardium, pneumoperitoneum, and pneumorhachis

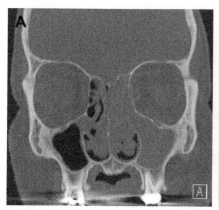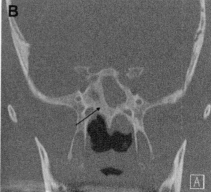

Fig. 6. Chronic sinusitis in an asthmatic patient. (*A*) Complete opacification of the left maxillary and ethmoid sinuses, and partial opacification of the right ethmoid sinus. (*B*) Thickening and sclerosis of the sphenoid sinus wall (*arrow*), consistent with sclerosis.

have been reported.[44,45] Spontaneous pneumomediastinum as triggered by bronchial asthma has an interesting mechanism, as described by Macklin and colleagues.[46] The Macklin effect describes an increase in alveolar pressure leading to alveolar rupture, with alveolar air subsequently dissecting through the pulmonary interstitium along the bronchovascular sheaths toward the hila and into the mediastinum. Asthma is but 1 described cause of spontaneous pneumomediastinum, and other associations should be considered, such as forceful diabetic ketoacidosis, inhalation of drugs, forceful strain during exercise, childbirth, and severe cough or vomiting.[46]

Chronic complications of asthma include ABPA, eosinophilic pneumonia, and eosinophilic granulomatosis with polyangiitis (EGPA) (Churg-Strauss syndrome). As discussed previously, bronchiectasis is an important feature of ABPA but is a finding that can also be seen in uncomplicated asthma. A more confident diagnosis of ABPA can be reached when the bronchiectasis involves 3 or more lobes, is moderate to severe, and is accompanied by mucus plugging and centrilobular nodules.[28] Ward and colleagues[28] found the bronchiectasis to be generally central in location (ie, involving segmental, subsegmental, and subsubsegmental airways), and a clear upper lobe preponderance is generally present.[26] Mucus-filled, dilated bronchi can manifest as tubular or branching opacities resembling fingers, the so-called finger-in-glove sign, which can be seen on both radiography and CT, and typically radiate from the hila towards the lung periphery[47] (**Fig. 7**). In approximately 25% to 30% of patients with ABPA, the mucus plugging is high in attenuation, greater than that of soft tissue,

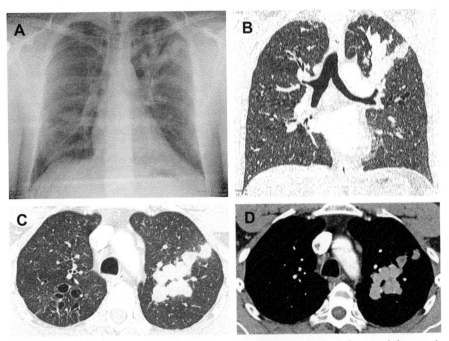

Fig. 7. (*A*) Chest radiograph shows tubular branching opacities in the left upper lobe, consistent with the finger-in-glove sign in a patient with ABPA. Coronal (*B*) and axial (*C*) lung windows show bilateral upper lung bronchiectasis, with mucous plugging in the left upper lobe accounting for the radiographic abnormality. (*D*) High density of the mucous plugging is a characteristic feature of ABPA.

secondary to the deposition of calcium salts.[48,49] Centrilobular nodules in ABPA presumably represent mucoid impaction in bronchi and bronchioles visualized in cross-section.[28] Other findings include fleeting alveolar opacities (typically earlier in the disease course), atelectasis, consolidation, and lung hyperinflation.[47,50]

Chronic eosinophilic pneumonia (CEP) is an indolent syndrome characterized by pulmonary infiltrates and both blood and tissue eosinophilia.[51] Approximately 50% of patients have coexisting asthma.[52] Peripheral, nonsegmental airspace consolidation, a finding referred to as the "photographic negative of pulmonary edema," is a characteristic radiographic finding of CEP but is seen in fewer than one-third of cases[53] and seems to be becoming less common with earlier detection and treatment of this condition. Typical findings at CT are peripheral predominant, patchy regions of airspace consolidation with or without ground-glass opacity[54] (Fig. 8). Ebara and colleagues[54] showed that CT features evolve at varying time intervals after onset of symptoms, for example, with nodules, streaky or bandlike opacities, and lobar atelectasis seen later in the disease course. A more recent study reported consolidation (74.4%), linear and reticular opacity (76.7%), and ground-glass opacity (65.1%) are the most frequently observed findings of CEP at CT, with parenchymal nodules rarely seen (4.7%).[55] Migratory opacities may be observed if serial radiographs or CT scans are acquired prior to diagnosis.[56] Pleural effusion is seen in fewer than 10% of cases.[57]

EGPA, also known as Churg-Strauss syndrome, is a complex disorder characterized by eosinophilic vasculitis, which can involve multiple organ systems, including the lungs, skin, heart, gastrointestinal tract, and nervous system.[51] Criteria adopted by the American College of Rheumatology define EGPA as the presence of 4 of the 6 following features: asthma, eosinophilia, pulmonary infiltrates, neuropathy,

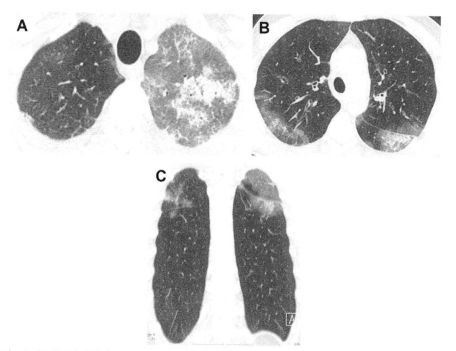

Fig. 8. (A, B) Axial CT through the upper lungs in a patient with with CEP shows patchy, peripheral ground-glass opacity and consolidation. (A) Septal thickening can be appreciated in the left upper lobe. (C) Coronal reformat shows the upper lung predominance of this abnormality.

paranasal sinus abnormality, and/or the presence of eosinophilic vasculitis.[58] In a study of 9 patients with EGPA, most common CT findings were ground-glass opacity, consolidation (which was mostly subpleural and surrounded by ground-glass), bronchial thickening, and centrilobular nodules[59] (**Fig. 9**). Less commonly observed findings included hyperinflation, larger nodules, interlobular septal thickening, medias-tinal, and hilar nodes, pleural effusion, and pericardial effusion.[59] In a more recent study, ground-glass opacity and consolidation were found at HRCT in 86.7% of pa-tients, although distribution was mixed between peripheral and random.[60] Radiographic and CT abnormalities are commonly migratory.

MIMICS

"All that wheezes is not asthma" is a quote made famous by Chevalier Jackson in the *Boston Medical Quarterly* in 1865, prompted by concern about an aspirated foreign body that caused wheezing being misdiagnosed as asthma.[61] This level of caution or skepticism should be maintained today when approaching a patient labeled with asthma, because misdiagnosis of nonasthmatic conditions as uncontrolled asthma is reported to be as high as 12% to 30%.[9] Therefore, both clinicians and radiologists reviewing the imaging of asthmatic patients are challenged to search for potential alternative diagnoses. Common conditions mimicking asthma include vocal cord dysfunction (VCD), tracheal or carinal obstruction, obliterative bronchiolitis (OB), and infiltrative disorders, such as sarcoidosis and hypersensitivity pneumonitis (HP). Diffuse idiopathic neuroendocrine cell hyperplasia (DIPNECH) is a female-predominant disorder that can potentially mimic asthma, which has interesting imag-ing features.

VCD is characterized by intermittent paradoxic motion of the vocal cords, mainly during inspiration, leading to airflow obstruction and dyspnea. VCD may mimic or coexist with asthma, resulting in overtreatment with corticosteroids.[62,63] The gold standard for diagnosing VCD is by direct visualization with flexible, transnasal laryn-goscopy.[64] There are no unique imaging manifestations of VCD, although this condi-tion may be suspected if radiographs or CT show lung hyperinflation in a severely symptomatic patient.[63]

Tracheal or carinal stenosis can result from various causes, including sequelae from previous intubation; benign or malignant neoplasm; aspirated foreign body; vascular rings; inflammatory disorders, such as Wegener granulomatosis, sarcoidosis, or

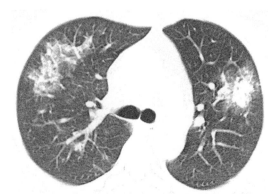

Fig. 9. Axial CT in a patient with Churg-Strauss syndrome showing peripheral (*right upper lobe*) ground-glass opacity and (*left upper lobe*) consolidation.

amyloidosis; idiopathic subglottic stenosis; and cartilaginous disorders, such as relapsing polychondritis or tracheobronchopathia osteochondroplastica.[65] Chest radiographs may show focal or diffuse narrowing of the tracheal air column depending on the underlying pathologic process. CT is the test of choice for further defining the site, extent, and severity of tracheal abnormality.[65] For example, a unique characteristic of tracheal involvement by Wegener granulomatosis is circumferential smooth or nodular thickening, including involvement of the posterior membrane[66] **(Fig. 10)**. This is readily depicted by CT and differentiates from disorders that spare the posterior tracheal membrane, such as relapsing polychondritis or tracheobronchopathia osteochondroplastica[66] **(Fig. 11)**.

OB is frequently characterized by an obstructive airflow pattern on PFT, with associated causes including autoimmune, postinfectious, exposure to inhalational toxins, and post-transplant.[67] It may be difficult clinically to distinguish between severe asthma and OB. Additionally, diffuse air trapping on expiratory imaging may be difficult to attribute to severe asthma versus OB.[63] A mosaic pattern, defined as alternating regions of varying lung attenuation on inspiratory imaging, seems most useful **(Fig. 12)**. In a study of the HRCT features of 14 patients with OB and 30 patients with severe asthma, Jensen and colleagues[68] showed a mosaic pattern in 50% of patients with OB compared with 3% in severe asthma. This proved the 1 key finding to provide confidence in differentiating between the 2 entities, because there was no significant difference between the 2 groups with other findings. Other common findings in OB include air trapping, bronchial thickening, decreased parenchymal attenuation, and bronchial dilation. Ground-glass opacity and centrilobular branching structures are less common.[68,69]

Infiltrative distal airways diseases, such as HP and sarcoidosis, are another cause of airways obstruction potentially mimicking asthma. HRCT is the superior imaging modality in characterizing the associated abnormality. For example, centrilobular nodules of ground-glass attenuation, which can be subtle, may be the predominant or only imaging abnormality of subacute HP at HRCT.[70] Accompanying lobular air trapping may be present, which is an indirect sign of bronchiolar obstruction[71] **(Fig. 13)**.

DIPNECH is a neuroendocrine cell proliferation predominately seen in middle-aged women, which presents with chronic cough and dyspnea and an obstructive pattern by PFTs.[72] Mosaic pattern, air trapping, bronchial thickening, and multiple pulmonary nodules are the HRCT findings described in previous studies.[73] Carr and colleagues[72] further defined the HRCT features in their retrospective review of a cohort of

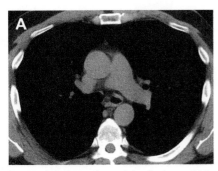
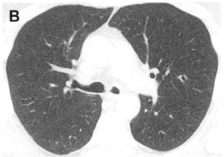

Fig. 10. (*A*) Circumferential soft tissue thickening of the left mainstem bronchus in a patient with Wegener granulomatosis. (*B*) Luminal stenosis can be appreciated on lung windows.

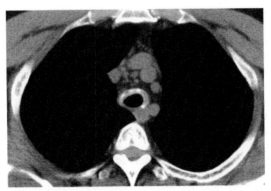

Fig. 11. Partially calcified thickening of the anterior and lateral tracheal walls in this patient with relapsing polychondritis. Note the sparing of the posterior membrane, a typical feature.

30 patients with DIPNECH, 26 of whom had HRCT. The most common findings were a mosaic pattern, air trapping involving greater than 50% of the lung, multiple pulmonary nodules (>20), and nodules measuring mostly between 6 mm and 10 mm.[72] The nodules tended to show a mid-lung and lower lung zonal preponderance and peribronchovascular or peripheral distribution[72] (**Fig. 14**).

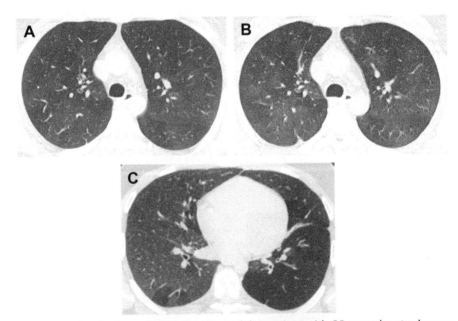

Fig. 12. Imaging findings of OB in 2 patients. (*A*) A patient with OB secondary to rheumatoid arthritis shows airway thickening and multifocal regions of low attenuation on inspiratory imaging. (*B*) Expiratory imaging shows these regions to remain lucent, consistent with air trapping. (*C*) A patient with OB related to previous childhood infection (Swyer-James syndrome) shows airway thickening and an inspiratory mosaic pattern, with the low attenuation most pronounced in the left lung.

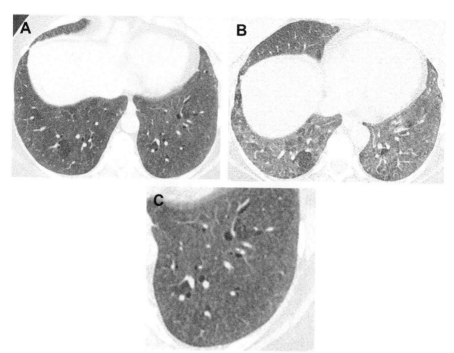

Fig. 13. (A) Inspiratory imaging of a patient with HP shows lobular foci of low attenuation, which remain lucent on (B) expiratory imaging, consistent with air trapping. (C) A magnified image of the left lower lobe depicts the background centrilobular nodularity.

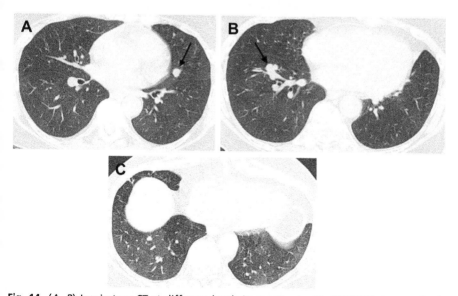

Fig. 14. (A, B) Inspiratory CT at different levels in a patient with DIPNECH shows a background mosaic pattern and multifocal pulmonary nodules (arrows). (C) Corresponding expiratory CT in the same patient shows areas of persistent lucency, consistent with air trapping. Note the normal lung parenchyma increases in density at expiration.

SUMMARY

Asthma is a common disorder with typical but nonspecific imaging findings. The primary role of imaging is not to make a diagnosis of asthma but to identify complications, such as ABPA, or mimics of asthma, such as HP.

REFERENCES

1. Paganin F, Trussard V, Seneterre E, et al. Chest radiography and high resolution computed tomography of the lungs in asthma. Am Rev Respir Dis 1992;146(4): 1084–7.
2. Lynch DA, Newell JD, Tschomper BA, et al. Uncomplicated asthma in adults: comparison of CT appearance of the lungs in asthmatic and healthy subjects. Radiology 1993;188(3):829–33.
3. Ismail Y, Loo CS, Zahary MK. The value of routine chest radiographs in acute asthma admissions. Singapore Med J 1994;35(2):171–2.
4. Lynch DA. Imaging of asthma and allergic bronchopulmonary mycosis. Radiol Clin North Am 1998;36(1):129–42.
5. White CS, Cole RP, Lubetsky HW, et al. Acute asthma. Admission chest radiography in hospitalized adult patients. Chest 1991;100(1):14–6.
6. Tsai TW, Gallagher EJ, Lombardi G, et al. Guidelines for the selective ordering of admission chest radiography in adult obstructive airway disease. Ann Emerg Med 1993;22(12):1854–8.
7. Buckmaster A, Boon R. Reduce the rads: a quality assurance project on reducing unnecessary chest X-rays in children with asthma. J Paediatr Child Health 2005; 41(3):107–11.
8. Gentile NT, Ufberg J, Barnum M, et al. Guidelines reduce x-ray and blood gas utilization in acute asthma. Am J Emerg Med 2003;21(6):451–3.
9. Chung KF, Wenzel SE, Brozek JL, et al. International ERS/ATS guidelines on definition, evaluation and treatment of severe asthma. Eur Respir J 2014;43(2): 343–73.
10. Aysola RS, Hoffman EA, Gierada D, et al. Airway remodeling measured by multidetector CT is increased in severe asthma and correlates with pathology. Chest 2008;134(6):1183–91.
11. Niimi A, Matsumoto H, Amitani R, et al. Airway wall thickness in asthma assessed by computed tomography. Relation to clinical indices. Am J Respir Crit Care Med 2000;162(4 Pt 1):1518–23.
12. Machado D, Pereira C, Teixeira L, et al. Thoracic high resolution computed tomography (HRCT) in asthma. Eur Ann Allergy Clin Immunol 2009;41(5):139–45.
13. Khadadah M, Jayakrishnan B, Abdulaziz M, et al. High resolution computed tomography in asthma. Oman Med J 2012;27(2):145–50.
14. McNamara AE, Müller NL, Okazawa M, et al. Airway narrowing in excised canine lungs measured by high-resolution computed tomography. J Appl Physiol (1985) 1992;73(1):307–16.
15. Okazawa M, Müller N, McNamara AE, et al. Human airway narrowing measured using high resolution computed tomography. Am J Respir Crit Care Med 1996; 154(5):1557–62.
16. Hoshino M, Matsuoka S, Handa H, et al. Correlation between airflow limitation and airway dimensions assessed by multidetector CT in asthma. Respir Med 2010; 104(6):794–800.
17. Lee KY, Park SJ, Kim SR, et al. Low attenuation area is associated with airflow limitation and airway hyperresponsiveness. J Asthma 2008;45(9):774–9.

18. Newman KB, Lynch DA, Newman LS, et al. Quantitative computed tomography detects air trapping due to asthma. Chest 1994;106(1):105–9.
19. Busacker A, Newell JD Jr, Keefe T, et al. A multivariate analysis of risk factors for the air-trapping asthmatic phenotype as measured by quantitative CT analysis. Chest 2009;135(1):48–56.
20. Coxson HO, Mayo JR, Behzad H, et al. Measurement of lung expansion with computed tomography and comparison with quantitative histology. J Appl Physiol (1985) 1995;79(5):1525–30.
21. Coxson HO, Rogers RM, Whittall KP, et al. A quantification of the lung surface area in emphysema using computed tomography. Am J Respir Crit Care Med 1999;159(3):851–6.
22. Harmanci E, Kebapci M, Metintas M, et al. High-resolution computed tomography findings are correlated with disease severity in asthma. Respiration 2002;69(5):420–6.
23. Takemura M, Niimi A, Minakuchi M, et al. Bronchial dilatation in asthma: relation to clinical and sputum indices. Chest 2004;125(4):1352–8.
24. Park CS, Müller NL, Worthy SA, et al. Airway obstruction in asthmatic and healthy individuals: inspiratory and expiratory thin-section CT findings. Radiology 1997;203(2):361–7.
25. Kim JS, Müller NL, Park CS, et al. Cylindrical bronchiectasis: diagnostic findings on thin-section CT. AJR Am J Roentgenol 1997;168(3):751–4.
26. Neeld DA, Goodman LR, Gurney JW, et al. Computerized tomography in the evaluation of allergic bronchopulmonary aspergillosis. Am Rev Respir Dis 1990;142(5):1200–5.
27. Mitchell TA, Hamilos DL, Lynch DA, et al. Distribution and severity of bronchiectasis in allergic bronchopulmonary aspergillosis (ABPA). J Asthma 2000;37(1):65–72.
28. Ward S, Heyneman L, Lee MJ, et al. Accuracy of CT in the diagnosis of allergic bronchopulmonary aspergillosis in asthmatic patients. AJR Am J Roentgenol 1999;173(4):937–42.
29. Harding SM, Richter JE. The role of gastroesophageal reflux in chronic cough and asthma. Chest 1997;111(5):1389–402.
30. Harding SM, Richter JE, Guzzo MR, et al. Asthma and gastroesophageal reflux: acid suppressive therapy improves asthma outcome. Am J Med 1996;100(4):395–405.
31. Field SK, Sutherland LR. Does medical antireflux therapy improve asthma in asthmatics with gastroesophageal reflux?: a critical review of the literature. Chest 1998;114(1):275–83.
32. Wiener GJ, Morgan TM, Copper JB, et al. Ambulatory 24-hour esophageal pH monitoring. Reproducibility and variability of pH parameters. Dig Dis Sci 1988;33(9):1127–33.
33. Mattox HE 3rd, Richter JE. Prolonged ambulatory esophageal pH monitoring in the evaluation of gastroesophageal reflux disease. Am J Med 1990;89(3):345–56.
34. Mittal RK, Holloway RH, Penagini R, et al. Transient lower esophageal sphincter relaxation. Gastroenterology 1995;109(2):601–10.
35. Schoeman MN, Tippett MD, Akkermans LM, et al. Mechanisms of gastroesophageal reflux in ambulant healthy human subjects. Gastroenterology 1995;108(1):83–91.
36. Berkovich GY, Levine MS, Miller WT Jr. CT findings in patients with esophagitis. AJR Am J Roentgenol 2000;175(5):1431–4.
37. Slavin RG. Asthma and sinusitis. J Allergy Clin Immunol 1992;90(3 Pt 2):534–7.

38. Aygun N, Uzuner O, Zinreich SJ. Advances in imaging of the paranasal sinuses. Otolaryngol Clin North Am 2005;38(3):429–37.
39. Mehta V, Campeau NG, Kita H, et al. Blood and sputum eosinophil levels in asthma and their relationship to sinus computed tomographic findings. Mayo Clin Proc 2008;83(6):671–8.
40. Stewart MG, Sicard MW, Piccirillo JF, et al. Severity staging in chronic sinusitis: are CT scan findings related to patient symptoms? Am J Rhinol 1999;13(3):161–7.
41. Bradley DT, Kountakis SE. Correlation between computed tomography scores and symptomatic improvement after endoscopic sinus surgery. Laryngoscope 2005;115(3):466–9.
42. Flinn J, Chapman ME, Wightman AJ, et al. A prospective analysis of incidental paranasal sinus abnormalities on CT head scans. Clin Otolaryngol Allied Sci 1994;19(4):287–9.
43. Bhattacharyya N. A comparison of symptom scores and radiographic staging systems in chronic rhinosinusitis. Am J Rhinol 2005;19(2):175–9.
44. van der Klooster JM, Grootendorst AF, Ophof PJ, et al. Pneumomediastinum: an unusual complication of bronchial asthma in a young man. Neth J Med 1998; 52(4):150–4.
45. Caramella D, Bulleri A, Battolla L, et al. Spontaneous epidural emphysema and pneumomediastinum during an asthmatic attack in a child. Pediatr Radiol 1997;27(12):929–31.
46. Murayama S, Gibo S. Spontaneous pneumomediastinum and Macklin effect: Overview and appearance on computed tomography. World J Radiol 2014; 6(11):850–4.
47. Martinez S, Heyneman LE, McAdams HP, et al. Mucoid impactions: finger-in-glove sign and other CT and radiographic features. Radiographics 2008;28(5): 1369–82.
48. Silva CI, Colby TV, Muller NL. Asthma and associated conditions: high-resolution CT and pathologic findings. AJR Am J Roentgenol 2004;183(3):817–24.
49. Logan PM, Muller NL. High-attenuation mucous plugging in allergic bronchopulmonary aspergillosis. Can Assoc Radiol J 1996;47(5):374–7.
50. Panchal N, Bhagat R, Pant C, et al. Allergic bronchopulmonary aspergillosis: the spectrum of computed tomography appearances. Respir Med 1997;91(4):213–9.
51. Wechsler ME. Pulmonary eosinophilic syndromes. Immunol Allergy Clin North Am 2007;27(3):477–92.
52. Fox B, Seed WA. Chronic eosinophilic pneumonia. Thorax 1980;35(8):570–80.
53. Jederlinic PJ, Sicilian L, Gaensler EA. Chronic eosinophilic pneumonia. A report of 19 cases and a review of the literature. Medicine (Baltimore) 1988;67(3): 154–62.
54. Ebara H, Ikezoe J, Johkoh T, et al. Chronic eosinophilic pneumonia: evolution of chest radiograms and CT features. J Comput Assist Tomogr 1994;18(5):737–44.
55. Arakawa H, Kurihara Y, Niimi H, et al. Bronchiolitis obliterans with organizing pneumonia versus chronic eosinophilic pneumonia: high-resolution CT findings in 81 patients. AJR Am J Roentgenol 2001;176(4):1053–8.
56. Marchand E, Cordier JF. Idiopathic chronic eosinophilic pneumonia. Semin Respir Crit Care Med 2006;27(2):134–41.
57. Jeong YJ, Kim KI, Seo IJ, et al. Eosinophilic lung diseases: a clinical, radiologic, and pathologic overview. Radiographics 2007;27(3):617–37 [discussion: 637–9].
58. Masi AT, Hunder GG, Lie JT, et al. The American College of Rheumatology 1990 criteria for the classification of Churg-Strauss syndrome (allergic granulomatosis and angiitis). Arthritis Rheum 1990;33(8):1094–100.

59. Choi YH, Im JG, Han BK, et al. Thoracic manifestation of Churg-Strauss syndrome: radiologic and clinical findings. Chest 2000;117(1):117–24.
60. Szczeklik W, Sokolowska B, Mastalerz L, et al. Pulmonary findings in Churg-Strauss syndrome in chest X-rays and high resolution computed tomography at the time of initial diagnosis. Clin Rheumatol 2010;29(10):1127–34.
61. Kaminsky DA. "All that wheezes is not asthma" (or COPD)! Chest 2015;147(2): 284–6.
62. Balkissoon R, Kenn K. Asthma: vocal cord dysfunction (VCD) and other dysfunctional breathing disorders. Semin Respir Crit Care Med 2012;33(6):595–605.
63. Woods AQ, Lynch DA. Asthma: an imaging update. Radiol Clin North Am 2009; 47(2):317–29.
64. Hicks M, Brugman SM, Katial R. Vocal cord dysfunction/paradoxical vocal fold motion. Prim Care 2008;35(1):81–103, vii.
65. Ryu JH, Scanlon PD. Obstructive lung diseases: COPD, asthma, and many imitators. Mayo Clin Proc 2001;76(11):1144–53.
66. Martinez F, Chung JH, Digumarthy SR, et al. Common and uncommon manifestations of Wegener granulomatosis at chest CT: radiologic-pathologic correlation. Radiographics 2012;32(1):51–69.
67. Barker AF, Bergeron A, Rom WN, et al. Obliterative bronchiolitis. N Engl J Med 2014;370(19):1820–8.
68. Jensen SP, Lynch DA, Brown KK, et al. High-resolution CT features of severe asthma and bronchiolitis obliterans. Clin Radiol 2002;57(12):1078–85.
69. Padley SP, Adler BD, Hansell DM, et al. Bronchiolitis obliterans: high resolution CT findings and correlation with pulmonary function tests. Clin Radiol 1993;47(4): 236–40.
70. Mohr LC. Hypersensitivity pneumonitis. Curr Opin Pulm Med 2004;10(5):401–11.
71. Silva CI, Churg A, Muller NL. Hypersensitivity pneumonitis: spectrum of high-resolution CT and pathologic findings. AJR Am J Roentgenol 2007;188(2): 334–44.
72. Carr LL, Chung JH, Duarte Achcar R, et al. The clinical course of diffuse idiopathic pulmonary neuroendocrine cell hyperplasia. Chest 2015;147(2):415–22.
73. Koo CW, Baliff JP, Torigian DA, et al. Spectrum of pulmonary neuroendocrine cell proliferation: diffuse idiopathic pulmonary neuroendocrine cell hyperplasia, tumorlet, and carcinoids. AJR Am J Roentgenol 2010;195(3):661–8.

Biomarkers in Severe Asthma

Xiao Chloe Wan, MD, Prescott G. Woodruff, MD, MPH*

KEYWORDS

- Severe asthma • Biomarker • Eosinophil • Periostin • Exhaled nitric oxide
- Endotype

KEY POINTS

- Asthma biomarkers can be broadly categorized as those that relate to type 2 inflammation and those that relate to other biological processes.
- Biomarkers of type 2 inflammation include sputum and blood eosinophils, exhaled nitric oxide levels, and serum periostin.
- In severe asthma, biomarkers are particularly useful in defining endotypes (ie, biologically related subtypes) and in predicting response to therapy.

INTRODUCTION

A biomarker is defined as "a characteristic that is objectively measured and evaluated as an indicator of normal biologic processes, pathogenic processes, or pharmacologic responses to a therapeutic intervention."[1] Biomarkers useful in respiratory disease can be obtained using several different types of clinical samples (**Box 1**). In this review, we restrict our discussion to biomarkers that can be measured in blood, sputum, or exhaled gas and those that are cellular, biochemical, or molecular in nature. There are several potential applications of biomarkers in the study and management of severe asthma (**Box 2**). Of these potential applications, significant advances have been made in biomarkers of endotypes (ie, biologically related subtypes) of asthma and in those that are predictive of response to therapy. In particular, biomarkers of type 2 inflammation (defined as inflammation driven by the Th2-cytokines, interleukin [IL]-4, IL-5, and IL-13) have proven valuable for endotyping in asthma. Here we review the current state of knowledge with respect to biomarkers in severe asthma, stratifying them by those that relate to type 2 inflammation and those that do not.

Division of Pulmonary, Critical Care, Sleep and Allergy, Department of Medicine and Cardiovascular Research Institute, University of California, San Francisco, 513 Parnassus Avenue, HSE 1305, San Francisco, CA 94143-0130, USA
* Corresponding author.
E-mail address: prescott.woodruff@ucsf.edu

Immunol Allergy Clin N Am 36 (2016) 547–557
http://dx.doi.org/10.1016/j.iac.2016.03.004　　　　　　**immunology.theclinics.com**

Box 1
Sample types of biomarker measurement in respiratory disease

- Bronchoscopic samples
- Induced sputum
- Blood
- Urine
- Exhaled gases

BIOMARKERS OF TYPE 2 INFLAMMATION
Sputum Eosinophils

Sputum eosinophils are obtained by sputum induction and are expressed as a percentage of inflammatory cells.[2] Upper limit of normal for sputum eosinophil differential is generally defined as approximately 1% to 2%,[2–4] with female gender and atopy associated with higher sputum eosinophil counts.[3] Sputum eosinophil count is increased in symptomatic individuals with asthma,[5] and elevated eosinophils can be found in 50% of corticosteroid-treated patients, and in 70% to 80% of corticosteroid-naive patients.[6] Sputum eosinophil count is elevated by allergen challenge and reduced by corticosteroids.[7,8] Studies of inhaled corticosteroid (ICS) reduction in patients with asthma show that an increase in sputum eosinophil count may be predictive of asthma exacerbation.[9–11]

Fractional Exhaled Nitric Oxide Concentration

Nitric oxide (NO) is synthesized by NO synthetases (NOSs).[12] Patients with asthma have high levels of NO in their exhaled breath, which is thought to be due to upregulation of inducible NOS (NOS2) in airway epithelial cells secondary to airway inflammation.[13] Chemiluminescence analyzers allow the measurement of NO concentration in gas phase.[14] A joint American Thoracic Society (ATS) and European Respiratory Society (ERS) guideline (last revised in 2005) recommends that fractional exhaled NO concentration (FeNO) in exhaled breath be expressed as parts per billion (ppb).[15] FeNO is elevated in asthma and decreased with inhaled steroids.[16] The distribution of FeNO value is skewed to the right with significant overlap between healthy controls and patients with asthma. Current smoking, atopy, and age influence the distribution of FeNO values.[17–22] The 2011 ATS clinical practice guideline on the interpretation of FeNO proposes cutoffs for clinical use of FeNO. It suggests that eosinophilic

---

Box 2
Potential applications of biomarkers in severe asthma

- Understanding the biology
- Diagnosis and screening
- Assessment of severity, control, or prognosis
- Identification of endotypes (biologically related subtypes of disease)
- Application in clinical trials and safety monitoring
  - Pharmacodynamic biomarkers
  - Predictive of response

---

inflammation is unlikely in symptomatic patients with low FeNO (<25 ppb in adults and <20 ppb in children), whereas high FeNO (>50 ppb in adults and >35 ppb in children) suggests airway eosinophilia and steroid-responsive inflammation.[13]

Blood Eosinophils

There has been growing interest in less-invasive alternatives to sputum induction. Blood eosinophil counts are a potential surrogate biomarker for eosinophilic inflammation in asthma and are relatively easy to obtain. Although studies of blood eosinophil count as predictors of high sputum eosinophils in eosinophilic asthma have yielded somewhat mixed results,[23–25] blood eosinophil counts have been useful in selection of patients for eosinophil-targeting agents as described later in this article. The cutoff used in the clinical trials to define high blood eosinophil counts have ranged between 150 and 300 cells/μL.[23–27]

Periostin

Periostin is a matricellular protein that is secreted by bronchial epithelial cells and lung fibroblasts in response to Th2 cytokines, IL-13, and IL-4.[28,29] Whether and how periostin may contribute to asthma pathogenesis is still unclear. Although some results are conflicting, mouse models suggest a role of periostin in subepithelial fibrosis, eosinophil recruitment, and mucus production from goblet cells.[30–32] A study of sputum and blood eosinophils, periostin, FeNO, and immunoglobulin E (IgE) in patients with severe asthma found that periostin was the strongest biomarker predictor of sputum and tissue eosinophilia.[33] The cutoff range to define periostin-high or periostin-low groups for prognostication of treatment response have not been precisely defined, with some clinical studies using the median periostin level of the study population[34–36] and others using 50 ng/mL as the cutoff.[37]

OTHER BIOMARKERS OF TYPE 2 INFLAMMATION

Dipeptidyl peptidase-4 (DPP4) is highly expressed in lung epithelial cells, endothelial cells, and submucosal glands. In rat models, its enzymatic activity increases in bronchoalveolar lavage (BAL) fluid and parenchymal tissue after an allergen challenge.[38] Like periostin, the role of DPP4 in asthma is uncertain. DPP4 inhibition has effects on airway inflammation in animal models that depend on the route of administration (oral, aerosolized, topical).[39] Studies of DPP4 in human airway inflammation are limited. Other potential biomarkers of type 2 inflammation include urinary bromotyrosine (BrTyr),[40,41] monocyte chemoattractant protein-4 (MCP4) , and eotaxin-2.[42,43]

BIOMARKERS UNRELATED TO TYPE 2 INFLAMMATION
Sputum Neutrophil

Using sputum induction and cytology, patients with asthma can be categorized as pauci-granulocytic, eosinophilic, neutrophilic, and mixed. Airway neutrophilia is well documented in severe exacerbations of asthma[44]; however, the prevalence of neutrophilia in severe asthma between exacerbations remains somewhat uncertain.

In healthy subjects, neutrophils and macrophages predominate in the induced sputum (median neutrophil percentage 37% [10th and 90th percentile, 11%–64%]).[3] Cigarette smoking, infection, ozone, and endotoxin all increase sputum neutrophil counts.[3] In asthma studies, the cutoffs for elevated sputum neutrophil count have ranged between 40% and 76%.[25,45,46]

Sputum neutrophilia may represent a stable phenotype of severe asthma or, alternatively, could reflect response to therapy. In cluster analyses from the Severe Asthma

Research Program (SARP), patients with the worst lung function despite maximal bronchodilator therapy had the highest sputum neutrophil count.[46] Conversely, other studies report that ICS use is associated with increased sputum neutrophils[47] and that, after tapering ICS, sputum neutrophilia was reduced. Combined increases in sputum eosinophils and neutrophils may identify patients with asthma with low lung function and increased symptoms.[45]

Interleukin-17

IL-17 can promote neutrophilic inflammation and plays a role in diseases such as psoriasis and ankylosing spondylitis.[48–51] Studies measuring IL-17 levels in induced sputum, BAL samples, and bronchial biopsies have found increased IL-17 levels in severe asthma.[52–55] Whether IL-17 plays a causative role in severe asthma is less certain, as a randomized trial of IL-17 blockade using Brodalumab, a humanized anti-IL17RA monoclonal antibody, in moderate to severe asthma was negative.[56] More recently, IL-17–producing cells and an IL-17–related gene expression signature were observed in severe asthma, and this IL-17 signature was orthogonal to type 2 inflammation.[57] One intriguing possibility raised by this data is the airway production of IL-17 may increase as type 2 inflammation is blocked in severe asthma. If so, a strategy that blocks both Th2 cytokines and IL-17 could be beneficial in severe asthma.

Other Non-Type 2 Inflammatory Biomarkers

Several other inflammatory biomarkers that are not associated with type 2 inflammation have been studied in severe asthma, including IL-6[58] and C-reactive protein.[59] Exhaled breath condensate pH may reflect underlying inflammatory process in the airway in asthma, as its levels may correlate with steroid treatment and asthma exacerbation.[60] More studies in these markers and others, including tumor necrosis factor α and biomarkers of oxidative stress are needed to better elucidate its role in asthma.

Special Considerations in Children

Periostin is a product of bone turnover and is elevated in children.[61] Thus, whether it will be useful as a biomarker of asthma in children is uncertain. Two recent studies show significantly higher periostin levels in children with asthma compared with healthy controls, suggesting that periostin may still have some value in this age group, although more studies are needed.[61,62] One study showed poor correlation between blood eosinophils and airway eosinophilia in children with severe asthma on high-dose ICS.[63] A BAL study of 69 children suggest that severe therapy-resistant asthma in children is characterized by eosinophilic, rather than neutrophilic predominant airways. However, there were no elevated cytokines in the BAL fluid suggestive of type 2 inflammation (IL-4, IL-5, IL-13) in these children compared with the control group.[64]

UTILITY IN SEVERE ASTHMA
Diagnosis

As asthma is heterogeneous with respect to type 2 inflammation, biomarkers such as FeNO are supportive rather than definitive for diagnosis of asthma.[13]

Prognosis

A study in SARP found no difference in FeNO level in severe as compared with nonsevere asthma; however, when the groups were subdivided further, high FeNO levels in severe asthma identified those with greatest airflow limitation and reversibility, highest sputum eosinophils, and most emergency department visits and intensive care unit admissions, suggesting that FeNO may be used to risk stratify.[65] Elevated sputum neutrophils with or without concurrent sputum eosinophilia have been associated with a more severe asthma phenotype.[66] In a multivariable analysis of 224 patients with asthma on ICS, high baseline serum periostin level ($\geq$95 ng/mL) was an independent risk factor for greater decline of lung function.[67] Furthermore, elevated levels of periostin have been found in aspirin-exacerbated respiratory disease and were again associated with more severe and eosinophilic asthma.[68]

Establishing a Baseline and Monitoring Control

How variable airway eosinophilia may be over time is uncertain. In one longitudinal study over 5 years, 70% of those with eosinophilic asthma (sputum eosinophils $\geq$2%) and 96% of those with noneosinophilic asthma retained their sputum phenotype.[69] However, one pro-con debate cited data from 40 patients with severe asthma, which showed that 60% of the patients changed their classification from eosinophilic (sputum eosinophils $\geq$2%) to noneosinophilic and vice versa.[70]

Endotyping

The observation that biomarkers of type 2 inflammation mark patients who have distinct immune cell infiltration, histological changes, and treatment response suggests that type 2 inflammation defines an endotype of asthma.[71] Formally, an endotype can be defined as patients who share a common underlying biology, and one review article suggested that investigation of a series of shared features could define an endotype (see **Box 2**).[72] Many of these proposed criteria for an endotype have been met for type 2 inflammation asthma, including association with treatment response. Those criteria that still require some investigation include studies of genetic predisposition and shared epidemiology.

Guiding Choice of Therapy in Severe Asthma

The concept of an endotype can inform precision medicine has been key in developing new therapies for severe asthma, especially because new therapies can be expensive and cumbersome and can have adverse effects.

The first example of using biomarkers to predict therapy in severe asthma comes from the development of mepolizumab, a humanized monoclonal antibody against IL-5. The first clinical trial of mepolizumab (in moderate asthma) did not use eosinophilia as inclusion criteria and failed to show benefit.[73] Subsequently, 2 studies in severe asthma that selected patients based on persistent sputum eosinophilia showed a remarkable benefit in reduction of exacerbations with mepolizumab.[74,75] Subsequent larger trials confirmed these observations, informed the use of blood eosinophils as a surrogate for sputum eosinophils, and identified optimized threshold values for prediction of clinical response. In the DREAM study, mepolizumab, reduced exacerbations in patients with severe asthma who had sputum eosinophil count $\geq$3%, FeNO $\geq$50 ppb, or blood eosinophil count $\geq$300 cells/μl. Furthermore, baseline blood eosinophil count correlated with the reduction in exacerbations.[76] Post hoc analysis of the DREAM study showed that blood eosinophils $\geq$150 cells/μl predicted response to mepolizumab and that a single measurement was predictive of future elevated blood eosinophil levels.[27] Mepolizumab also reduced exacerbations, improved asthma symptoms, and had oral steroid-sparing effects in patients with eosinophilic inflammation (prerandomization blood eosinophil count $\geq$300 cells/μl, or 150 cells/μl during optimization phase) who required chronic oral steroids for their asthma.[77] In November 2015, the Food and Drug Administration approved mepolizumab for treatment of severe asthma in patients 12 years and older with an eosinophilic phenotype. Similarly, reslizumab, an anti-IL5 humanized monoclonal antibody, has also been demonstrated to improve lung function and quality of life in poorly controlled asthma with sputum eosinophilia $\geq$3% or blood eosinophil count $\geq$400/μL.[78,79]

An alternative approach to using biomarkers of type 2 inflammation to guide the use of biologics for severe asthma was the development of periostin as a predictive biomarker for response to lebrikizumab, an anti-IL-13 humanized monoclonal antibody. In a phase II study (MILLY study), lebrikizumab significantly improved lung function but not exacerbation rates when stratifying patients by elevated periostin levels.[35] Subsequently, 2 pooled phase IIb studies (LUTE and VERSE studies) demonstrated both improved lung function and reduced exacerbation in patients with periostin-high severe asthma.[37] The efficacy of lebrikizumab in mild asthma is less clear, as a study of patients with mild asthma not on ICS showed no significant clinical benefit with lebrikizumab.[36] Similarly, a phase IIb study of tralokinumab, a humanized anti-IL-13 monoclonal antibody, in severe asthma showed no decrease in asthma exacerbations, except in post hoc subgroup analysis, in which asthma exacerbations decreased in those with high periostin level and lung function improved in those with elevated DPP-4 level.[80]

Finally, post hoc analysis of a clinical trial of omalizumab, a widely used anti-IgE monoclonal antibody, identified potential biomarkers of response (reduction in exacerbations).[81] This is particularly interesting in that patients were already selected for those with a positive skin test or in vitro response to a relevant perennial aeroallergen. The investigators found that FeNO and blood eosinophils at baseline predicted response to omalizumab and that there was a trend for improved response in those with increased baseline levels of serum periostin.

Guide Dosing of Inhaled Corticosteroid

Randomized trials have demonstrated that the use of sputum eosinophil to guide ICS therapy can reduce asthma exacerbations without increasing the total amount of ICS used.[82,83] One meta-analysis showed that the use of sputum eosinophils to titrate asthma treatment reduced exacerbations, whereas the use of FeNO reduced ICS dose in adults but failed to show significant improvement in asthma control.[84] In children with severe asthma, the use of sputum eosinophils to guide management was not shown to decrease asthma exacerbations or overall control compared with standard symptom-based management.[85] The use of FeNO to guide therapy in children resulted in somewhat higher ICS use without significant improvement in clinical outcomes.[84,86] The ATS/ERS guideline on severe asthma recommends that in adults, clinical criteria and sputum eosinophil counts, but not FeNO, be used for guiding therapy.[87]

Assess Adherence

According to collective experience of investigators in the ATS guideline, one of the most common causes of persistently elevated FeNO despite therapy is likely poor compliance.[13]

SUMMARY

Biomarkers have been critical for studies of disease pathogenesis and the development of new therapies in severe asthma. In particular, biomarkers of type 2 inflammation have proven valuable for endotyping and targeting new biological agents. Because of these successes in understanding and marking type 2 inflammation, lack of knowledge regarding non–type 2 inflammatory mechanisms in asthma will soon be the major obstacle to the development of new treatments and management strategies in severe asthma. Biomarkers can play a role in these investigations as well by providing insight into the underlying biology in human studies of patients with severe asthma.

REFERENCES

1. Biomarkers Definitions Working Group. Biomarkers and surrogate endpoints: preferred definitions and conceptual framework. Clin Pharmacol Ther 2001; 69(3):89–95.
2. Reddel HK, Taylor DR, Bateman ED, et al. An official American Thoracic Society/European Respiratory Society Statement: asthma control and exacerbations. Am J Respir Crit Care Med 2009;180(1):59–99.
3. Belda J, Leigh R, Parameswaran K, et al. Induced sputum cell counts in healthy adults. Am J Respir Crit Care Med 2000;161(2 Pt 1):475–8.
4. Spanevello A, Confalonieri M, Sulotto F, et al. Induced sputum cellularity. Am J Respir Crit Care Med 2000;162(3):1172–4.
5. Pizzichini E, Pizzichini MM, Efthimiadis A, et al. Indices of airway inflammation in induced sputum: reproducibility and validity of cell and fluid-phase measurements. Am J Respir Crit Care Med 1996;154(2 Pt 1):308–17.
6. Haldar P, Pavord ID. Noneosinophilic asthma: a distinct clinical and pathologic phenotype. J Allergy Clin Immunol 2007;119(5):1043–52 [quiz: 1053–4].
7. Pin I, Freitag AP, O'Byrne PM, et al. Changes in the cellular profile of induced sputum after allergen-induced asthmatic responses. Am Rev Respir Dis 1992; 145(6):1265–9.
8. Pizzichini MM, Pizzichini E, Clelland L, et al. Sputum in severe exacerbations of asthma: kinetics of inflammatory indices after prednisone treatment. Am J Respir Crit Care Med 1997;155(5):1501–8.
9. Leuppi JD, Salome CM, Jenkins CR, et al. Predictive markers of asthma exacerbation during stepwise dose reduction of inhaled corticosteroids. Am J Respir Crit Care Med 2001;163(2):406–12.
10. Jatakanon A, Lim S, Barnes PJ. Changes in sputum eosinophils predict loss of asthma control. Am J Respir Crit Care Med 2000;161(1):64–72.
11. Deykin A, Lazarus SC, Fahy JV, et al. Sputum eosinophil counts predict asthma control after discontinuation of inhaled corticosteroids. J Allergy Clin Immunol 2005;115(4):720–7.
12. Stuehr DJ. Mammalian nitric oxide synthases. Biochim Biophys Acta 1999; 1411(2–3):217–30.
13. Dweik RA, Boggs PB, Erzurum SC, et al. An official ATS clinical practice guideline: interpretation of exhaled nitric oxide levels (FENO) for clinical applications. Am J Respir Crit Care Med 2011;184(5):602–15.
14. Gustafsson LE, Leone AM, Persson MG, et al. Endogenous nitric oxide is present in the exhaled air of rabbits, guinea pigs and humans. Biochem Biophys Res Commun 1991;181(2):852–7.
15. American Thoracic Society, European Respiratory Society. ATS/ERS recommendations for standardized procedures for the online and offline measurement of exhaled lower respiratory nitric oxide and nasal nitric oxide, 2005. Am J Respir Crit Care Med 2005;171(8):912–30.
16. Silkoff PE, McClean P, Spino M, et al. Dose-response relationship and reproducibility of the fall in exhaled nitric oxide after inhaled beclomethasone dipropionate therapy in asthma patients. Chest 2001;119(5):1322–8.

17. Jackson DJ, Virnig CM, Gangnon RE, et al. Fractional exhaled nitric oxide measurements are most closely associated with allergic sensitization in school-age children. J Allergy Clin Immunol 2009;124(5):949–53.

18. Kovesi T, Kulka R, Dales R. Exhaled nitric oxide concentration is affected by age, height, and race in healthy 9- to 12-year-old children. Chest 2008;133(1):169–75.

19. Steerenberg PA, Janssen NAH, de Meer G, et al. Relationship between exhaled NO, respiratory symptoms, lung function, bronchial hyperresponsiveness, and blood eosinophilia in school children. Thorax 2003;58(3):242–5.

20. Schilling J, Holzer P, Guggenbach M, et al. Reduced endogenous nitric oxide in the exhaled air of smokers and hypertensives. Eur Respir J 1994;7(3):467–71.

21. Kharitonov SA, Robbins RA, Yates D, et al. Acute and chronic effects of cigarette smoking on exhaled nitric oxide. Am J Respir Crit Care Med 1995;152(2):609–12.

22. Robbins RA, Millatmal T, Lassi K, et al. Smoking cessation is associated with an increase in exhaled nitric oxide. Chest 1997;112(2):313–8.

23. Wagener AH, de Nijs SB, Lutter R, et al. External validation of blood eosinophils, FE(NO) and serum periostin as surrogates for sputum eosinophils in asthma. Thorax 2015;70(2):115–20.

24. Hastie AT, Moore WC, Li H, et al. Biomarker surrogates do not accurately predict sputum eosinophil and neutrophil percentages in asthmatic subjects. J Allergy Clin Immunol 2013;132(1):72–80.

25. Schleich FN, Manise M, Sele J, et al. Distribution of sputum cellular phenotype in a large asthma cohort: predicting factors for eosinophilic vs neutrophilic inflammation. BMC Pulm Med 2013;13:11.

26. Nadif R, Siroux V, Oryszczyn M-P, et al. Heterogeneity of asthma according to blood inflammatory patterns. Thorax 2009;64(5):374–80.

27. Katz LE, Gleich GJ, Hartley BF, et al. Blood eosinophil count is a useful biomarker to identify patients with severe eosinophilic asthma. Ann Am Thorac Soc 2014; 11(4):531–6.

28. Takayama G, Arima K, Kanaji T, et al. Periostin: a novel component of subepithelial fibrosis of bronchial asthma downstream of IL-4 and IL-13 signals. J Allergy Clin Immunol 2006;118(1):98–104.

29. Sidhu SS, Yuan S, Innes AL, et al. Roles of epithelial cell-derived periostin in TGF-β activation, collagen production, and collagen gel elasticity in asthma. Proc Natl Acad Sci U S A 2010;107(32):14170–5.

30. Gordon ED, Sidhu SS, Wang Z-E, et al. A protective role for periostin and TGF-β in IgE-mediated allergy and airway hyperresponsiveness. Clin Exp Allergy 2012; 42(1):144–55.

31. Sehra S, Yao W, Nguyen ET, et al. Periostin regulates goblet cell metaplasia in a model of allergic airway inflammation. J Immunol 2011;186(8):4959–66.

32. Blanchard C, Mingler MK, McBride M, et al. Periostin facilitates eosinophil tissue infiltration in allergic lung and esophageal responses. Mucosal Immunol 2008; 1(4):289–96.

33. Jia G, Erickson RW, Choy DF, et al. Periostin is a systemic biomarker of eosinophilic airway inflammation in asthmatic patients. J Allergy Clin Immunol 2012; 130(3):647–54.e10.

34. Scheerens H, Arron JR, Zheng Y, et al. The effects of lebrikizumab in patients with mild asthma following whole lung allergen challenge. Clin Exp Allergy 2014;44(1): 38–46.

35. Corren J, Lemanske RF, Hanania NA, et al. Lebrikizumab treatment in adults with asthma. N Engl J Med 2011;365(12):1088–98.

36. Noonan M, Korenblat P, Mosesova S, et al. Dose-ranging study of lebrikizumab in asthmatic patients not receiving inhaled steroids. J Allergy Clin Immunol 2013; 132(3):567–74.e12.

37. Hanania NA, Noonan M, Corren J, et al. Lebrikizumab in moderate-to-severe asthma: pooled data from two randomised placebo-controlled studies. Thorax 2015;70(8):748–56.

38. Schade J, Stephan M, Schmiedl A, et al. Regulation of expression and function of dipeptidyl peptidase 4 (DP4), DP8/9, and DP10 in allergic responses of the lung in rats. J Histochem Cytochem 2008;56(2):147–55.

39. Stephan M, Suhling H, Schade J, et al. Effects of dipeptidyl peptidase-4 inhibition in an animal model of experimental asthma: a matter of dose, route, and time. Physiol Rep 2013;1(5):e00095.

40. Cowan DC, Taylor DR, Peterson LE, et al. Biomarker-based asthma phenotypes of corticosteroid response. J Allergy Clin Immunol 2015;135(4):877–83.e1.

41. Wedes SH, Wu W, Comhair SAA, et al. Urinary bromotyrosine measures asthma control and predicts asthma exacerbations in children. J Pediatr 2011;159(2): 248–55.e1.

42. Provost V, Larose M-C, Langlois A, et al. CCL26/eotaxin-3 is more effective to induce the migration of eosinophils of asthmatics than CCL11/eotaxin-1 and CCL24/eotaxin-2. J Leukoc Biol 2013;94(2):213–22.

43. Lamkhioued B, Garcia-Zepeda EA, Abi-Younes S, et al. Monocyte chemoattractant protein (MCP)-4 expression in the airways of patients with asthma. Am J Respir Crit Care Med 2000;162(2):723–32.

44. Ordoñez CL, Shaughnessy TE, Matthay MA, et al. Increased neutrophil numbers and IL-8 levels in airway secretions in acute severe asthma. Am J Respir Crit Care Med 2000;161(4):1185–90.

45. Hastie AT, Moore WC, Meyers DA, et al. Analyses of asthma severity phenotypes and inflammatory proteins in subjects stratified by sputum granulocytes. J Allergy Clin Immunol 2010;125(5):1028–36.e13.

46. Moore WC, Meyers DA, Wenzel SE, et al. Identification of asthma phenotypes using cluster analysis in the severe asthma research program. Am J Respir Crit Care Med 2010;181(4):315–23.

47. Cowan DC, Cowan JO, Palmay R, et al. Effects of steroid therapy on inflammatory cell subtypes in asthma. Thorax 2010;65(5):384–90.

48. Chesné J, Braza F, Mahay G, et al. IL-17 in severe asthma. Where do we stand? Am J Respir Crit Care Med 2014;190(10):1094–101.

49. Krueger JG, Fretzin S, Suárez-Fariñas M, et al. IL-17A is essential for cell activation and inflammatory gene circuits in subjects with psoriasis. J Allergy Clin Immunol 2012;130(1):145–54.e9.

50. Baeten D, Baraliakos X, Braun J, et al. Anti-interleukin-17A monoclonal antibody secukinumab in treatment of ankylosing spondylitis: a randomised, double-blind, placebo-controlled trial. Lancet 2013;382(9906):1705–13.

51. Mease PJ, Genovese MC, Greenwald MW, et al. Brodalumab, an anti-IL17RA monoclonal antibody, in psoriatic arthritis. N Engl J Med 2014;370(24):2295–306.

52. Nanzer AM, Chambers ES, Ryanna K, et al. Enhanced production of IL-17A in patients with severe asthma is inhibited by 1α,25-dihydroxyvitamin D3 in a glucocorticoid-independent fashion. J Allergy Clin Immunol 2013;132(2): 297–304.e3.

53. Irvin C, Zafar I, Good J, et al. Increased frequency of dual-positive TH2/TH17 cells in bronchoalveolar lavage fluid characterizes a population of patients with severe asthma. J Allergy Clin Immunol 2014;134(5):1175–86.e7.

54. Kim HY, Lee HJ, Chang Y-J, et al. Interleukin-17-producing innate lymphoid cells and the NLRP3 inflammasome facilitate obesity-associated airway hyperreactivity. Nat Med 2014;20(1):54–61.

55. Bullens DMA, Truyen E, Coteur L, et al. IL-17 mRNA in sputum of asthmatic patients: linking T cell driven inflammation and granulocytic influx? Respir Res 2006; 7:135.

56. Busse WW, Holgate S, Kerwin E, et al. Randomized, double-blind, placebo-controlled study of brodalumab, a human anti–IL-17 receptor monoclonal antibody, in moderate to severe asthma. Am J Respir Crit Care Med 2013;188(11): 1294–302.

57. Choy DF, Hart KM, Borthwick LA, et al. TH2 and TH17 inflammatory pathways are reciprocally regulated in asthma. Sci Transl Med 2015;7(301):301ra129.

58. Konno S, Taniguchi N, Makita H, et al. Distinct phenotypes of cigarette smokers identified by cluster analysis of patients with severe asthma. Ann Am Thorac Soc 2015;12(12):1771–80. Available at. http://dx.doi.org/10.1513/AnnalsATS.201507-407OC.

59. De Lima Azambuja R, da Costa Santos Azambuja LS, Costa C, et al. Adiponectin in asthma and obesity: protective agent or risk factor for more severe disease? Lung 2015;193(5):749–55.

60. Kostikas K, Koutsokera A, Papiris S, et al. Exhaled breath condensate in patients with asthma: implications for application in clinical practice. Clin Exp Allergy 2008;38(4):557–65.

61. Anderson WC 3rd, Szefler SJ. New and future strategies to improve asthma control in children. J Allergy Clin Immunol 2015;136(4):848–59.

62. Song J-S, You J-S, Jeong S-I, et al. Serum periostin levels correlate with airway hyper-responsiveness to methacholine and mannitol in children with asthma. Allergy 2015;70(6):674–81.

63. Ullmann N, Bossley CJ, Fleming L, et al. Blood eosinophil counts rarely reflect airway eosinophilia in children with severe asthma. Allergy 2013;68(3):402–6.

64. Bossley CJ, Fleming L, Gupta A, et al. Pediatric severe asthma is characterized by eosinophilia and remodeling without TH2 cytokines. J Allergy Clin Immunol 2012;129(4):974–82.e13.

65. Dweik RA, Sorkness RL, Wenzel S, et al. Use of exhaled nitric oxide measurement to identify a reactive, at-risk phenotype among patients with asthma. Am J Respir Crit Care Med 2010;181(10):1033–41.

66. Moore WC, Hastie AT, Li X, et al. Sputum neutrophil counts are associated with more severe asthma phenotypes using cluster analysis. J Allergy Clin Immunol 2014;133(6):1557–63.e5.

67. Kanemitsu Y, Matsumoto H, Izuhara K, et al. Increased periostin associates with greater airflow limitation in patients receiving inhaled corticosteroids. J Allergy Clin Immunol 2013;132(2):305–12.e3.

68. Kim M-A, Izuhara K, Ohta S, et al. Association of serum periostin with aspirin-exacerbated respiratory disease. Ann Allergy Asthma Immunol 2014;113(3): 314–20.

69. Van Veen IH, Ten Brinke A, Gauw SA, et al. Consistency of sputum eosinophilia in difficult-to-treat asthma: a 5-year follow-up study. J Allergy Clin Immunol 2009; 124(3):615–7, 617.e1–2.

70. Peters SP. Counterpoint: is measuring sputum eosinophils useful in the management of severe asthma? No, not for the vast majority of patients. Chest 2011; 139(6):1273–5 [discussion: 1275–8].

71. Woodruff PG, Modrek B, Choy DF, et al. T-helper type 2–driven inflammation defines major subphenotypes of asthma. Am J Respir Crit Care Med 2009;180(5): 388–95.
72. Lötvall J, Akdis C, Bacharier L, et al. Asthma endotypes: a new approach to classification of disease entities within the asthma syndrome. J Allergy Clin Immunol 2011;127(2):355–60.
73. Flood-Page P, Swenson C, Faiferman I, et al. A study to evaluate safety and efficacy of mepolizumab in patients with moderate persistent asthma. Am J Respir Crit Care Med 2007;176(11):1062–71.
74. Haldar P, Brightling CE, Hargadon B, et al. Mepolizumab and exacerbations of refractory eosinophilic asthma. N Engl J Med 2009;360(10):973–84.
75. Nair P, Pizzichini MM, Kjarsgaard M, et al. Mepolizumab for prednisone-dependent asthma with sputum eosinophilia. N Engl J Med 2009;360(10): 985–93.
76. Pavord ID, Korn S, Howarth P, et al. Mepolizumab for severe eosinophilic asthma (DREAM): a multicentre, double-blind, placebo-controlled trial. Lancet 2012; 380(9842):651–9.
77. Bel EH, Wenzel SE, Thompson PJ, et al. Oral glucocorticoid-sparing effect of mepolizumab in eosinophilic asthma. N Engl J Med 2014;371(13):1189–97.
78. Castro M, Mathur S, Hargreave F, et al. Reslizumab for poorly controlled, eosinophilic asthma: a randomized, placebo-controlled study. Am J Respir Crit Care Med 2011;184(10):1125–32.
79. Castro M, Zangrilli J, Wechsler ME, et al. Reslizumab for inadequately controlled asthma with elevated blood eosinophil counts: results from two multicentre, parallel, double-blind, randomised, placebo-controlled, phase 3 trials. Lancet Respir Med 2015;3(5):355–66.
80. Brightling C, Chanez P, Leigh R, et al. Efficacy and safety of tralokinumab in patients with severe uncontrolled asthma: a randomised, double-blind, placebo-controlled, phase 2b trial. Lancet Respir Med 2015;3(9):692–701.
81. Hanania N, Wenzel S, Rosén K, et al. Exploring the effects of omalizumab in allergic asthma. Am J Respir Crit Care Med 2013;187(8):804–11.
82. Jayaram L, Pizzichini MM, Cook RJ, et al. Determining asthma treatment by monitoring sputum cell counts: effect on exacerbations. Eur Respir J 2006;27(3): 483–94.
83. Green RH, Brightling CE, McKenna S, et al. Asthma exacerbations and sputum eosinophil counts: a randomised controlled trial. Lancet 2002;360(9347): 1715–21.
84. Petsky HL, Cates CJ, Lasserson TJ, et al. A systematic review and meta-analysis: tailoring asthma treatment on eosinophilic markers (exhaled nitric oxide or sputum eosinophils). Thorax 2012;67(3):199–208.
85. Fleming L, Wilson N, Regamey N, et al. Use of sputum eosinophil counts to guide management in children with severe asthma. Thorax 2012;67(3):193–8.
86. Lu M, Wu B, Che D, et al. FeNO and asthma treatment in children: a systematic review and meta-analysis. Medicine 2015;94(4):e347.
87. Chung K, Wenzel S, Brozek J, et al. International ERS/ATS guidelines on definition, evaluation and treatment of severe asthma. Eur Respir J 2013;43(2):343–73.

Eosinophilic Endotype of Asthma

Fernando Aleman, MD[a], Hui Fang Lim, MBBS, MRCP(UK)[b],
Parameswaran Nair, MD, PhD, FRCP, FRCPC[c],*

KEYWORDS

• Asthma • Eosinophil • Sputum • Airway inflammation • Endotype

KEY POINTS

• Eosinophilic asthma is an endotype whereby eosinophils play a central effector role in the pathophysiology of the condition rather than being just one of many cells that may be present in the airway.

• Although there is no general consensus, a diagnosis of eosinophilic asthma may be made if the absolute eosinophil count is 400/μL or greater in blood or 3% or greater in sputum on more than one occasion, particularly during exacerbations.

• At the moment, sputum examination is the most reliable and valid method to identify the eosinophilic endotype and can be effectively used to monitor asthma control and guide therapeutic decisions.

• When persistently elevated ($\geq$400/μL), blood eosinophil counts may also be used to identify eosinophilic asthma and predict the response to corticosteroids. However, there is still insufficient evidence to recommend the use of fraction of exhaled nitric oxide (FeNO), immunoglobulin E, or periostin to guide decisions in clinical practice.

• Inflammatory phenotyping of severe asthmatic patients is essential for therapy optimization. Identification of eosinophilic asthma allows provision of targeted therapies to suppress eosinophilic inflammation, which effectively improve lung function and reduce symptoms and exacerbations.

Asthma is a chronic disorder characterized by variable airflow limitation and airway hyperresponsiveness and an associated chronic inflammation of the airways. As our understanding of the pathophysiological mechanisms that lead to these processes advances, we recognize several clinical endotypes, particularly depending on the type of airway inflammation, severity, and response to treatment.[1] The most predominant and clearly described endotype is eosinophilic asthma, which accounts for

Dr P. Nair is supported by a Canada Research Chair in Airway Inflammometry.
[a] Division of Respirology, St Joseph's Healthcare Hamilton, McMaster University, Hamilton, Ontario, Canada; [b] Department of Respiratory Medicine, National University of Singapore, Singapore, Singapore; [c] Division of Respirology, St Joseph's Healthcare Hamilton, McMaster University, 50 Charlton Avenue East, Hamilton, Ontario L8N 4A6, Canada
* Corresponding author.
E-mail address: parames@mcmaster.ca

approximately 50% to 60% of the total asthma population. Most of these patients can be controlled on moderate to high doses of inhaled corticosteroids (ICS), but 5% to 10% have severe disease that requires oral corticosteroids to control the eosinophilic airway inflammation.[1] This article is a brief overview of the definition, identification, natural history, and implications of treatment of eosinophilic asthma. The mechanisms that contribute to airway eosinophilia are not discussed in detail in this article.

DEFINITION OF EOSINOPHILIC ASTHMA

The definition is arbitrary. It is probably best considered as an endotype whereby eosinophils play a central effector role in the development of the physiological abnormalities that characterize the condition rather than being just one of many cells that may be present in the airway. It may be difficult to establish this; the main indication that eosinophils are the dominant cells responsible for the pathophysiological changes of the disease in a particular patient may be the demonstration that eosinophils are persistently increased and activated in the blood and airway (sputum, broncho alveolar lavage, or bronchial mucosa or submucosa) when asthma is severe or uncontrolled[2] and that treatments aimed at decreasing the number and activity of eosinophils in the airways improve lung function and reduce symptoms and exacerbations.[3] There is no general consensus on what defines *persistence* and what the appropriate cutoff levels are in various body compartments. It seems reasonable to consider a demonstration of an absolute eosinophil count of 400/µL or greater in blood or 3% or greater in sputum on more than one occasion, particularly at the time of an exacerbation, to consider an eosinophilic endotype of asthma. It is logical that these numbers that represent the upper-limit-of-normal values are determined by the dose corticosteroids that these patients are on at the time of assessment.

DIAGNOSIS OF EOSINOPHILIC ASTHMA

Demonstration of eosinophils in the airways would be the most direct evidence of an eosinophilic endotype of asthma. This presence can be demonstrated in the tissue (bronchial mucosa or submucosa) or in the lumen (in bronchial wash, bronchoalveolar lavage, or in sputum).

Bronchial Mucosal and BAL Eosinophils

The histopathologic examination of a bronchial-biopsy specimen would perhaps be the most accurate method to demonstrate the presence of eosinophils in the airway epithelium and submucosa. However, because this involves an invasive procedure, it is impractical in routine clinical practice for monitoring over periods of time and to evaluate patients at the time of exacerbations. The correlation between eosinophils in the various airway compartments is poor.[4] This poor correlation is not surprising given that BAL samples the peripheral airways, whereas bronchial wash and sputum represent a mixture of small and more proximal larger airways. Further, the quantification of eosinophils in BAL and in bronchial submucosa is not standardized and, therefore, difficult to compare between laboratories. More or less, if the BAL and tissue show abundant eosinophil numbers, they are likely to be increased in sputum as well. The converse may not be true.[5] More importantly, sputum (airway luminal) eosinophil numbers correlated more with clinical parameters of asthma control, for example, the number of exacerbations, than tissue eosinophil numbers.[5] This correlation is perhaps not surprising, given that eosinophils are activated when they move from one compartment to another and are more activated in the airway lumen than in tissue (or in circulation).[6]

Sputum Eosinophil

The development and implementation of techniques to safely and reliably induce and examine sputum have provided opportunities to study the characteristics of airway inflammation in clinical patients, emphasizing the heterogeneity of airway inflammation in asthma.[1] Sputum examination is currently the most comprehensive and noninvasive method for measuring airway inflammation.[7] Sputum induction with hypertonic saline is safe even in patients with a forced expiratory volume in the first second of expiration as low as 0.9L,[8] and it is successful in approximately 80% of patients with asthma.[1,9] The method for sputum collection,[10] processing and quantification of cell counts,[11] is well described and standardized; its reliability, validity, and responsiveness have been proven.[12] Normal values have been established for sputum cell counts, and guidelines for adjusting treatment based on sputum examination are available.[13] Although the 90th percentile in normal individuals is 1.2%, a sputum percentage of 3% or greater is often considered to be clinically relevant. In addition to the intact cell differential, perhaps markers of activation, such as eosinophil free granules, or the level of granular proteins (eg, eosinophil peroxidase) are just as or more important; this requires further investigation.[14]

Blood Eosinophil Counts

The relationship between blood and sputum eosinophil counts has been recently reviewed.[15] If the blood eosinophil counts are consistently elevated (the consensus seems to be $\geq 400/\mu L$), this probably indicates a pathobiological and clinical relevance. Indeed, this level of eosinophilia seems to relate to more asthma-related events,[16] response to therapy with corticosteroids,[17] and to more specific anti–interleukin 5 (IL-5) directed therapies.[18–21]

Circulating eosinophil numbers and their correlation with airway eosinophils and clinical relevance may depend on the dose of corticosteroids that patients are on and the time of sampling (given the significant diurnal variation).[22] Although blood eosinophils may be correlated with sputum eosinophils in mild to moderate asthma, the same may not be true in severe asthma. It is traditionally thought that eosinophils are produced in the bone marrow and then travel through the blood to reach inflammatory sites, guided by cytokines, such as IL-5. Although this may be true in mild to moderate steroid-responsive eosinophilic asthma, recent studies suggest that local differentiation, maturation, and activation of eosinophils in the airways, driven by IL-5 and IL-13 that are locally produced by relatively steroid-insensitive type 2 innate lymphoid cells (ILC-2s), may contribute to persistent sputum eosinophilia in severe prednisone-dependent patients who may have normal blood eosinophils. This finding may be true even in patients who may be on anti–IL-5 therapy if the dose of the drug is inadequate.[23]

Other Methods to Identify the Eosinophilic Phenotype

FeNO is possibly the most widely used method in clinical practice for the evaluation of airway inflammation because of the availability of a Food and Drug Administration–approved device (NIOX, Aerocrine, Sweden) that made it possible to standardize the method.[13] Although, FeNO has been suggested as a potential biomarker for eosinophilic bronchitis, the degree of correlation between FeNO and sputum eosinophils is usually low[24]; a cutoff value of 42 ppb or greater (determined to have the best combination of sensitivity and specificity) still has a modest positive predictive value (74%) and overall accuracy (78%) to detect a sputum cell count of greater than 3%.[22] However, FeNO could potentially be more accurate when identifying patients who have both sputum and blood eosinophilia.[9] In any case, there is insufficient evidence to suggest that FeNO can be used to optimize therapy and improve outcomes in asthma in the more severe patients, who are those who need biomarkers to guide their therapy. A systematic review found that tailoring treatment based on FeNO failed to reduce the number of exacerbations, both in adults and children, and could potentially be harmful, as it was associated with higher ICS doses in the pediatric studies.[25]

Periostin

Periostin is a matricellular protein that is secreted by bronchial epithelial cells in response to several stimuli, notably IL-13.[26] It has been suggested as a biomarker for eosinophilic asthma, based on observations that periostin is significantly correlated with sputum eosinophils and that serum levels greater than 25 ng/mL have a positive predictive value of 93% to detect tissue or luminal eosinophilia.[27,28] However, another study[22] was unable to replicate those results but suggested that periostin could be used to identify phenotypes that have a T2-high cytokine profile and not necessarily the classic Th2-high signature that would be characterized by the persistent sputum and blood eosinophil at cutoff levels that have been discussed in this review with eosinophils being a major effector cell in those patients. A lower level of eosinophils, in association with increased periostin or FeNO (a reflection of increased epithelia inducible nitric oxide synthase activity), may be surrogates of an epithelial dysfunction with eosinophils not being the major effector cell or IL-5 not being the dominant cytokine.

Metabolomics

Metabolomics is the study of biochemical molecules derived from cellular metabolic pathways. It is currently being developed and evaluated for application in routine clinical practice as a noninvasive method to assess airway inflammation. So far, it has been used in research settings for the analysis of exhaled breath volatile organic compounds (VOCs) and urine metabolites.[13] Several recent studies have obtained promising results. Van der Schee and colleagues[29] found that an electronic nose, by analyzing exhaled breath VOC profiles, could differentiate between asthmatic patients and healthy controls with almost the same accuracy of FeNO and sputum eosinophils and had greater accuracy to predict the response to steroid treatment. Similarly, Wedes and colleagues[30] found that urine bromotyrosine, a byproduct of eosinophil peroxidase activity, was associated with asthma control and was able to predict exacerbations more accurately than other parameters, such as FeNO.

Gene Expression Biomarkers

This technique is another novel method that can be used in asthma to identify an eosinophil endotype. Baines and colleagues[31] found a 6-gene expression biomarker signature that can accurately identify the eosinophilic phenotype and is superior to sputum eosinophils in predicting responsiveness to ICS treatment. Further development of this polymerase chain reaction–based method might provide a fast, simple, and readily available test for the identification of eosinophilic asthma. In addition, special efforts have been made to develop point-of-care tests that will be able to identify eosinophilic asthma in the clinical setting and aid in the management of patients. The Unbiased Biomarkers for the Prediction of Respiratory Disease Outcomes (U-BIO-PRED) aims to identify a series of biomarkers that would allow classifying patients into different asthma phenotypes. The application of these handprints, together with the development of new technologies, may allow the development of quick tests that would be applicable in routine clinical practice.

PREVALENCE, STABILITY, AND NATURAL HISTORY OF THE EOSINOPHILIC ASTHMA PHENOTYPE

Eosinophilic asthma accounts for approximately 50% to 60% of the total severe asthma population and is, therefore, the most common phenotype (**Fig. 1**).[1,32,33] There are conflicting data on the stability of asthma phenotypes over time. A prospective cohort revealed that eosinophilia was a persistent feature in 70% of the patients over a period of 5 years.[34] Similarly, a longitudinal study on 3320 asthmatic adults using cluster-based methods showed that stability persisted in 54% to 88% of the clusters after 10 years.[35]

However, a retrospective survey revealed that, in patients who had 2 or more sputum examinations, the inflammatory phenotype remained consistent in only 23% of patients.[2] Large cohort studies, such as the Pan-European BIOAIR cohort[36] and the British Thoracic Society (BTS) Severe Asthma Registry,[37] similarly reported that only 40% to 50% of asthma phenotypes remained stable overtime. The stability of the severe asthma phenotype defined by physiological parameters seemed to be more stable than those defined by biomarkers such as sputum or blood eosinophil and FeNO (48.6% vs 30.0%).[36] Similarly the BTS data showed that overall phenotype stability was 52%, ranging from 25% in the late-onset with obesity cluster to 71% late-onset eosinophilic cluster. Hence, it would seem that the stability of asthma phenotypes depends largely on the methods used to define the phenotype. Further, the use of corticosteroids may change the prevalence of the eosinophilic phenotype. As demonstrated by Cowan and colleagues,[38] most patients would develop airway eosinophilia when the dose of steroids is reduced. However, as discussed earlier, this does not necessarily mean that in those patients eosinophils are the key effector cells contributing to symptoms and exacerbations. Additionally, the type of bronchitis can change during exacerbations, as observed by D'Silva and colleagues.[39] Therefore, patients with eosinophilic asthma can still develop neutrophilic bronchitis during exacerbations, if the cause is a bronchial infection.

McGrath and colleagues[40] assessed the prevalence of eosinophilic asthma in patients who underwent multiple sputum examinations and found that 22% of the patients had eosinophilia on every occasion (persistent eosinophilia), 31% had eosinophilia on at least 1 occasion (intermittent eosinophilia), and 47% never had eosinophilia (persistent noneosinophilia). Overall, 53% had eosinophilia on at least 1 sputum examination, which would be consistent with the prevalence of 40% to 50% that was reported for eosinophilic asthma by previous studies. However,

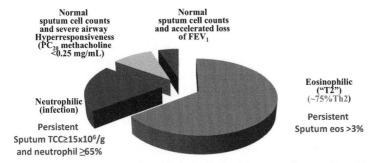

Fig. 1. Prevalence of endotypes (defined by sputum quantitative cell counts) in 132 patients with severe asthma at the Firestone Institute for Respiratory Health in Hamilton, ON. 67% patients had persistent sputum eosinophils. 15% patients has persistent intense sputum neutrophilia (5% of these were associated with eosinophils). The rest has normal sputum cell counts on multiple occasions, a proportion of whom has severe airway hyperresponsiveness.

eosinophilic asthma is defined in this review as eosinophilic bronchitis on at least 2 occasions. McGrath and colleagues[40] did not provide information on the proportion of patients who had eosinophilic bronchitis on at least 2 occasions, so it is difficult to ascertain the prevalence of the eosinophilic endotype based on the definition provided in this review. In any case, intermittent eosinophilic asthma is still included within the spectrum of eosinophilic asthma, but it may represent a milder form of the disease. This study highlighted the importance of performing measurements on multiple occasions, particularly at the time of exacerbations. McGrath and colleagues[40] also reported a high prevalence of neutrophilic bronchitis within the persistently noneosinophilic group, both in steroid-treated and steroid-untreated patients. Currently, there is still debate on whether neutrophils are involved in the pathophysiology of noneosinophilic asthma or whether they are only present as a consequence of infections or the use of corticosteroids.[41]

It is not currently known if persistent eosinophilic bronchitis can lead to fixed airflow obstruction (chronic obstructive pulmonary disease). Previous studies have found an association between persistent sputum eosinophilia and chronic airflow limitation, suggesting that persistent inflammation can lead to narrowing of the airways.[42] In fact, eosinophils may play a role in the remodeling process in the airways by secreting molecule, such as eosinophilic cationic protein, transforming growth factor (TGF-β), and other cytokines.[43] At least one study found that steroid-unresponsive eosinophilic inflammation, and the subsequent high concentrations of TGF-β, correlated with the thickness of the basement membrane in airway biopsy specimens.[44] If demonstrated, the implication of persistent eosinophilic inflammation in the development of fixed airflow obstruction could have important implications for the management and prognosis of eosinophilic asthma. It remains to be seen whether aggressive treatment to control eosinophilic inflammation can slow down the decline in lung function.

MECHANISMS THAT MAY CONTRIBUTE TO A PERSISTENT EOSINOPHILIC ENDOTYPE

Traditionally, asthma is thought to be a disease driven by T-helper type 2 (T_H2), associated with allergic sensitization and adaptive immunity pathways driven by cytokines, such as IL-4, IL-5, and IL-13, finally converging on the end-target cell, the eosinophil.[45] In recent years, mounting evidence suggests that other pathways and cells might contribute to the recruitment of eosinophils into blood and airway. Cells associated with the innate immunity, such as ILCs, have been discovered to express both IL-5 and IL-13[23]; they are intrinsically steroid resistant. The T_H17 pathway was traditionally thought to be associated with steroid-resistant neutrophilic inflammation and negatively regulated by T_H2 cytokines. However, Choy and colleagues[46] demonstrated in a cross-sectional study that T_H2 and T_H17 gene expression were mutually exclusive; T_H2 and T_H17 signatures were both associated with eosinophilic inflammation. Importantly, treatment targeting both pathways in a murine model conferred greater therapeutic efficacy than by simply targeting the T_H2 pathway. Hence, the eosinophil is not simply the representative target of a T_H2-driven pathway and should be thought of as a marker of steroid-sensitive disease that may be due to ILC and T_H17 cells and their mediators.

Other cells have the ability to produce cytokines that have been traditionally associated with T_H2 cells. For this reason, type 2 asthma has emerged as a new nomenclature, in order to acknowledge the substantial production of type 2 cytokines by cells such as natural killer lymphocytes,[47] invariant T cells, eosinophil and basophil progenitor cells, and ILC-2s, in addition to the classic Th2 cells. Therefore, under this new concept Th2 cells have become a part of type 2 inflammation. By secreting cytokines, such as IL-4, IL-13, IL-5, IL-9, and IL-10, these cells contribute to the development of the features that characterize type 2 asthma, such as elevated FeNO and high immunoglobulin E (IgE) and periostin levels.[48]

The Clinical Relevance of Identifying an Eosinophilic Endotype

Most of the current therapeutic recommendations are based on assessment of symptoms and spirometry, even when these correlate poorly with the type or degree of airway inflammation.

Inflammatory phenotyping of asthmatic patients is important for therapy optimization.[25] Although the eosinophilic phenotype of asthma responds well to corticosteroid treatment, noneosinophilic asthma has little or no response.[49] Strategies that are based on sputum examination to guide treatment decisions have been effective in improving lung function and decreasing asthma symptoms and exacerbations, and this has been achieved without increasing the dose of ICS or oral corticosteroid.[25] By tailoring corticosteroid treatment according to the level of eosinophilic bronchitis, sputum examination allows to avoid overtreatment in patients who do not have airway eosinophils and increase the dose of steroids in patients who do have uncontrolled eosinophilic bronchitis, both during clinically stable conditions and during exacerbations. In addition, sputum examination can detect an increase in airway eosinophils up to 3 months before the development of a clinical exacerbation.[50] This ability allows opportunely adjusting steroid treatment and, thus, preventing eosinophilic exacerbations.[51] Sputum eosinophil count also provides an effective method to identify patients who will benefit from targeted therapy with anti–IL-5 monoclonal antibodies (mAbs).[3,52] The effectiveness of a treatment strategy based on assessment of airway inflammation was not as clear in patients with mild asthma, suggesting that sputum examination may be only necessary in moderate to severe asthma.[25,51]

Corticosteroids are currently the mainstay of treatment of asthma, so it is recommended to commence all asthmatic patients on ICS. Patients who remain uncontrolled and have blood eosinophils of 400/μL or greater should be assessed for noncompliance, inadequate inhaler technique, ongoing allergen exposure, and comorbidities (chronic rhinosinusitis, vocal cord dysfunction, gastroesophageal reflux disease). If all causes for uncontrolled asthma are ruled out and blood eosinophils are persistently elevated, the ICS dose should be increased. Patients who remain uncontrolled on high-dose ICS should be assessed for airway eosinophilia (Th2) and other T2 markers, such as serum periostin, IgE, and FeNO. If blood and sputum eosinophils are elevated despite high-dose ICS, prednisone should be considered; these patients would be potential candidates for anti–IL-5 mAb therapies. In some instances, blood and sputum eosinophils will remain controlled, but T2 markers, such as periostin, will be elevated. These patients may be considered for anti–IL-13 mAb therapies, but at the moment there is insufficient evidence to support this recommendation.

SUMMARY

In recent years, advances in the knowledge about the pathophysiology of airway diseases have revealed that asthma is a complex and heterogeneous disease. For this reason, it is helpful to classify patients with moderate to severe refractory asthma into endotypes, with the intention to provide therapies that will specifically target the pathophysiological abnormalities of their disease.

Although there is no consensus on a specific definition of the eosinophilic endotype, a particular patient can be determined to have eosinophilic asthma if there is documented evidence of elevated sputum (>3%) and/or blood ($\geq$400/μL) eosinophils on at least 2 occasions (particularly when the symptoms are severe or uncontrolled) and if treatment strategies aimed at suppressing eosinophils (ICS, oral corticosteroids, or anti–IL-5 mAbs) are effective in controlling symptoms and exacerbations. This information would be considered as proof that eosinophils play a central role in the pathophysiology of the disease, which is ultimately what characterizes the eosinophilic endotype of asthma.

Currently, the most sensitive and reliable method to diagnose eosinophilic asthma is eosinophil counts on sputum examination. If this is not available, peripheral blood eosinophil counts may be useful, particularly if they are elevated ($\geq 400/\mu L$). However, it is important to keep in mind that normal blood eosinophils do not rule out eosinophilic bronchitis. This is particularly true in patients with severe asthma, who are more likely to have dissociation between blood and sputum eosinophil counts. Other biomarkers may also have the ability to identify patients with T2 inflammation, but at the moment there is insufficient evidence to advocate for their use in clinical practice. In addition, the emergence of new technologies has allowed for the development of proteomics and gene expression biomarkers, among others, which have yielded promising results. In the future, these technologies may give rise to point-of-care tests that would facilitate the identification and management of asthmatic patients in routine clinical practice.

REFERENCES

1. D'Silva L, Hassan N, Wang HY, et al. Heterogeneity of bronchitis in airway diseases in tertiary care clinical practice. Can Respir J 2011;18(3):144–8.
2. Bousquet J, Chanez P, Lacoste JY, et al. Eosinophilic inflammation in asthma. N Engl J Med 1990;323(15):1033–9.
3. Nair P, Pizzichini M, Kjarsgaard M. Mepolizumab for prednisone-dependent asthma with sputum eosinophilia. N Engl J Med 2009;360:985–93.
4. Pavord I, Pizzichini MM, Pizzichini E, et al. The use of induced sputum to investigate airway inflammation. Thorax 1997;52(6):498–501.
5. Lemiere C, Ernst P, Olivenstein R, et al. Airway inflammation assessed by invasive and noninvasive means in severe asthma: eosinophilic and noneosinophilic phenotypes. J Allergy Clin Immunol 2006;118(5):1033–9.
6. Persson C, Uller L. Primary lysis of eosinophils as a major mode of activation of eosinophils in human diseased tissues. Nat Rev Immunol 2013;13(12):902.
7. Djukanović R, Sterk PJ, Fahy JV, et al. Standardised methodology of sputum induction and processing. Eur Respir J 2002;20(37 Suppl):1s–2s.
8. Vlachos-Mayer H, Leigh R, Sharon RF, et al. Success and safety of sputum induction in the clinical setting. Eur Respir J 2000;16(5):997–1000.
9. Schleich FN, Chevremont A, Paulus V, et al. Importance of concomitant local and systemic eosinophilia in uncontrolled asthma. Eur Respir J 2014;44(1):97–108.
10. Popov TA. Some technical factors influencing the induction of sputum for cell analysis. Eur Respir J 1995;8:559–65.
11. Kelly MM, Efthimiadis A, Hargreave FE. Induced sputum : selection method. Methods Mol Med 2001;56:77–91.
12. Djukanovic R. Standardized methodology of sputum induction and processing. Eur Respir J Suppl 2002;37:1s–2s.
13. Nair P. Update on clinical inflammometry for the management of airway diseases. Can Respir J 2013;20(2):117–20.
14. Persson C, Uller L. Theirs but to die and do: primary lysis of eosinophils and free eosinophil granules in asthma. Am J Respir Crit Care Med 2014;189(6):628–33.

15. Mukherjee M, Nair P. Blood or sputum eosinophils to guide asthma therapy? Lancet Respir Med 2015;3(11):824–5.
16. Price DB, Rigazio A, Campbell JD, et al. Blood eosinophil count and prospective annual asthma disease burden: a UK cohort study. Lancet Respir Med 2015; 3(11):849–58.
17. Brightling CE, Green RH, Pavord ID. Biomarkers predicting response to corticosteroid therapy in asthma. Treat Respir Med 2005;4(5):309–16.
18. Bel EH, Wenzel SE, Thompson PJ, et al. Oral glucocorticoid-sparing effect of mepolizumab in eosinophilic asthma. N Engl J Med 2014;371(13):1189–97.
19. Castro M, Mathur S, Hargreave F, et al. Reslizumab for poorly controlled, eosinophilic asthma. Am J Respir Crit Care Med 2011;184(10):1125–32.
20. Castro M, Wenzel SE, Bleecker ER, et al. Benralizumab, an anti-interleukin 5 receptor α monoclonal antibody, versus placebo for uncontrolled eosinophilic asthma: a phase 2b randomised dose-ranging study. Lancet Respir Med 2014; 2(11):879–90.
21. Castro M, Zangrilli J, Wechsler M, et al. Reslizumab for inadequately controlled asthma with elevated blood eosinophil counts: results from two multicentre, parallel, double-blind, randomised, placebo-controlled, phase 3 trials. Lancet Respir Med 2015;3:355–66.
22. Wagener AH, de Nijs SB, Lutter R, et al. External validation of blood eosinophils, FENO and serum periostin as surrogates for sputum eosinophils in asthma. Thorax 2015;70(2):115–20.
23. Smith SG, Chen R, Kjarsgaard M, et al. Increased numbers of activated group 2 innate lymphoid cells in the airways of patients with severe asthma and persistent airway eosinophilia. J Allergy Clin Immunol 2016;137(1):75–86.e8.
24. Hastie AT, Moore WC, Li H, et al. Biomarker surrogates do not accurately predict sputum eosinophil and neutrophil percentages in asthmatic subjects. J Allergy Clin Immunol 2013;132(1):72–80.
25. Petsky HL, Cates CJ, Lasserson TJ, et al. A systematic review and meta-analysis: tailoring asthma treatment on eosinophilic markers (exhaled nitric oxide or sputum eosinophils). Thorax 2012;67(3):199–208.
26. Sidhu SS, Yuan S, Innes AL, et al. Roles of epithelial cell-derived periostin in TGF-beta activation, collagen production, and collagen gel elasticity in asthma. Proc Natl Acad Sci U S A 2010;107(32):14170–5.
27. Woodruff PG, Boushey HA, Dolganov GM, et al. Genome-wide profiling identifies epithelial cell genes associated with asthma and with treatment response to corticosteroids. Proc Natl Acad Sci U S A 2007;104(40):15858–63.
28. Jia G, Erickson RW, Choy DF, et al. Periostin is a systemic biomarker of eosinophilic airway inflammation in asthmatic patients. J Allergy Clin Immunol 2012; 130(3):647–54.e10.
29. van der Schee MP, Palmay R, Cowan JO, et al. Predicting steroid responsiveness in patients with asthma using exhaled breath profiling. Clin Exp Allergy 2013; 43(11):1217–25.
30. Wedes SH, Wu W, Comhair SA, et al. Urinary bromotyrosine measures asthma control and predicts asthma exacerbations in children. J Pediatr 2011;159(2): 248–55.e1.
31. Baines KJ, Simpson JL, Wood LG, et al. Sputum gene expression signature of 6 biomarkers discriminates asthma inflammatory phenotypes. J Allergy Clin Immunol 2014;133:997–1007.
32. Wenzel SE. Asthma: defining of the persistent adult phenotypes. Lancet 2006; 368(9537):804–13.

33. Haldar P, Pavord ID. Noneosinophilic asthma: a distinct clinical and pathologic phenotype. J Allergy Clin Immunol 2007;119(5):1043–52 [quiz: 1053–4].

34. van Veen IH, Wu W, Comhair SA, et al. Consistency of sputum eosinophilia in difficult-to-treat asthma: a 5-year follow-up study. J Allergy Clin Immunol 2009; 124(3):615–7, 617.e1–2.

35. Boudier A, Curjuric I, Basagaña X, et al. Ten-year follow-up of cluster-based asthma phenotypes in adults. A pooled analysis of three cohorts. Am J Respir Crit Care Med 2013;188(5):550–60.

36. Kupczyk M, Dahlén B, Sterk PJ, et al. Stability of phenotypes defined by physiological variables and biomarkers in adults with asthma. Allergy 2014;69(9): 1198–204.

37. Newby C, Heaney LG, Menzies-Gow A, et al. Statistical cluster analysis of the British Thoracic Society severe refractory asthma registry: clinical outcomes and phenotype stability. PLoS One 2014;9(7):e102987.

38. Cowan DC, Cowan JO, Palmay R, et al. Effects of steroid therapy on inflammatory cell subtypes in asthma. Thorax 2010;65(5):384–90.

39. D'Silva L, Cook RJ, Allen CJ, et al. Changing pattern of sputum cell counts during successive exacerbations of airway disease. Respir Med 2007;101(10):2217–20.

40. McGrath KW, Icitovic N, Boushey HA, et al. A large subgroup of mild-to-moderate asthma is persistently noneosinophilic. Am J Respir Crit Care Med 2012;185(6): 612–9.

41. Nair P, Aziz-Ur-Rehman A, Radford K. Therapeutic implications of 'neutrophilic asthma'. Curr Opin Pulm Med 2015;21(1):33–8.

42. ten Brinke A, Zwinderman AH, Sterk PJ, et al. Factors associated with persistent airflow limitation in severe asthma. Am J Respir Crit Care Med 2001;164(5):744–8.

43. Kay AB, Phipps S, Robinson DS. A role for eosinophils in airway remodelling in asthma. Trends Immunol 2004;25(9):477–82.

44. Wenzel SE, Schwartz LB, Langmack EL, et al. Evidence that severe asthma can be divided pathologically into two inflammatory subtypes with distinct physiologic and clinical characteristics. Am J Respir Crit Care Med 1999;160:1001–8.

45. Pelaia G, Vatrella A, Maselli R. The potential of biologics for the treatment of asthma. Nat Rev Drug Discov 2012;11(12):958–72.

46. Choy DF, Hart KM, Borthwick LA, et al. TH2 and TH17 inflammatory pathways are reciprocally regulated in asthma. Sci Transl Med 2015;7(301):301ra129.

47. Umetsu DT, DeKruyff RH. A role for natural killer T cells in asthma. Nat Rev Immunol 2006;6(12):953–8.

48. Hinks TS, Zhou X, Staples KJ, et al. Innate and adaptive T cells in asthmatic patients: relationship to severity and disease mechanisms. J Allergy Clin Immunol 2015;136(2):323–33.

49. Pizzichini MM, Pizzichini E, Parameswaran K. Non-asthmatic chronic cough: no effect of treatment with an inhaled corticosteroid in patients without sputum eosinophilia. Can Respir J 1999;6(4):323–30.

50. Deykin A, Lazarus SC, Fahy JV, et al. Sputum eosinophil counts predict asthma control after discontinuation of inhaled corticosteroids. J Allergy Clin Immunol 2005;115(4):720–7.

51. Jayaram L, Pizzichini MM, Cook RJ, et al. Determining asthma treatment by monitoring sputum cell counts: effect on exacerbations. Eur Respir J 2006;27(3): 483–94.

52. Haldar P, Brightling CE, Hargadon B, et al. Mepolizumab and exacerbations of refractory eosinophilic asthma. N Engl J Med 2009;360(10):973–84.

Neutrophilic and Pauci-immune Phenotypes in Severe Asthma

Reynold A. Panettieri Jr, MD*

KEYWORDS

- Irreversible airway obstruction • Airway remodeling • Nonatopic asthma
- Steroid insensitivity • Intrinsic asthma

KEY POINTS

- Although T-helper type 2 inflammation evokes airway hyperresponsiveness and narrowing, neutrophilic or pauci-immune asthma accounts for significant asthma morbidity.
- Viruses, toxicants, environmental tobacco smoke exposure, and bacterial infections induce asthma exacerbations that are mediated by neutrophilic inflammation or by neurogenic, nonimmune mechanisms.
- Neutrophilic and pauci-immune phenotypes manifest steroid insensitivity.

INTRODUCTION

Airway obstruction, inflammation, and hyperresponsiveness define asthma. This complex syndrome, however, manifests marked heterogeneity in characterizing disease severity and in response to therapy. About 61% of adult patients with asthma exhibit allergen sensitivities or atopy, and 39% manifest little evidence of allergic disease.[1] Surprisingly, the precise mechanisms that regulate nonallergic asthma, traditionally known as intrinsic asthma, remain an enigma.

Asthma exacerbations substantially contribute globally to morbidity, mortality, and health care costs.[2] Allergens, viruses, environmental tobacco smoke (ETS), and air pollution exposure commonly trigger exacerbations. Some but not all triggers respond to conventional therapy that includes oral glucocorticoids (GCs).[3,4] After allergen exposure, T-helper type 2 (T_H2) inflammation orchestrated by trafficking CD4 positive lymphocytes and eosinophils and by activation of mast cells induces airway obstruction that reverses on treatment with GCs. Other triggers, such as ETS, ozone, or viruses, induce neutrophilic inflammation or directly modulate airway epithelial,

Clinical & Translational Science, Rutgers Institute for Translational Medicine & Science, Robert Wood Johnson Medical School, University of Pennsylvania, Philadelphia, PA, USA
* Child Health Institute of New Jersey, Rutgers, The State University of New Jersey, 89 French Street, Suite 4210, New Brunswick, NJ 08901.
E-mail address: rp856@ca.rutgers.edu

Immunol Allergy Clin N Am 36 (2016) 569–579
http://dx.doi.org/10.1016/j.iac.2016.03.007   immunology.theclinics.com
0889-8561/16/$ – see front matter © 2016 Elsevier Inc. All rights reserved.

smooth muscle, or neural cell function to evoke airway hyperresponsiveness (AHR) and obstruction that is steroid insensitive.[2,5,6] Presumably, the direct effects of these triggers on airway structural cells may not induce typical T_H2 inflammatory responses. The lack of airway inflammatory cells or biomarkers in the presence of airway obstruction and AHR defines pauci-immune or pauci-granulocytic asthma.[7] Characterization of novel therapeutic approaches targeting neutrophilic or pauci-immune asthma may have a profound impact on decreasing asthma exacerbations.

Using unbiased statistical approaches, evidence now suggests that patients with asthma can be grouped into specific clusters. Cluster analyses organize patient data (blood samples, pulmonary function testing, and so forth) in a manner that demonstrates that some groups of patients are more similar than others according to mean vector connectivity (k-means algorithm).[7] Investigators have identified asthma clusters manifested by predominant neutrophilic inflammation, pauci-immune asthma, and steroid insensitivity disease.[7] Collectively, evidence suggests that some asthma exacerbations and specific asthma cohorts at baseline manifest predominantly neutrophilic or pauci-immune phenotypes.

PATHOPHYSIOLOGY
Neutrophilic Asthma

Neutrophilic asthma characterizes a clinical syndrome manifested by limited numbers of eosinophils in the airways or peripheral circulation, nonatopy, rhinosinusitis with sleep disturbances, ETS exposure, and gastroesophageal reflux disease.[8–10] Diagnostically, total sputum cell counts and neutrophil numbers are increased in comparison with those of healthy patients or patients with atopic asthma. Sputum neutrophil numbers, however, poorly correlate with methacholine responsiveness, whereas neutrophil numbers inversely correlate with pulmonary function.[10,11] In bronchial alveolar lavage (BAL) and bronchial biopsies, numbers of neutrophils increase with more severe disease.[12–15] Evidence also suggests that sputum neutrophil numbers are associated with a progressive loss of lung function.[10,11] Because GCs increase neutrophil numbers in tissue and peripheral blood, the diagnosis can be complicated when patients are prescribed high-dose inhaled or oral steroids.[16] Given the efficacy of steroids to increase neutrophilia, this can serve as a biomarker of oral steroid adherence.

Sputum analyses unfortunately require sophisticated training, and limited availability hampers their clinical use. Discovery of novel biomarkers to identify patients with neutrophilic asthma will foster precision approaches to improve therapy. Levels of neutrophil-derived mediators (leukotriene B_4 [LTB_4], granulocyte-macrophage colony-stimulating factor [GM-CSF], tumor necrosis factor α [TNFα], interleukin [IL]-17A, IL-8, elastase, or matrix metalloproteinase 9 [MMP-9]) are detectable in BAL fluid and plasma in patients with severe neutrophilic asthma.[13,15,17–19] Unlike eosinophilic asthma, systemic inflammation as measured by increased blood levels of IL-8, IL-6, C-reactive protein, and IL-17A was also reported in patients with severe neutrophilic asthma.[20] Although such blood levels hold promise, to date there exist no valid or reliable serum biomarkers to diagnose neutrophilic asthma.

Neutrophils play pivotal roles in innate immunity.[16] Conventional thought suggests that neutrophils primarily traffic to inflamed sites and then secrete granular enzymes, reactive oxygen species, and proteins to eliminate invading bacteria, fungal elements, and viruses. The 6- to 8-hour limited life span of the circulating neutrophil is consistent with this immune-surveillance function.[21] Evidence also shows that some neutrophils survive much longer with life spans of 3 to 5 days, especially in tissue.[14,22,23] Further, neutrophils can return to the circulation via lymphatics and reverse migration through vascular endothelium.[24–26] These observations suggest a more complex role of the neutrophil in modulating local inflammatory responses apart from host defense as shown in **Fig. 1**.

The differential life span of tissue and circulating neutrophils suggests that these cells manifest varied functional phenotypes as shown in **Table 1**. Tissue-based neutrophils have decreased apoptosis, mediated in part by granulocyte–CSF, GM-CSF, interferon (IFN)-γ, IL-13, LTB_4, and lipopolysaccharide (LPS).[14] Pertinent to severe asthma, some neutrophil subsets express FcγRIII (CD16) and FcϵRI and inhibit T-cell proliferation in a Mac-1- and H_2O_2-dependent manner.[27,28] These neutrophils still retain key innate effector cell functions, such as eliminating microbes.[29] Recruitment and retention of mucosal neutrophils are also facilitated by T_H17 cells, a subset of T helper lymphocytes releasing IL-17 that induces secretion of IL-8 by airway epithelium.[30] Interestingly, IL-17 and IL-8 secretion is insensitive to GCs, a hallmark of severe neutrophilic asthma.[25] In mice, neutrophils also transdifferentiate to express CD11a, CD11b, CD11c, HLA-DR, CD80, and CD86, acquiring an antigen-presenting cell phenotype (neutrophil/dendritic hybrid).[31] Whether such a transitional phenotype exists in severe asthma remains unknown. Collectively, these observations suggest that neutrophils can modulate adaptive responses and provide novel therapeutic targets for further exploration.

In chronic disease, repetitive injury of the airways from allergens, viruses, and toxicants in asthma evokes remodeling that increases matrix deposition, airway smooth muscle (ASM) mass, mucus gland hypertrophy, and angiogenesis.[2,5,6] Whether these remodeling events induce irreversible airway obstruction remains controversial.[6] Activated neutrophils secrete TGF-β, MMP-9, elastase and myeloperoxidase.[11] In the BAL, MMP-9 levels correlate with neutrophil counts in asthma.[32] Conceptually, neutrophils may play a role in promoting airway remodeling, but this remains unclear.

Pauci-immune Asthma

Considerable research efforts have focused on studying the molecular mechanisms regulating eosinophilic and allergic asthma, whereas less is known regarding neutrophilic asthma; the pathogenesis of pauci-immune asthma remains unexplored. The availability of trafficking cells and soluble mediators provides investigators with a platform to study allergic and neutrophilic asthma, whereas pauci-immune disease may involve intrinsic alterations in structural cell function (epithelium, smooth muscle, vessels, and nerves) that pose experimental challenges.

Although intrinsic abnormalities of airway epithelium and smooth muscle in asthma remain controversial, compelling evidence suggests that airway epithelium, smooth muscle, and nerves can orchestrate and perpetuate airway inflammation.[2,6] Airway epithelium and smooth muscle also secrete a variety of paracrine or autocrine factors that modulate cellular functions, such as agonist-induced shortening, secretion, and migration.[5] Conceivably, an intrinsic alteration in structural cells may promote a phenotype consistent with pauci-immune asthma. Using cultured airway epithelium or smooth muscle from patients with severe asthma, these cells retain attributes of hypersecretion and hyperresponsiveness. ASM derived from fatal asthma subjects as compared with age- and sex-matched controls manifests greater proliferation to growth factors and shortening in response to agonists.[33–35] Importantly, the ASM growth is insensitive to GCs. Cultured airway epithelium from patients with asthma also manifests a dysfunctional repair mechanism.[36] Epithelium and ASM secrete a plethora of cytokines, chemokines, prostaglandins, and eicosanoids that potentially modulates airway function. In ASM, TNFα and type 1 and 2 IFN evoke secretion of

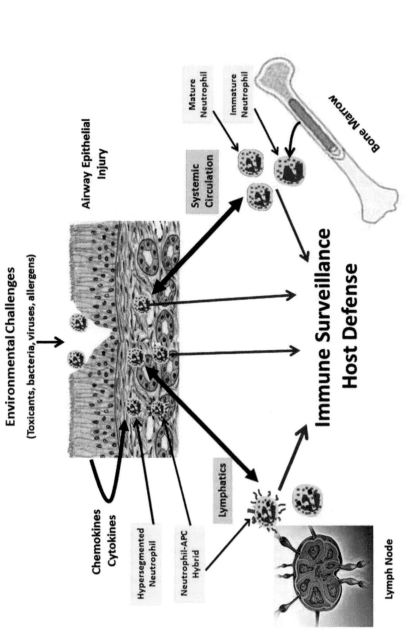

Fig. 1. Neutrophil subsets mediate immune surveillance and host defense. Evidence suggests that neutrophil subsets may mediate differential effects on immune surveillance and microbial killing. A variety of epithelial insults (ozone, bacteria, and viruses) induce secretion of chemokines and cytokines that promote neutrophil trafficking. Most circulating neutrophils are a mature phenotype (neu-2). On injury, other phenotypes appear, namely, neu-1, the immature or band neutrophil, and neu-3, the hypersegmented neutrophil. During asthma exacerbations, the presence of chemokines and cytokines (IL-8, IL-17A, and so forth) prolongs the life span of the neutrophil and modulates T₂ and innate immune responses. The prolonged life span also

Table 1 Neutrophil subsets manifest specific phenotypes			
Neutrophil Attributes	**Immature**	**Mature**	**Hypersegmented**
Nuclei morphology	Band	Segmented	Multilobed
L-selectin (CD62L)[a]	+	+	−
FcγRIII (CD16)[a]	−	+	+
T-cell suppression	−	−	+
Life span	Hours	Hours	Days
Neutrophil-APC hybrid	−	−	+
Activated*	−	−	+
Microbial killing	−	+	+

Abbreviation: APC, antigen-presenting cell.
 * Activated: Capable of endocytosis, neutrophil extracellular net formation, and MPO and MMP-9 production.
 [a] Cell surface expression.

IL-6 and IL-8 that is insensitive to GCs.[37–40] In airway epithelium and ASM, cytokine stimulation of intracellular adhesion molecule 1 (ICAM-1) expression is also steroid insensitive; ICAM-1 is the primary cell surface receptor for rhinovirus infectivity.[2,37–41] The steroid insensitivity of chemokine and cytokine expression in these structural cells parallels that described in neutrophilic asthma. Although little is known concerning the pathogenesis of pauci-immune asthma, mounting evidence in vitro and ex vivo suggests that intrinsic abnormalities exist in structural cells in asthma. The lack of efficacy of GCs in modulating structural cell function highlights the need for novel, non-GC therapeutic targets to manage pauci-immune asthma.

Therapeutic Approaches

To date, there are no approved therapies for neutrophilic and pauci-immune asthma. Traditionally, clinicians prescribe combined therapies of inhaled GCs and long-acting bronchodilators as a cornerstone of medical management. Unfortunately, conventional approaches often fail to improve pulmonary function or functional status in these patients; both syndromes are steroid insensitive.[42]

In neutrophilic asthma, the presence of submucosal or airway neutrophils implies that targeting the trafficking or activation state of the neutrophil would be therapeutically advantageous. Strategies to modulate neutrophil function include inhibition of chemokine receptors (CXCR2 antagonists); blockade of TNFα, IL-6, or IL-17; kinase inhibition (p38MAPK, PI3K-δ/γ, JAK, or PDE4); or macrolides. Most of these approaches remain investigational.

Neutrophil migration is orchestrated by chemokines (CXCL1 [GRO-a], CXCL5 [ENA-78], CXCL8 [IL-8], and LTB_4) that activate G-protein coupled receptors CXCR2 or, in the case of LTB_4, the LTB_4 receptor 2.[16] Conceptually, inhibition of these receptors would decrease neutrophil trafficking and inflammation. In chronic obstructive pulmonary disease (COPD), CXCR2 inhibition significantly decreased sputum neutrophils but only modestly decreased mild exacerbations and had little effect on pulmonary function.[43] In severe asthma, CXCR2 inhibition induced significant decreases in circulating neutrophils but had no effect on pulmonary function or quality-of-life measures.[44] To date, inhibition of 5-lipoxygenase that generates LTB_4 and LTD_4 offers therapeutic benefit in triad asthma associated with aspirin sensitivity and nasal polyps; the relative contribution of LTB_4 and LTD_4 in improving patients' outcomes in neutrophilic asthma remains unknown. Despite the attractiveness of inhibiting neutrophil chemotaxis, the lack of clinical improvements and the possibility for neutropenia with immunosuppression limit the therapeutic value of this target in asthma.

Levels of TNFα, IL-6, or IL-17 are increased in either the blood or sputum of patients with neutrophilic asthma.[11,16] Accordingly, binding free circulating cytokines or inhibition of the cognate receptor could improve clinical outcomes in neutrophilic asthma. Using monoclonal antibodies targeting either TNFα or IL-17, there were marginal therapeutic benefits in the treatment of severe asthma.[45-47] Whether these agents would be effective in neutrophilic asthma remains unknown because the clinical trials were not designed to assess efficacy in this cohort of subjects.

Intracellular kinases (p38MAPK, JNK, PI3K-δ/γ, and JAK) and phosphodiesterases (PDEs) amplify extracellular signals via a variety of receptors to modulate cell proliferation, chemokine and cytokine production, apoptosis, and steroid sensitivity. Each of these kinases or PDEs selectively modulates neutrophil secretion, diapedesis, and apoptosis.[11,16] Although most intracellular kinase inhibitors are being developed for COPD, these agents may also have value in neutrophilic asthma.[42] Evidence suggests that p38MAPK and JNK1 also phosphorylate the GC receptor and impair its translocation into the nucleus that is necessary to mediate GCs' antiinflammatory effects.[42] Using in vitro model systems, inhibition of p38MAPK or JNK1 reverses steroid insensitivity.[42] Whether these mechanisms are physiologically relevant in neutrophilic asthma remains hypothetical. Given the ubiquitous expression of intracellular kinases, inhibition of p38MAPK, JNK, PI3K-δ/γ, and JAK may evoke undesirable consequences, such as immunosuppression or malignancy.

PDEs degrade cAMP or cGMP and decrease activation of protein kinase A or G, respectively. In some cells, cAMP or cGMP act intracellularly as antiinflammatory signaling molecules; accordingly, inhibition of PDEs that increase cAMP and cGMP levels would enhance antiinflammatory responses.[42] In neutrophils, T cells, and macrophages, PDE4 are the dominant isoform. Studies in COPD showed that roflumilast, a PDE4 inhibitor, improved neutrophil-mediated airway inflammation and decreased exacerbations[48]; whether such effects would have therapeutic benefit in neutrophilic asthma remains unknown.

In patients with severe asthma, macrolide antibiotics used to treat chronic indolent infections with atypical bacteria (Mycoplasma pneumonia or Chlamydia pneumonia) improved patient-reported outcomes.[49,50] Whether neutrophilic asthma, however, is due to chronic infection remains controversial. Apart from the antiinfective actions of macrolide antibiotics, these agents potentially act as antiinflammatory agents. Evidence suggests that macrolides inhibit nuclear factor–κB activation and secretion of CXCL8 and promote phagocytosis.[51,52] In severe asthma with neutrophilic inflammation, azithromycin reduced sputum neutrophil counts and CXCL8 levels with improved patient-reported outcomes.[53,54] Overall, the current speculation that macrolide antibiotics may be beneficial in neutrophilic asthma and the low risk of complications justify a 6-month clinical trial in select patients prone to exacerbations.

The therapeutic benefit of combined long-acting beta agonists and anticholinergic agents is now established in COPD. Recent evidence also supports the addition of antimuscarinic agents in the treatment of severe asthma.[42] Whether these approaches would have preferential effects in neutrophilic or pauci-immune asthma as compared with those in eosinophilic asthma remains unknown. Few if any studies have focused on therapeutic approaches in pauci-immune asthma. Over the past 5 years, the use of bronchial thermoplasty (BT) in severe asthma has gained significant interest. BT segmentally delivers thermal energy to the airway in a manner that ultimately decreases ASM mass in the proximal airways.[55] The therapeutic improvement in exacerbations was sustained for at least 5 years.[56] Other studies now show that BT also modulates mucosal inflammatory responses and collagen deposition.[57–59] Because patients who undergo BT are poor candidates for T_H2 or immunoglobulin E monoclonal antibody therapies or have failed such approaches, BT may become the treatment of choice for neutrophilic or pauci-immune severe asthma. Further prospective studies, however, are needed to demonstrate efficacy in these cohorts.

Current Controversies

Despite research efforts to therapeutically target neutrophilic asthma, few approaches have substantially improved patient outcomes.[11,16,42] Further, clinicians, when challenged by a refractory patient, often prescribe oral GCs to improve control. Unfortunately, this approach promotes neutrophil survival and increases neutrophil numbers, resulting in a diagnostic conundrum. Our failure to show therapeutic efficacy of novel agents in neutrophilic asthma poses interesting hypotheses that the global inhibition of neutrophils in the circulation or airways may be inappropriate. As discussed in this review, compelling evidence suggests that subsets of neutrophils can serve a negative homeostatic function to suppress inflammation, whereas other subsets may promote antigen presentation and amplify T_H2 inflammation.[11,16] A greater appreciation for the heterogeneity of neutrophil responses and subsets may foster awareness that global targeting of neutrophil activation or trafficking will be futile. Potentially, improved phenotyping of patients with neutrophilic asthma will identify those whose diseases are driven by specific neutrophil subsets to predict therapeutic responses.

Our lack of understanding of the pathogenesis, therapy, and prognosis of pauci-immune asthma represents a profound unmet need. Challenges exist in characterizing structural cell function in asthma that impedes research progress; improved noninvasive imaging may provide opportunities to deep phenotype patients to devise and predict responses to new therapeutic agents.

FUTURE CONSIDERATIONS/SUMMARY

Asthma manifests as a heterogeneous syndrome characterized in part by reversible airway obstruction and inflammation. Although our understanding of eosinophil- and T_H2-mediated inflammation in asthma has improved, our knowledge remains inadequate regarding neutrophilic or pauci-immune disease. The recognition that the neutrophil may play an important role in mediating the asthma diathesis has identified novel therapeutic targets to mitigate neutrophil activation or migration. Although some drugs are early in development, evidence suggests that these targets may not uniformly offer therapeutic efficacy in neutrophilic asthma. Because heterogeneity exists among neutrophil subsets, research paradigms must consider that the global inhibition of neutrophil activation and migration may be inadequate to address the unmet therapeutic need. Improved characterization of neutrophil subsets and the development of accurate biomarkers to predict response to treatment will likely improve clinical outcomes. In pauci-immune asthma, the challenge of studying structural cell abnormalities, which are likely pivotal in mediating this syndrome, poses obstacles to our understanding of the pathogenesis and development of precision therapeutic approaches. Because neutrophilic and pauci-immune asthma are steroid insensitive, the increased use of inhaled or systemic steroids may have little therapeutic benefit while inducing significant adverse effects.

REFERENCES

1. Knudsen TB, Thomsen SF, Nolte H, et al. A population-based clinical study of allergic and non-allergic asthma. J Asthma 2009;46(1):91–4.
2. Koziol-White CJ, Panettieri RA Jr. Airway smooth muscle and immunomodulation in acute exacerbations of airway disease. Immunol Rev 2011;242:178–85.
3. Athens JW, Haab OP, Raab SO, et al. Leukokinetic studies. IV. The total blood, circulating and marginal granulocyte pools and the granulocyte turnover rate in normal subjects. J Clin Invest 1961;40:989–95.
4. Hetherington SV, Quie PG. Human polymorphonuclear leukocytes of the bone marrow, circulation, and marginated pool: function and granule protein content. Am J Hematol 1985;20:235–46.
5. Damera G, Panettieri RA Jr. Does airway smooth muscle express an inflammatory phenotype in asthma? Br J Pharmacol 2011;163(1):68–80.
6. Damera G, Panettieri RA. Irreversible airway obstruction in asthma: what we lose, we lose early. Allergy Asthma Proc 2014;35(2):111–8.
7. Chung KF. Defining phenotypes in asthma: a step towards personalized medicine. Drugs 2014;74(7):719–28.
8. Baines KJ, Simpson JL, Wood LG, et al. Systemic upregulation of neutrophil alpha-defensins and serine proteases in neutrophilic asthma. Thorax 2011; 66(11):942–7.
9. Douwes J, Gibson P, Pekkanen J, et al. Non-eosinophilic asthma: importance and possible mechanisms. Thorax 2002;57(7):643–8.
10. Simpson JL, Baines KJ, Ryan N, et al. Neutrophilic asthma is characterised by increased rhinosinusitis with sleep disturbance and GERD. Asian Pac J Allergy Immunol 2014;32(1):66–74.
11. Shaw DE, Berry MA, Hargadon B, et al. Association between neutrophilic airway inflammation and airflow limitation in adults with asthma. Chest 2007;132(6): 1871–5.
12. Louis R, Lau LC, Bron AO, et al. The relationship between airways inflammation and asthma severity. Am J Respir Crit Care Med 2000;161(1):9–16.
13. Teran LM, Campos MG, Begishvilli BT, et al. Identification of neutrophil chemotactic factors in bronchoalveolar lavage fluid of asthmatic patients. Clin Exp Allergy 1997;27(4):396–405.
14. Uddin M, Nong G, Ward J, et al. Prosurvival activity for airway neutrophils in severe asthma. Thorax 2010;65(8):684–9.
15. Wenzel SE, Szefler SJ, Leung DY, et al. Bronchoscopic evaluation of severe asthma. Persistent inflammation associated with high dose glucocorticoids. Am J Respir Crit Care Med 1997;156(3 Pt 1):737–43.
16. Bruijnzeel PL, Uddin M, Koenderman L. Targeting neutrophilic inflammation in severe neutrophilic asthma: can we target the disease-relevant neutrophil phenotype? J Leukoc Biol 2015;98(4):549–56.
17. Jatakanon A, Uasuf C, Maziak W, et al. Neutrophilic inflammation in severe persistent asthma. Am J Respir Crit Care Med 1999;160(5 Pt 1):1532–9.
18. Simpson JL, Grissell TV, Douwes J, et al. Innate immune activation in neutrophilic asthma and bronchiectasis. Thorax 2007;62(3):211–8.
19. Uddin M, Lau LC, Seumois G, et al. EGF-induced bronchial epithelial cells drive neutrophil chemotactic and anti-apoptotic activity in asthma. PLoS One 2013; 8(9):e72502.
20. Wood LG, Baines KJ, Fu J, et al. The neutrophilic inflammatory phenotype is associated with systemic inflammation in asthma. Chest 2012;142(1):86–93.

21. Shi J, Gilbert GE, Kokubo Y, et al. Role of the liver in regulating numbers of circulating neutrophils. Blood 2001;98(4):1226–30.

22. Dancey JT, Deubelbeiss KA, Harker LA, et al. Neutrophil kinetics in man. J Clin Invest 1976;58(3):705–15.

23. Pillay J, Kamp VM, van Hoffen E, et al. A subset of neutrophils in human systemic inflammation inhibits T cell responses through Mac-1. J Clin Invest 2012;122(1): 327–36.

24. Buckley CD, Ross EA, McGettrick HM, et al. Identification of a phenotypically and functionally distinct population of long-lived neutrophils in a model of reverse endothelial migration. J Leukoc Biol 2006;79(2):303–11.

25. Bullens DM, Truyen E, Coteur L, et al. IL-17 mRNA in sputum of asthmatic patients: linking T cell driven inflammation and granulocytic influx? Respir Res 2006;7:135.

26. Woodfin A, Voisin MB, Beyrau M, et al. The junctional adhesion molecule JAM-C regulates polarized transendothelial migration of neutrophils in vivo. Nat Immunol 2011;12(8):761–9.

27. Gounni AS, Lamkhioued B, Koussih L, et al. Human neutrophils express the high-affinity receptor for immunoglobulin E (Fc epsilon RI): role in asthma. FASEB J 2001;15(6):940–9.

28. Maletto BA, Ropolo AS, Alignani DO, et al. Presence of neutrophil-bearing antigen in lymphoid organs of immune mice. Blood 2006;108(9):3094–102.

29. Geng S, Matsushima H, Okamoto T, et al. Emergence, origin, and function of neutrophil-dendritic cell hybrids in experimentally induced inflammatory lesions in mice. Blood 2013;121(10):1690–700.

30. Cosmi L, Annunziato F, Galli MIG, et al. CRTH2 is the most reliable marker for the detection of circulating human type 2 Th and type 2 T cytotoxic cells in health and disease. Eur J Immunol 2000;30(10):2972–9.

31. Matsushima H, Geng S, Lu R, et al. Neutrophil differentiation into a unique hybrid population exhibiting dual phenotype and functionality of neutrophils and dendritic cells. Blood 2013;121(10):1677–89.

32. Mann BS, Chung KF. Blood neutrophil activation markers in severe asthma: lack of inhibition by prednisolone therapy. Respir Res 2006;7:59.

33. Banerjee A, Damera G, Bhandare R, et al. Vitamin D and glucocorticoids differentially modulate chemokine expression in human airway smooth muscle cells. Br J Pharmacol 2008;155(1):84–92.

34. Black JL, Panettieri RA Jr, Banerjee A, et al. Airway smooth muscle in asthma: just a target for bronchodilation? Clin Chest Med 2012;33(3):543–58.

35. Damera G, Fogle HW, Lim P, et al. Vitamin D inhibits growth of human airway smooth muscle cells through growth factor-induced phosphorylation of retinoblastoma protein and checkpoint kinase 1. Br J Pharmacol 2009;158:1429–41.

36. Davies DE. Epithelial barrier function and immunity in asthma. Ann Am Thorac Soc 2014;11(Suppl 5):S244–51.

37. Amrani Y, Lazaar AL, Panettieri RA Jr. Up-regulation of ICAM-1 by cytokines in human tracheal smooth muscle cells involves an NF-kB-dependent signaling pathway that is only partially sensitive to dexamethasone. J Immunol 1999;163: 2128–34.

38. Bhandare R, Damera G, Banerjee A, et al. Glucocorticoid receptor interacting protein-1 restores glucocorticoid responsiveness in steroid-resistant airway structural cells. Am J Respir Cell Mol Biol 2010;42(1):9–15.

39. Tliba O, Panettieri RA Jr, Tliba S, et al. TNF-a differentially regulates the expression of pro-inflammatory genes in human airway smooth muscle cells by activation of IFN-b-dependent CD38 pathway. Mol Pharmacol 2004;66:322–9.
40. Tliba O, Tliba S, Huang CD, et al. TNFalpha modulates airway smooth muscle function via the autocrine action of Ifnbeta. J Biol Chem 2003;278(50):50615–23.
41. Ammit AJ, Lazaar AL, Irani C, et al. Tumor necrosis factor-a-induced secretion of RANTES and interleukin-6 from human airway smooth muscle cells: modulation by glucocorticoids and b-agonists. Am J Respir Cell Mol Biol 2002;26:465–74.
42. Barnes PJ. Therapeutic approaches to asthma-chronic obstructive pulmonary disease overlap syndromes. J Allergy Clin Immunol 2015;136(3):531–45.
43. Magnussen H, Watz H, Sauer M, et al. Safety and efficacy of SCH527123, a novel CXCR2 antagonist, in patients with COPD. Eur Respir J 2010;36(Suppl):38S.
44. Nair P, Gaga M, Zervas E, et al. Safety and efficacy of a CXCR2 antagonist in patients with severe asthma and sputum neutrophils: a randomized, placebo-controlled clinical trial. Clin Exp Allergy 2012;42(7):1097–103.
45. Al-Ramli W, Prefontaine D, Chouiali F, et al. T(H)17-associated cytokines (IL-17A and IL-17F) in severe asthma. J Allergy Clin Immunol 2009;123(5):1185–7.
46. Chesne J, Braza F, Mahay G, et al. IL-17 in severe asthma. Where do we stand? Am J Respir Crit Care Med 2014;190(10):1094–101.
47. Wenzel SE, Barnes PJ, Bleecker ER, et al. A randomized, double-blind, placebo-controlled study of tumor necrosis factor-alpha blockade in severe persistent asthma. Am J Respir Crit Care Med 2009;179(7):549–58.
48. Calverley PM, Rabe KF, Goehring UM, et al. Roflumilast in symptomatic chronic obstructive pulmonary disease: two randomised clinical trials. Lancet 2009;374(9691):685–94.
49. Kraft M, Cassell GH, Pak J, et al. Mycoplasma pneumoniae and Chlamydia pneumoniae in asthma: effect of clarithromycin. Chest 2002;121(6):1782–8.
50. Sutherland ER, King TS, Icitovic N, et al. A trial of clarithromycin for the treatment of suboptimally controlled asthma. J Allergy Clin Immunol 2010;126(4):747–53.
51. Hodge S, Hodge G, Brozyna S, et al. Azithromycin increases phagocytosis of apoptotic bronchial epithelial cells by alveolar macrophages. Eur Respir J 2006;28(3):486–95.
52. Kobayashi Y, Wada H, Rossios C, et al. A novel macrolide solithromycin exerts superior anti-inflammatory effect via NF-kappaB inhibition. J Pharmacol Exp Ther 2013;345(1):76–84.
53. Brusselle GG, Vanderstichele C, Jordens P, et al. Azithromycin for prevention of exacerbations in severe asthma (AZISAST): a multicentre randomised double-blind placebo-controlled trial. Thorax 2013;68(4):322–9.
54. Simpson JL, Powell H, Boyle MJ, et al. Clarithromycin targets neutrophilic airway inflammation in refractory asthma. Am J Respir Crit Care Med 2008;177(2):148–55.
55. Castro M, Rubin AS, Laviolette M, et al. Effectiveness and safety of bronchial thermoplasty in the treatment of severe asthma: a multicenter, randomized, double-blind, sham-controlled clinical trial. Am J Respir Crit Care Med 2010;181(2):116–24.
56. Wechsler ME, Laviolette M, Rubin AS, et al. Bronchial thermoplasty: long-term safety and effectiveness in patients with severe persistent asthma. J Allergy Clin Immunol 2013;132(6):1295–302.
57. Chakir J, Haj-Salem I, Gras D, et al. Effects of bronchial thermoplasty on airway smooth muscle and collagen deposition in asthma. Ann Am Thorac Soc 2015;12:1612–8.

58. Denner DR, Doeing DC, Hogarth DK, et al. Airway inflammation after bronchial thermoplasty for severe asthma. Ann Am Thorac Soc 2015;12(9):1302–9.
59. Panettieri RA Jr. Bronchial thermoplasty: targeting structural cells in severe persistent asthma. Ann Am Thorac Soc 2015;12(11):1593–4.

Traditional Therapies for Severe Asthma

Eileen Wang, MD, MPH[a,b], Flavia C.L. Hoyte, MD[a,b],*

KEYWORDS

- Severe asthma • Controller therapies • Add-on therapies • Guidelines
- Nonbiologic therapies • Expert Panel Report 3 (EPR-3)
- Global Initiative for Asthma (GINA)
- European Respiratory Society and American Thoracic Society (ERS/ATS)

KEY POINTS

- Management of severe asthma can be difficult and requires consideration of multiple contributing factors, including adherence and comorbidities.
- Choosing therapies for severe asthma is not straightforward, in large part because therapeutic trials often target mild to moderate asthmatics and because there are frequently conflicting data for the application of these therapies in severe asthmatics.
- Severe asthma is a heterogeneous disease. As various phenotypes and endotypes are better understood, tailored and/or targeted therapies should help improve disease outcomes, efficacy, and cost-effectiveness.

INTRODUCTION

The European Respiratory Society and American Thoracic Society (ERS/ATS) guidelines define severe asthma for patients 6 years or older as "asthma which requires treatment with high-dose inhaled corticosteroids (ICSs) plus a second controller [for the previous year] or systemic corticosteroids [for 50% or more of the previous year] to prevent it from becoming 'uncontrolled' or which remains 'uncontrolled' despite this therapy." This definition includes patients who previously received these therapies but discontinued them secondary to inadequate response. These guidelines define uncontrolled asthma as poor symptom control, frequent severe exacerbations, serious exacerbations, and/or airflow limitation.[1]

Disclosure Statement: The authors have no relevant financial or nonfinancial relationships to disclose.
[a] Division of Allergy and Clinical Immunology, Department of Medicine, National Jewish Health, 1400 Jackson Street, Denver, CO 80206, USA; [b] Division of Allergy and Clinical Immunology, Department of Internal Medicine, University of Colorado Hospital, 1635 Aurora Court, Aurora, CO 80045, USA
* Corresponding author. National Jewish Health, 1400 Jackson Street, Denver, CO 80206.
E-mail address: hoytef@njhealth.org

Immunol Allergy Clin N Am 36 (2016) 581–608
http://dx.doi.org/10.1016/j.iac.2016.03.013   immunology.theclinics.com
0889-8561/16/$ – see front matter © 2016 Elsevier Inc. All rights reserved.

Consideration and evaluation of comorbidities and contributory factors are integral in the assessment and management of patients with severe asthma. These include the asthma–chronic obstructive pulmonary disease (COPD) overlap syndrome (see Putcha N, Wise RA: Asthma COPD Overlap Syndrome: Nothing New Under the Sun, in this issue), chronic rhinosinusitis and aspirin-exacerbated respiratory disease (see Katial RK: Chronic Rhinosinusitis and Aspirin Exacerbated Respiratory Disease, in this issue), obesity, chronic infection (see Carr TF, Kraft M: Chronic Infection and Severe Asthma, in this issue), obstructive sleep apnea, vocal cord dysfunction, and gastroesophageal reflux disease (see Rogers L: Role of Sleep Apnea and Gastroesophageal Reflux in Severe Asthma, in this issue). When identified, these conditions must be adequately treated to maximize asthma control for patients with severe asthma. Furthermore, assessment of adherence to therapies and inhaler technique, which can be challenging, are necessary to determine treatment failures and/or inadequate response.[2–4] In addition, cigarette smoking can reduce inhaled[5] and oral corticosteroid (OCS) effectiveness[6] and is associated with worse lung function[7,8] and asthma symptoms.[9] As a result, smoking cessation is an integral part of asthma care. Preventative vaccinations, such as influenza and pneumococcal polysaccharide vaccines, are recommended in patients with asthma.[10]

The National Heart, Lung, and Blood Institute and the World Health Organization collaborated to create the Global Initiative for Asthma (GINA) in 1993. GINA's report, "Global Strategy for Asthma Management and Prevention,"[11] provides recommendations based on review of scientific evidence, is annually updated, and is the foundation of clinical practice guidelines in many countries. In 2014, the report underwent major revisions, which included presenting evidence-based recommendations in a practice-oriented and practical manner, amending the definition of asthma to reflect its heterogeneity, and framing therapeutic options based on phenotypes, patient preference, and risk factors.[11,12]

The Expert Panel Report 3 (EPR-3), commissioned by the National Asthma Education and Prevention Program (NAEPP), was released in 2007 and provides updated recommendations for the management of asthma and asthma exacerbations. EPR-3 details 4 components of asthma: assessment and monitoring, patient education, control of factors contributing to asthma severity, and pharmacologic therapy—the last of which is the focus of this article. Although determination of asthma severity guides initial therapy choices, the report highlights a conceptual shift to focus on the assessment and monitoring of asthma control when adjusting therapy thereafter. The assessment of asthma control is based on 2 factors: impairment—defined as the "frequency and intensity of symptoms and functional limitations" currently or recently experienced—and risk—defined as "the likelihood of either asthma exacerbations, progressive decline in lung function, or risk of adverse effects from medication." As a result, the goals of asthma therapy center on reduction of these 2 factors. Reducing impairment from asthma includes the following: preventing chronic symptoms, reducing need for short-acting β-agonists (SABAs), achieving normal pulmonary function, maintaining the ability to perform normal activity levels, and meeting patients' expectations regarding asthma care. Reduction of risk includes prevention of recurrent exacerbations and loss of lung function, along with reduction of adverse effects of therapy.[13,14]

EPR-3 details stepwise treatment recommendations based on 3 different age groups: 0 to 4 years, 5 to 11 years, and 12 years and older. For the oldest group, steps 5 and 6 reflect the group of patients identified by the ERS/ATS definition of severe asthma (**Tables 1** and **2**). These patients require high-dose ICS (**Table 3**) plus a second controller or systemic corticosteroids. As noted in **Table 3**, per the EPR-3, the classification of high-dose ICS is related to the potential for increased adverse effects rather than increased efficacy.[1] GINA guidelines also contain a table based on similar principles but with some variation of the doses.[11] Preferred therapy for step 5 is high-dose ICS with a long-acting β-agonist (LABA) and consideration of omalizumab for allergic patients. For step 6, preferred therapy is high-dose ICS, LABA, and OCS therapy with consideration of omalizumab for allergic patients.[13,14] **Tables 1** and **2** provide a summary of recommendations from EPR-3, the ERS/ATS guidelines, and GINA for severe asthmatics.

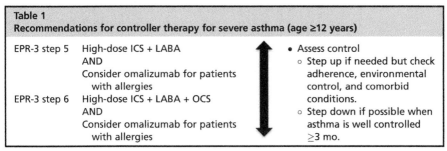

Table 1
Recommendations for controller therapy for severe asthma (age ≥12 years)

EPR-3 step 5	High-dose ICS + LABA AND Consider omalizumab for patients with allergies	• Assess control ○ Step up if needed but check adherence, environmental control, and comorbid conditions.
EPR-3 step 6	High-dose ICS + LABA + OCS AND Consider omalizumab for patients with allergies	○ Step down if possible when asthma is well controlled ≥3 mo.

Abbreviations: ICS, inhaled corticosteroid; OCS, oral corticosteroid; LABA, long-acting beta agonists.
Data from National Asthma Education Prevention Program. Expert Panel Report 3 (EPR-3): guidelines for the diagnosis and management of asthma-summary report 2007. J Allergy Clin Immunol 2007;120(5 Suppl):S94–138.

COMBINATION INHALED CORTICOSTEROID AND LONG-ACTING β-AGONIST THERAPY

For severe asthmatics, NAEPP and GINA guidelines recommend controller therapy to include combination IHC and LABA. Although most of the studies on this class of medications were conducted in patients with moderate asthma, the recommendations have been extrapolated and applied to severe asthmatics. In 1997, the Formoterol and Corticosteroids Establishing Therapy International Study Group conducted a double-blind, randomized trial, which showed that addition of formoterol, a LABA, to budesonide therapy reduced both mild and severe asthma exacerbations.[15] Faurschou and colleagues[16] studied the efficacy and safety of adding on inhaled salmeterol therapy to ICS in asthmatic patients who were not well controlled on high doses of ICS. This multicenter, double-blind, randomized, parallel-group study found that addition of salmeterol improved lung function and reduced asthma symptom scores over addition of albuterol used daily. In 2004, further supporting this data, the Gaining Optimal Asthma Control study—a 1-year, multicenter, international, stratified, randomized, double-blind, parallel-group study—found that subjects with uncontrolled asthma achieved control more rapidly and at a lower corticosteroid dose with combination fluticasone/salmeterol therapy compared with those on fluticasone therapy alone. Furthermore, the combination fluticasone/salmeterol group had lower rates of exacerbations, improved quality-of-life scores, and greater increases in forced expiratory volume in 1 second (FEV_1).[17]

In stable asthma patients on maintenance ICS, Nielson and colleagues[18] showed that addition of salmeterol to ICS therapy resulted in reduced minimal acceptable dose of ICS and less as-needed SABA use. Nelson and colleagues[19] compared combination fluticasone propionate/salmeterol with a combination of fluticasone propionate and oral montelukast and showed better control in the combination ICS/LABA group.

Table 2
Comparison of recommendations for controller therapy for severe asthma (age ≥12 years)

Therapeutic Options	Expert Panel Report 3[13,14]	European Respiratory Society/American Thoracic Society[1]	Global Initiative for Asthma[11]
Combination ICS/LABA	High-dose ICS + LABA are recommended in steps 5 and 6.	Recommend the stepwise increase in the dose of ICS, in combination with a LABA, for improved control.	Recommend optimization of ICS/LABA dose, including considering higher doses of ICS than are routinely recommended for general use. Given the increased risk of systemic side effects, attempt to step down slowly at 3–6 mo intervals.
Long-acting anticholinergic/muscarinic antagonist therapy	—	Note that for adults, tiotropium bromide improved lung function and symptoms in moderate to severe asthmatics not controlled on ICS. Addition of tiotropium bromide improved lung function, decreased SABA use, reduced risk of severe exacerbations in patients on high-dose combination ICS/LABA. Studies lacking in children.	Add-on therapy showed improved lung function and increased time to first exacerbation.
Omalizumab	Consider for patient with allergies.	Recommend a trial in adults and children with severe uncontrolled allergic asthma.	Severe allergic asthmatics with elevated IgE levels may benefit.
Systemic corticosteroids	Before maintenance dose of OCS initiated in step 6, consider a 2-wk course of OCS to confirm clinical reversibility.	Note that optimal timing for addition of OCS therapy and whether continuous low-dose vs multiple discontinuous bursts are better for controlling exacerbations are not well understood.	Some severe asthmatics may benefit from low-dose maintenance OCS treatment, but monitor for and take preventative measures against potential long-term side effects.

Theophylline	Before OCS is introduced in step 6, a trial of adding on theophylline may be considered, although data are lacking.	Note that in moderate asthmatics, theophylline improved asthma control when added to ICS. Possibility that theophylline may improve corticosteroid insensitivity, but no such studies performed in children or adults with severe asthma.	In the small number of available studies, add-on therapy seems of limited benefit.
Antileukotrienes	Before OCS is introduced in step 6, a trial of adding on an antileukotriene may be considered, although data are lacking.	Note that in moderate asthmatics, ICS + montelukast not as effective as ICS + LABA in reducing rate of exacerbations or improving symptoms. In moderate to severe asthma, some studies show addition of antileukotriene to ICS improves lung function and this effect seen in aspirin-sensitive asthma. Conflicting data, however, in another study on asthmatics that did not show benefit with addition of montelukast to ICS and additional therapy.	LTRAs may be helpful for patients found to be aspirin sensitive but otherwise seem of limited benefit.
Allergen immunotherapy	In allergic asthmatics, consider SCIT for steps 2–4 (nonsevere asthma).	—	Potential benefits of SCIT or SLIT must be weighed against the risk of adverse effects, inconvenience, and cost.
Macrolide antibiotics	—	Not recommended in adults or children with severe asthma for treatment of asthma	—
Bronchial thermoplasty	—	Recommend performing in adults with severe asthma only in institutional review board–approved independent systematic registry or clinical study	May be helpful in selected patients with uncontrolled severe asthma despite use of recommended therapeutic regimens, but more studies are needed to identify its efficacy and long-term safety in broader severe asthma populations.

Abbreviations: ICS, inhaled corticosteroid; LTRA, leukotriene receptor antagonists; LABA, long-acting beta agonists; OCS, oral corticosteroid; SABA, short-acting beta agonists; SCIT, subcutaneous immunotherapy; SLIT, sublingual immunotherapy.
Data from Refs.[1,11,13,14]

Table 3
Inhaled corticosteroids

Medication	Formulations	Small-Particle Inhaled Corticosteroids	High Daily Dose (Expert Panel Report 3)[13]	
			5–11 y Old	≥12 y Old
Beclomethasone	40 μg or 80 μg/actuation HFA MDI (QVAR)	✔	>320 μg	>480 μg
Budesonide	90 μg, 180 μg, or 200 μg/ actuation DPI (Pulmicort Flexhaler)	—	>800 μg	>1200 μg
	0.25 mg, 0.5 mg, or 1 mg/2 mL inhalation suspension for nebulization (Pulmicort Respules)	—	2.0 mg	N/A
Ciclesonide	80 μg or 160 μg/actuation HFA (Alvesco)	✔	>160 μg[a,11]	>320 μg[a,11]
Flunisolide	80 μg/actuation HFA MDI with attached spacer (Aerospan)	✔	≥640 μg	>640 μg
Fluticasone propionate	44 μg, 110 μg, or 220 μg/ actuation HFA/MDI (Flovent)	—	>352 μg	>440 μg
	50 μg, 100 μg, or 250 μg/ inhalation DPI (Flovent Diskus)	—	>400 μg	>500 μg
Fluticasone furoate	100 μg or 200 μg/actuation DPI (Arnuity Ellipta)	—	N/A	[b]
Mometasone	110 μg or 220 μg/actuation DPI (Asmanex Twisthaler)	—	≥440 μg[11,a]	>400 μg
	100 μg or 200 μg/actuation HFA MDI (Asmanex)	—	N/A	[b]

Note: Per EPR-3, based on data from comparative clinical trials, "the high dose is the dose that appears likely to be the threshold beyond which significant hypothalamic-pituitary adrenal (HPA) axis suppression is produced, and, by extrapolation, the risk is increased for other clinically significant systemic effects if used for prolonged periods of time."[13]

Abbreviations: DPI, dry powder inhaler; HFA, hydrofluoroalkanes; MDI, metered-dose inhaler; N/A, not applicable either because not approved or indicated for this age.

[a] Data not available from EPR-3.

[b] No data from EPR-3 or GINA.

Data from Global Strategy for Asthma Management and Prevention, Global Initiative for Asthma (GINA). 2015; and National Asthma Education and Prevention Program. Expert Panel Report 3: Guidelines for the Diagnosis and Management of Asthma. Full Report 2007.

Formulations and dosing of combination ICS/LABA inhalers are listed in **Table 4**. All ICS/LABA inhalers require twice-daily dosing except for the Breo Ellipta (fluticasone furoate/vilanterol), which was approved by the US Food and Drug Administration (FDA) in April 2015 for once-daily therapy for asthma in adults, without mention of asthma severity.

Beyond controller therapy, studies have looked at the use of combination ICS/LABA therapy for both controller and rescue therapy, although not currently approved by the FDA for use in the United States. The STAY study was a double-blind, randomized, placebo-group study that looked at children and adults with asthma on ICS therapy and compared 3 groups, 2 of which used terbutaline as rescue therapy (1 with budesonide and the other with budesonide/formoterol as controller therapy) and the last of

Table 4 Combination inhaled corticosteroid/long-acting β-agonist inhalers		
Medication	Formulations	Dosing
Budesonide/formoterol	80 μg/4.5 μg, 160 μg/4.5 μg/ actuation HFA MDI (Symbicort)	2 Puffs twice daily
Fluticasone propionate/ salmeterol	45 μg/21 μg, 115 μg/21 μg, 230 μg/ 21 μg/actuation HFA MDI (Advair)	2 Puffs twice daily
	100 μg/50 μg, 250 μg/50 μg, 500 μg/ 50 μg/actuation DPI (Advair Diskus)	1 Inhalation twice daily
Mometasone/formoterol	100 μg/5 μg, 200 μg/5 μg/actuation HFA MDI (Dulera)	2 Puffs twice daily
Fluticasone furoate/ vilanterol[a]	100 μg/25 μg, 200 μg/25 μg/ actuation DPI (Breo Ellipta)[a]	1 Inhalation once daily

Abbreviations: DPI, dry powder inhaler; HFA, hydrofluoroalkanes; MDI, metered-dose inhaler.
[a] Approved only for adults age 18 and older.

which used combination budesonide/formoterol as both controller and rescue therapy. The latter group demonstrated lower rates of severe exacerbations, increased time to first exacerbation, and improved lung function and symptoms scores.[20,21] In patients receiving budesonide/formoterol maintenance therapy, Rabe and colleagues[22] compared 3 reliever strategies: SABA (terbutaline), rapid-onset LABA (formoterol), and budesonide/formoterol in a randomized, double-blind, parallel-group study. They found increased time to first severe exacerbation, decreased rates of severe exacerbations, decreased nighttime awakenings, decreased reliever use, and decreased mean asthma symptom scores for those using budesonide/formoterol for relief compared with both terbutaline and formoterol.

Numerous studies have also looked at adjustable maintenance dosing of combination ICS/LABA therapy, which allows patients to step up and step down therapy based on control of symptoms. In comparison with fixed maintenance dosing, they noted that adjustable maintenance dosing of combination ICS/LABA therapy resulted in various clinical outcomes, including a lower rate of exacerbations, lower costs, decreased use of ICS/LABA therapy, improved health-related quality of life, and decreased nocturnal awakenings.[23–29] In contrast, a randomized, multicenter study by Busse and colleagues[30] did not show any difference in control or lung function comparing adjustable versus fixed-dose budesonide/formoterol and fixed-dose fluticasone propionate/salmeterol. Although not adopted in the United States, use of ICS/LABA for maintenance and relief has been adopted in other countries and is part of the GINA guidelines.[11]

Although data supporting the efficacy of combination ICS/LABA maintenance therapy in severe asthmatics have been robust, there remains concern regarding the safety of LABA therapy. The Salmeterol Multicenter Asthma Research Trial (SMART), which began in 1996 and published its results in 2006, studied the safety of salmeterol xinafoate when added to usual asthma care. It was a 28-week, randomized, double-blind, placebo-controlled, observational study with 26,355 subjects. The study found a small but significant increase in respiratory-related deaths and asthma-related deaths in subjects receiving salmeterol compared with placebo. The increased risk was predominantly found in African Americans in the subgroup analysis.[31]

As a result, in 2005, the FDA issued a black box warning on salmeterol (Serevent) and combination fluticasone/salmeterol (Advair) regarding the SMART study's findings of a small but significantly increased risk of asthma-related deaths. Review of various case-control, retrospective, and prospective studies, however, including the SMART study, by experts, such as Dr Harold Nelson, the SMART study's first author, raised questions as to the nature of this association. He noted that the findings were in asthmatics on LABA without ICS and there was insufficient evidence in those on combination ICS/LABA therapy.[32,33] To further evaluate the safety of LABAs in combination with ICS for the treatment of asthma, the FDA has required manufacturers of LABAs to conduct 5 randomized, double-blind, controlled clinical trials comparing the addition of LABAs to ICS versus ICS alone. The trials, 4 of which are in adolescent and adult subjects and 1 of which is in the pediatric population, started in 2011, with expected results in 2017.[34]

LONG-ACTING ANTICHOLINERGIC/MUSCARINIC ANTAGONIST THERAPY

Tiotropium is a long-acting muscarinic antagonist that is widely used in COPD patients. In September 2014, Spiriva Respimat (tiotropium) was accepted by the regulatory authorities in the European Union as an add-on maintenance bronchodilator therapy in adult asthmatics already on ICS/LABA therapy but still uncontrolled with 1 or more severe exacerbations in the previous year. Subsequently, in September 2015, the FDA approved Spiriva Respimat for once-daily, maintenance treatment of asthma in patients 12 years of age and older in the United States. Addition of tiotropium in patients with moderate to severe asthma not adequately controlled by ICS or ICS/LABA has been shown to improve lung function and decrease rates of exacerbations.[35–37] A study by Kerstjens and colleagues[38] found significantly increased baseline FEV_1, increased time to first exacerbation, and decreased risk of severe exacerbations with addition of tiotropium to poorly controlled asthmatics on combination ICS/LABA therapy.

OMALIZUMAB

Omalizumab is a recombinant DNA-derived humanized IgG1k monoclonal anti-IgE antibody, administered subcutaneously and approved by the FDA in 2003 for use in patients with moderate to severe asthma age 12 and older. It is indicated for patients with an IgE level of 30 to 700 IU/mL, positive allergen skin or specific IgE testing to a perennial allergen, and incomplete symptom control with high-dose ICS therapy. Examples of perennial allergens include dust mite, animal dander, cockroach, and molds. Dosing, which can be every 2 or 4 weeks, is based on body weight and total serum IgE levels. EPR-3 recommends consideration of omalizumab for both steps 5 and 6 in severe asthmatic patients who are allergic.[14]

In allergic asthmatics with frequent exacerbations and poor lung function despite high-dose ICS or combination ICS/LABA, omalizumab as an add-on therapy has been shown to improve quality of life and reduce the rate of exacerbations, emergency department visits, use of rescue medications, and required dose of IHCs.[39–45] A study analyzing biomarkers of fractional exhaled nitric oxide, peripheral blood eosinophil count, and serum periostin found greater reduction in the frequency of exacerbations with the administration of omalizumab for those with higher levels for each of the 3 biomarkers.[46] Another study by Busse and colleagues[47] showed a significant reduction in exacerbation rates in those subjects with baseline peripheral eosinophil counts of 300/µL or greater when receiving omalizumab compared with placebo. In contrast, those with baseline eosinophil counts less than 300/µL did not show any improvement in exacerbation rates on omalizumab versus placebo. In a pooled analysis of 7 randomized controlled omalizumab trials, however, determining predictors for which patients will respond to or derive the most benefit from omalizumab was difficult and did not reveal consistent results.[48]

Although the incidence of adverse events in clinical trials was not found to be increased for those receiving omalizumab therapy,[41,49] there have been subsequent reports of adverse reactions to include episodes of anaphylaxis. As a result, the American Academy of Allergy, Asthma & Immunology and the American College of Allergy, Asthma and Immunology formed a joint task force to review the data from clinical trials and postmarketing surveillance on omalizumab-associated anaphylaxis. The results were published in 2007 and revealed an anaphylaxis-reporting rate of 0.09%, with 66% of those reactions with known time frame occurring in the first 2 hours after 1 of the first 3 doses. Therefore, the task force recommended an observation period of 2 hours for the first 3 doses, monitoring of subsequent doses for 30 minutes, educating patients about the risk of immediate or delayed allergic reactions at any point in the course of therapy, and prescribing all patients an epinephrine autoinjector with instructions on its use. The mechanism of anaphylactic reactions and methods to identify patients at risk are unknown.[50] Furthermore, early data showed an association between omalizumab therapy and malignancy but subsequent analyses, including a 5-year prospective cohort study[51] and a retrospective pooled analysis of more than 10,000 patients,[52] did not support this finding. Lastly, in a 5-year observational cohort study assessing long-term safety comparing omalizumab-treated and nonomalizumab-treated moderate to severe allergic asthmatics, the omalizumab cohort had a higher incidence rate of overall cardiovascular and cerebrovascular serious events. As a result, the FDA issued a safety announcement detailing this increased risk, although the data have not yet been published.[53] Because omalizumab is in a new class of agents, continued surveillance remains important.[54] There are ongoing clinical trials for a new high-affinity anti-IgE agent.[55,56]

SYSTEMIC CORTICOSTEROIDS

Maintenance doses of OCSs are recommended in severe persistent asthmatics at step 6 in the EPR-3 guidelines. Prior to initiation, however, these guidelines recommend consideration of adding on either theophylline or an antileukotriene to ICS/LABA combination therapy, although there is currently insufficient evidence for this approach. Furthermore, these guidelines recommend a 2-week course of OCS to confirm clinical reversibility and response.[14] Clinical studies of systemic corticosteroids as part of maintenance therapy are limited. A double-blind, placebo-controlled, crossover study with two 3-month treatment periods separated by a 3-month washout period in severe asthmatics compared high-dose intramuscular triamcinolone with low-dose daily prednisone. The study revealed increased peak expiratory flow rate (PEFR), lower rates of exacerbations, and lower total steroid doses, including during exacerbations, but more significant rates of adverse effects in the high-dose intramuscular triamcinolone group. Improved adherence was noted to be an advantage of the intramuscular triamcinolone group and likely contributed to the results.[57] Patients with a history of steroid resistance—defined as those who demonstrate continued airway obstruction and inflammation despite systemic corticosteroid therapy—should be evaluated for misdiagnosis, poor adherence or technique to their medications, pharmacokinetic abnormalities in steroid absorption or elimination, comorbid conditions, and persistent allergen

Table 5 Corticosteroid adverse effects	
System	**Adverse Effects**
Bone health	Decreased bone density Avascular necrosis
Gastrointestinal	Peptic ulceration
Endocrinologic	Adrenal suppression Hyperglycemia
Ophthalmic	Cataracts Glaucoma
Musculoskeletal	Myopathy (ventilated patients particularly at risk)[68]
Infectious	Increased risk of infections Delayed wound healing
Dermatologic	Dermal thinning Ecchymosis Striae
Morphologic	Cushingoid changes Truncal obesity Moon facies Buffalo hump
Cardiovascular	Increased risk of myocardial infarction Increased risk of cerebrovascular disease Elevated blood pressure
Psychiatric	Insomnia Anxiety Agitation Mood lability Mania Depression Aggression Psychosis

exposure. The pathogenesis of steroid-resistant asthma continues to be an ongoing area of research.[58–61]

In acute exacerbations, the EPR-3 guidelines recommends short courses of systemic corticosteroids until 80% of PEFR or resolution of symptoms.[14] A Cochrane review of 12 studies involving 863 subjects with acute asthma exacerbations revealed that use of corticosteroids within 1 hour of presentation to an emergency department reduced admission rates with no increase in adverse effects.[62] Other studies have demonstrated the utility of systemic corticosteroid therapy during acute exacerbations in reducing relapse rates[63,64] and mortality.[65]

Particularly for long-term or frequent use, adverse reactions of systemic corticosteroids are numerous and affect multiple organ systems (**Table 5**).[66–68] Minimizing utilization when possible or tapering down to the lowest efficacious dose is important to reduce the risk of developing steroid adverse effects.

ADDITIONAL ADD-ON THERAPIES

Per the EPR-3 guidelines, prior to addition of OCS, trials of adding an antileukotriene or theophylline to combination ICS/LABA therapy may be considered, although there is a lack of clinical trials evaluating these approaches. Furthermore, other add-on therapies, such as allergen immunotherapy, bronchial thermoplasty (BT), macrolide antibiotics, and small-particle IHCs have been postulated. Many of these therapies are implemented with the goal of decreasing dependence on chronic OCS.

Theophylline

Not only does theophylline (dimethylxanthine) have bronchodilator effects through the inhibition of phosphodiesterase 3 but also it is thought to have antiinflammatory effects. Also, there is some evidence that it may reduce corticosteroid insensitivity; however, further clinical studies are needed.[1,69] It has been used for the treatment of asthma since 1922.[70] Because of the high doses required, subsequent side effects, and required blood level monitoring, the use of theophylline as a bronchodilator in obstructive lung diseases declined with the increased use of β_2-agonists.[70]

There are some data showing that using theophylline at a lower dose decreases the risk of adverse effects and removes the need for blood level monitoring while maintaining its anti-inflammatory effects.[71] In a study of patients with poor asthma control, however, addition of low-dose theophylline did not improve control except in subjects who were not on ICS therapy.[72] Conversely, studies on the withdrawal of theophylline therapy in asthmatic patients on high-dose ICS or systemic corticosteroids showed increased symptoms and worsened lung function.[73,74]

Antileukotrienes

In the United States, available formulations of antileukotrienes include montelukast (Singulair) and zafirlukast (Accolate), which are leukotriene receptor antagonists (LTRAs), and zileuton (Zyflo), a 5-lipoxygenase inhibitor. After the activation of inflammatory cells, such as mast cells and eosinophils, leukotrienes, which are proinflammatory mediators, are generated by 5-lipoxygenation of arachidonic acid and induce bronchoconstriction, vasodilation, mucus secretion, recruitment of eosinophils, and decreased ciliary motility. Corticosteroid therapy does not block cysteinyl leukotriene synthesis, suggesting a role for targeting this pathway directly with this class of medications.[75]

There is limited evidence supporting LTRAs as add-on therapy to combination ICS/LABA. Most studies that showed benefit, such as improved lung function and symptoms scores, were conducted in asthmatic patients on ICS therapy alone[76–78] (**Table 6**). In contrast, a study of asthmatics on ICS and additional therapies did not show any significant change of symptom scores, lung function, or SABA use with addition of montelukast, though the period of therapy was only 14 days.[79] Furthermore, in studies comparing the addition of either a LABA or LTRA to ICS therapy, adding a LABA demonstrated greater improvements in lung function, symptoms scores, and rates of exacerbation but also mildly increased serious adverse effects.[80] There is some evidence, however, for targeting antileukotriene therapy for those with allergic asthma[77] and aspirin-intolerant asthma.[81]

Zileuton inhibits leukotrienes B_4, C_4, D_4, and E_4 formation as a specific inhibitor of 5-lipoxygenase. It comes in immediate-release and controlled-release formulations. Unlike the LTRAs montelukast and zafirlukast, zileuton therapy requires routine monitoring for transaminitis because early studies noted a small number of patients with an increase in alanine aminotransferase and aspartate aminotransferase levels that resolved with drug withdrawal.[82,83] As a result, the approved package insert for zileuton immediate-release recommends monitoring of hepatic transaminases prior to initiation and during therapy. Most studies of zileuton have been limited to patients with mild to moderate asthma only on β-agonist therapy and did not include severe asthmatics. In these studies, zileuton immediate-release and controlled-release formulations were found to improve lung function, decrease rescue SABA use, and reduce

Table 6
Representative examples of antileukotriene studies

Study, Year	Population Studied	Study Characteristics	Findings	Results Supportive of Therapy
LTRAs				
Virchow et al,[76] 2000	Adult asthmatics on ICS therapy	Randomized, double-blind, parallel-group, multicenter study	Addition of zafirlukast compared with placebo improved lung function and symptoms scores while decreasing rates of exacerbations and SABA use.	Yes (as addition to ICS)
Robinson et al,[79] 2001	Adult asthmatics on ICS and additional therapies	Randomized, double-blind, placebo-controlled, crossover study	Addition of montelukast for 14 d did not result in any significant change of symptom scores, lung function, or SABA use.	Not supportive
Price et al,[78] 2003	Adult asthmatics inadequately controlled on inhaled budesonide	Randomized, double-blind, parallel-group, noninferiority, multicenter study	Addition of montelukast to inhaled budesonide was as efficacious as doubling the dose of budesonide.	Yes (as addition to ICS)
Price et al,[77] 2006	Adult asthmatics with allergic rhinitis inadequately controlled on inhaled budesonide (COMPACT subgroup analysis)	—	Asthmatic patients with allergic rhinitis had greater improvement in lung function with montelukast and budesonide vs doubling the dose of budesonide.	Yes (as addition to ICS in allergic asthmatics)
Dahlén et al,[81] 2002	Adults with asthma, chronic rhinosinusitis, and aspirin intolerance. Most were on ICS and/or OCS	Randomized, double-blind, placebo-controlled, multicenter study	Montelukast therapy improved FEV_1, reduced asthma symptoms, and decreased exacerbation rates.	Yes (for aspirin-intolerant asthmatics)
Chauhan & Ducharme,[80] 2014	Adults or children with recurrent asthma on ICS and LABA or LTRA for minimum of 4 wk	Cochrane review of randomized controlled trials (18 total with 7208 participants)	Compared with ICS + LTRA, ICS + LABA resulted in greater improvements in lung function, symptoms scores, and rates of exacerbation but also mildly increased serious adverse effects.	Not supportive

Zileuton

Study	Population	Study design	Outcomes	Steroid sparing?
Israel et al,[82] 1996	Adults with mild to moderate asthma on inhaled β-agonists only.	Randomized, double-blind, parallel-group, multicenter study	Zileuton therapy resulted in decreased exacerbation rates and improved quality of life scores; 8 patients had increases in liver function tests that resolved with drug withdrawal.	Yes (study in patients on β-agonists only)
Nelson et al,[83] 2007	Patients age 12 and older with moderate asthma on SABA only	Phase 3, randomized, placebo-controlled, multicenter study	Zileuton therapy resulted in increased FEV_1, decreased SABA use, decreased rates of exacerbations, and similar rates of adverse events compared with placebo. Elevations of aminotransferase levels seen in zileuton groups that resolved with drug withdrawal.	Yes (study in patients on β-agonists only)
Liu et al,[84] 1996	Adults with mild to moderate asthma on inhaled β-agonists only.	Randomized, double-blind, parallel-group, placebo-controlled, multicenter study.	Zileuton therapy improved FEV_1 and morning PEFR, reduced blood eosinophil levels, decreased asthma symptoms and β-agonist use.	Yes (study in patients on β-agonists only)
Dahlén et al,[85] 1998	Adults with asthma, chronic nasal mucosal disease, and NSAID intolerance. All but 1 were on ICS or OCS.	Randomized, double-blind placebo-controlled, crossover, multicenter study	Zileuton therapy improved FEV_1, reduced nasal symptoms, decreased bronchial responsiveness to inhaled aspirin and histamine and basal urinary excretion of LTE_4.	Yes (for aspirin-intolerant asthmatics)

Abbreviations: COMPACT, Clinical Outcomes with Montelukast as a Partner Agent to Corticosteroid Therapy; LTE_4, leukotriene E_4; NSAID, nonsteroidal anti-inflammatory drug.

rate of exacerbations.[82–84] Another study in aspirin-intolerant asthmatics showed improved lung function, reduced rhinitis symptoms, and decreased rescue SABA use with addition of zileuton therapy.[85]

Allergen Immunotherapy

The EPR-3 guidelines recommend consideration of immunotherapy for mild to moderate asthma in steps 2 to 4, particularly when there is a clear relationship between symptoms and allergen exposure. Also, these guidelines state that the strongest evidence is for immunotherapy with single allergens and that there is better evidence for house dust mites, animal danders, and pollens compared with molds and cockroaches.[14] Meta-analyses of subcutaneous immunotherapy (SCIT) compared with placebo in asthmatic patients demonstrated improvements in asthma symptoms and lung function along with reductions in medication use and bronchial hyperreactivity.[86,87] For both SCIT and sublingual immunotherapy (SLIT), the randomized controlled studies that demonstrate efficacy are evaluating single-allergen immunotherapy. In contrast, studies of multiallergen immunotherapy are limited and have conflicting data. As a result, more studies are needed in this area.[88] In severe asthma patients, risks – particularly of anaphylaxis, which can be more severe in a poorly controlled asthmatic – must be weighed against possible benefits. Frequently, poor lung function and asthma control preclude adding on immunotherapy.

Macrolide Antibiotics

There are some data regarding the utility of macrolide antibiotics in severe asthma based on their antimicrobial and anti-inflammatory actions (see Carr TF, Kraft M: Chronic Infection and Severe Asthma, in this issue).

Bronchial Thermoplasty

A recent addition to the therapeutic options available for patients with severe asthma is BT, approved by the FDA in 2010. This therapy targets the airway smooth muscle (ASM), which plays a major role in the pathophysiology of asthma. In addition to the hypertrophy and hyperplasia of these cells noted on histologic evaluation of the asthmatic airway and contributing to bronchoconstriction of the airways,[89] there is evidence that these cells promote inflammation through the release of cytokines and chemokines.[90]

To reduce the ASM burden, BT involves 3 sequential bronchoscopies, each 3 weeks apart, that target the right lower lobe, left lower lobe, and bilateral upper lobes, respectively. During these bronchoscopies, the Alair System is used to deliver multiple pulses of monopolar radiofrequency thermal energy at 65°C for 10 seconds at a time, resulting in a maximum of 18 watts of power with each pulse. This is done repeatedly while gradually withdrawing the bronchoscope by 5 mm at a time to treat the entire airway of the specific lobe or lobes being targeted.[91]

There have been three phase 3 clinical trials evaluating the efficacy and safety of BT: the Asthma Intervention Research (AIR), Research in Severe Asthma (RISA), and AIR2 trials (**Table 7**).[92–94] Of these, RISA was the only one to include subjects dependent on chronic OCSs, which constituted approximately half of subjects enrolled. After BT, these subjects were analyzed after a period where their steroid dose remained stable and again after a steroid-weaning phase.[93] The most recent of these trials, AIR2, was unique because it is the only BT study that was blinded and included a sham control, which is especially important because both the BT group and the sham control showed significant improvements in Asthma Quality

Table 7
Phase 3 clinical trials for bronchial thermoplasty

Clinical Trial	Year	Major Inclusion Criteria (All Were Age 18–65 and Had Airway Hyper-responsiveness)	Type of Study (Number of Subjects)	Findings of Bronchial Thermoplasty Group Compared with Control Group	Findings at 5 y (In Addition to Stable Respiratory Events, FEV$_1$ and FVC, Chest Imaging)

AIR[94]	2007	• Moderate to severe persistent asthma
		• FEV$_1$ 60%–85% predicted
		• Worsening asthma symptoms on LABA withdrawal
		• Stable for prior 6 wk
			Randomized controlled study (n = 112)	• Improved
				  ○ Frequency of mild exacerbations (primary endpoint) at 3 and 12 mo, but not at 6 mo
				  ○ Symptom-free days
				  ○ ACQ scores
				  ○ AQLQ scores
				  ○ Morning PEFR
				  ○ Rescue medication use
				• No difference in
				  ○ FEV$_1$
				  ○ AHR
					• Compared with controls[96]
					  ○ Improved
					    ▪ AHR
					  ○ No difference in
					    ▪ Frequency of OCS bursts
					    ▪ Frequency of hospitalizations
					    ▪ Frequency of ED visits

RISA[93]	2007	• Severe persistent asthma
		• FEV$_1$ ≥50% predicted
		• Half of subjects on chronic OCS
			Randomized controlled study (n = 32)	• Improved
				  ○ ACQ scores
				  ○ AQLQ scores
				  ○ Prebronchodilator FEV$_1$% predicted only during steroid stable phase
				  ○ β-Agonist use
				• No difference in
				  ○ Symptom-free days
				  ○ PEFR
				  ○ OCS/ICS dosing
				  ○ AHR
					• Compared with baseline prior to BT[a,95]
					  ○ Improved
					    ▪ Frequency of hospitalizations
					    ▪ Frequency of ED visits

(continued on next page)

Table 7
(continued)

Clinical Trial	Year	Major Inclusion Criteria (All Were Age 18–65 and Had Airway Hyper-responsiveness)	Type of Study (Number of Subjects)	Findings of Bronchial Thermoplasty Group Compared with Control Group	Findings at 5 y (In Addition to Stable Respiratory Events, FEV_1 and FVC, Chest Imaging)

AIR2[92]	2010	• Severe persistent asthma
		• FEV_1 ≥60% predicted
		• AQLQ ≤6.25
		• Important exclusion criteria
		  ○ ≥4 OCS bursts for asthma in prior year
		  ○ ≥3 Asthma hospitalization in prior year
		  ○ Chronic sinusitis
			Randomized, double-blind, sham-controlled study (n = 288)	• Improved
				  ○ AQLQ scores compared with pre-BT baseline (primary endpoint)
				  ○ Frequency of severe exacerbations (↓32%)
				  ○ Frequency of ED visits (↓84%)
				  ○ Days lost from work/school due to asthma (↓66%)
				• No difference in
				  ○ AQLQ change compared with sham control group
				  ○ ACQ score
				  ○ PEFR
				  ○ Symptom-free days
				  ○ Rescue medication use
				  ○ Frequency of hospitalizations
					• Compared with controls[97]
					  ○ Improved
					    ■ Frequency of severe exacerbations
					    ■ Frequency of ED visits

Abbreviations: ACQ, Asthma Control Questionnaire; AHR, airway hyper-responsiveness; ED, emergency department; FVC, forced vital capacity.
[a] For the RISA trial, only those subjects receiving BT had follow-up at 5 years.
Data from Refs.[92–97]

of Life Questionnaire (AQLQ) scores, which were the primary endpoint. As a result, the difference in the increase of AQLQ scores between the 2 groups was small and not significant, suggesting the possibility of a large placebo effect associated with BT.[92] AIR2 excluded subjects with FEV_1 less than or equal to 60% of predicted and those with greater than or equal to 4 OCS bursts for asthma or greater than or equal to 3 asthma hospitalization in the prior year, thereby excluding many severe asthmatics for whom practitioners might consider BT as a therapeutic option.

During the treatment period of each of these 3 studies, increases in the frequency of hospitalizations and adverse events were noted, but these effects did not persist.[92–94] As shown in **Table 7**, long-term effects of BT have been analyzed from each of these studies with variable results, although all 3 studies indicate long-term safety out to 5 years based on stable lung function and imaging.[95–97]

Small-Particle Inhaled Corticosteroids

Small-particle ICS therapy, thought to have improved delivery to the small airways, can be added with the goal of targeting small airway inflammation. More studies need to be done, however, to evaluate its impact and efficacy (see Finkas LK, Martin R: Role of Small Airways in Asthma, in this issue). **Table 3** identifies available ICS therapies considered to be small-particle ICS.

SPECIAL POPULATIONS
Pediatrics

This discussion of severe asthma therapy applies to patients 12 and over. In children younger than 12, the same principles of step-up and step-down therapy, as guided by the EPR-3 guidelines, apply. One caveat is that the use of these medications is often off-label because only some of them are FDA approved for children younger than 12, usually at lower doses than for adults (**Table 8**).

Although the only combination ICS/LABA inhaler approved by the FDA for children under 4 is the 100-μg/50-μg strength of salmeterol/fluticasone, the EPR-3 guidelines call for high-dose ICS with either montelukast or LABA as the treatment of choice for severe asthmatics less than 4 years old who fall into step 5 of the EPR-3 guidelines. For children ages 5 to 12, the preferred treatment for step 5 is a high-dose ICS/LABA combination, based on extrapolation of data from adolescents and adults. These older children have leukotriene antagonists and theophylline as alternative but not preferred, add-on therapy. For both age groups, step 6 involves the addition of maintenance OCSs.[14]

One consideration unique to the pediatric population is the adverse effect on growth that can arise from long-term corticosteroid use, including OCS and/or ICS. Effect on growth has been studied for low-dose and medium-dose ICSs. Several studies have demonstrated approximately 1-cm reduction in growth velocity during the first year of therapy that is not progressive over time.[98–100] It is unclear whether higher doses of ICS would lead to a greater loss of growth velocity. At least 1 of these studies suggests, however, that the effect may be dose-dependent because growth in children using steroids only intermittently rather than regularly was similar to the placebo group.[100] Concerns over this and other systemic corticosteroid side effects, shown in **Table 5**, are behind the EPR-3 recommendation to first add nonsteroid alternatives before increasing the steroid dose when there is poor control in children. As in adults, however, the benefit of ICS is thought to outweigh the risks in children with severe asthma.[13,14]

Table 8
Age of Food and Drug Administration approval for pediatric asthma medications

Medication	Formulation	Approved Ages
ICSs		
Budesonide	Nebulizer suspension	≥1 y of age
	DPI	≥6 y of age
Beclomethasone	MDI HFA	≥5 y of age
Ciclesonide	MDI HFA	≥12 y of age
Flunisolide	MDI HFA	≥6 y of age
Fluticasone furoate	DPI	≥12 y of age
Fluticasone propionate	DPI	≥4 y of age
	MDI HFA	
Mometasone	DPI	≥4 y of age
	MDI HFA	≥12 y of age
Combination ICS/LABAs		
Budesonide/formoterol	MDI HFA	≥12 y of age
Mometasone/formoterol	MDI HFA	≥12 y of age
Salmeterol/fluticasone	DPI 100-μg/50-μg strength	≥4 y of age
	MDI HFA	≥12 y of age
Antileukotrienes		
Montelukast	4-mg granules	≥1 y of age
	4-mg chewable tablet	2–5 y of age
	5-mg chewable tablet	≥6 y of age
	10-mg tablet	≥15 y of age
Zafirlukast	10-mg tablet	≥5 y of age
	20-mg tablet	≥12 y of age
Zileuton	600-mg tablet	≥12 y of age
	600-mg ER tablet	
SABAs		
Albuterol	Nebulizer suspension	≥2 y of age
	MDI HFA	≥4 y of age
	DPI[a]	≥12 y of age
Levalbuterol	Nebulizer suspension	≥6 y of age
	MDI HFA	≥4 y of age
Other		
Cromolyn nebulizer	—	≥2 y of age
Omalizumab	—	≥12 y of age
Theophylline	—	No lower limit
Tiotropium Respimat	—	≥12 y of age

Abbreviations: DPI, dry powder inhaler; ER, extended release; HFA, hydrofluoroalkanes; MDI, metered-dose inhaler.
[a] The company is currently petitioning the FDA for a lower age of approval.
Data from Lexi-comp and product package inserts.

Pregnancy and Lactation

In a report published in 2005, the NAEPP emphasizes the importance of asthma control during pregnancy.[101] Maternal asthma, particularly when severe or poorly controlled, increases the risk of perinatal mortality, preeclampsia, preterm birth, and low-birth-weight infants.[102–107] As such, this group concludes that treating pregnant women with asthma medications is safer than risking asthma symptoms and exacerbations, even though few of these medications have actually been studied in pregnant women (**Table 9**). Based on available safety data, albuterol is the preferred SABA and budesonide is the preferred ICS. The NAEPP notes, however, that there are no data to indicate that other ICS formulations are unsafe during pregnancy,[101] suggesting that a patient who is maintaining good control on a particular ICS could continue this therapy rather than switch to a budesonide-containing formulation. LABAs lack safety data in pregnancy, and consequently all ICS/LABA formulations are category C in pregnancy. OCS has been found to increase the risk of cleft lip development when taken during the first trimester, although the number of steroid-dependent women studied was

Table 9 Asthma medications in pregnancy and lactation		
Medication	Pregnancy Category	Manufacturers' Recommendation During Lactation
SABAs		
Albuterol	C	Caution
Levalbuterol	C	Caution
ICSs		
Budesonide	B	Caution
Beclomethasone	C	Not recommended
Ciclesonide	C	Caution
Flunisolide	C	Caution
Fluticasone furoate	C	Caution
Fluticasone propionate	C	Caution
Mometasone	C	Caution
Combination ICS/LABAs[a]		
Budesonide/formoterol	C	Not recommended
Fluticasone furoate/vilanterol	C	Caution
Fluticasone propionate/salmeterol	C	Caution
Mometasone/formoterol	C	Caution
Antileukotrienes		
Montelukast	B	Caution
Zafirlukast	B	Not recommended
Zileuton	C	Not recommended
Other		
OCSs	C	Caution
Omalizumab	B	Caution
Cromolyn sodium	B	Caution
Theophylline	C	Caution

Note: relevant pregnancy categories are defined as follows: category B – animal reproduction studies have failed to demonstrate a risk to the fetus and there are no adequate and well-controlled human studies; category C – animal reproduction studies have shown an adverse effect on the fetus and there are no adequate and well-controlled human studies, but potential benefits may warrant use of the drug in pregnant women despite potential risks.
[a] All LABA formulations are category C in pregnancy.
Data from Lexi-comp and product package inserts.

very low.[108] Pregnant women requiring OCS also have higher rates of preeclampsia, preterm delivery, cesarean sections, diabetic complications of pregnancy, and low-birth-weight infants. It is unclear what contribution comes from OCS therapy versus severe or uncontrolled asthma, which predisposes to many of these same outcomes.[108–111] Baseline asthma severity can change during pregnancy: severity increases for one-third of women, decreases for another one-third, and stays the same in the remaining one-third. It is, therefore, crucial to closely monitor pregnant women and to step up or down therapy accordingly.

Extensive lactation safety data are lacking for most asthma medications. As such, manufacturers generally recommend the use of caution when using their medications during lactation, or avoidance altogether. The NAEPP and American Academy of Pediatrics, however, explicitly state that ICS, prednisone, theophylline, β-agonists, and cromolyn are not contraindications to breastfeeding.[101,112] A study of 8 infants exposed to steroids in breast milk, with their asthmatic mothers on 200 μg or 400 μg of daily inhaled budesonide, showed negligible systemic exposure.[113]

Obesity

Obesity seems to be a predisposing factor for severe asthma, with up to 48% of some severe asthma cohorts being obese.[114,115] Obese patients tend to have more difficulty controlling asthma and demonstrate decreased response to conventional asthma therapies, including ICS.[116–119] Recent thinking suggests that obese asthmatics may represent a unique phenotype of asthma, but further studies are needed to delineate exactly which factors set this group apart and make these patients more severe or difficult to control.

Specific Racial and Ethnic Groups

Asthma control and severity vary among racial and ethnic groups, often related to socioeconomic and cultural factors but also thought related to biological and pathophysiologic differences. Regarding therapy, patients of African racial background have less responsiveness to SABAs compared with Mexican Americans and Puerto Ricans.[120] African Americans have also been noted to have more treatment failures on LABAs, discussed previously with regard to increased deaths in the SMART trial concentrated among African American subjects.[31,121] In addition, polymorphisms in the genes encoding receptors for ICS, LTRA, and β-agonists vary between different ethnic groups, although the clinical implications of such variations with regard to therapeutic response have yet to be fully elucidated.[122] Ultimately, the effect of race and ethnicity on asthma severity is complex, and tailoring therapies to specific ethnic or racial groups will require more research to determine the exact interplay of epidemiology, genetics, and pathophysiology driving differences between these groups.

SUMMARY AND FUTURE CONSIDERATIONS

Severe asthma is a heterogeneous disease and includes uncontrolled asthma refractory to current available therapies. Many of these therapies require further research and investigation into their efficacy as add-on therapies and determining which populations would garner most benefit. In addition to the detailed traditional therapies in this article, immunomodulatory medications and biologics, including the recently approved mepolizumab, have been studied in the treatment of severe asthma (see Pavord ID, Hilvering B, Shrimanker R: Emerging Biologics in Severe Asthma, in this issue).

Because of the complex nature and heterogeneity of managing severe asthma, personalized medicine – based on identifying phenotypes and endotypes of asthma – becomes pivotal in selecting targeted add-on or novel therapies.[123] Some types of clinical phenotypes include corticosteroid-resistant asthma, asthma with frequent severe exacerbations, and asthma with fixed airflow obstruction. Inflammatory phenotypes include eosinophilic, neutrophilic, and paucigranulocytic asthma.[1,124] Endotypes are classified based on specific causal mechanisms. Examples include aspirin-sensitive asthma, allergic bronchopulmonary mycosis, and severe late-onset hypereosinophilic asthma.[124] As asthma endotypes and phenotypes are better understood and characterized, targeting therapy for each individual patient through personalized medicine should help improve disease outcomes, efficacy, and cost-effectiveness.

REFERENCES

1. Chung KF, Wenzel SE, Brozek JL, et al. International ERS/ATS guidelines on definition, evaluation and treatment of severe asthma. Eur Respir J 2014; 43(2):343–73.

2. Feehan M, Ranker L, Durante R, et al. Adherence to controller asthma medications: 6-month prevalence across a US community pharmacy chain. J Clin Pharm Ther 2015;40(5):590–3.

3. Keemink YS, Klok T, Brand PL. Long-term adherence to daily controller medication in children with asthma: the role of outpatient clinic visits. Pediatr Pulmonol 2015;50(11):1060–4.

4. Klok T, Kaptein AA, Duiverman EJ, et al. Long-term adherence to inhaled corticosteroids in children with asthma: observational study. Respir Med 2015; 109(9):1114–9.

5. Chalmers GW, Macleod KJ, Little SA, et al. Influence of cigarette smoking on inhaled corticosteroid treatment in mild asthma. Thorax 2002;57(3):226–30.

6. Chaudhuri R, Livingston E, McMahon AD, et al. Cigarette smoking impairs the therapeutic response to oral corticosteroids in chronic asthma. Am J Respir Crit Care Med 2003;168(11):1308–11.

7. Apostol GG, Jacobs DR Jr, Tsai AW, et al. Early life factors contribute to the decrease in lung function between ages 18 and 40: the Coronary Artery Risk Development in Young Adults study. Am J Respir Crit Care Med 2002;166(2): 166–72.

8. Lange P, Parner J, Vestbo J, et al. 15-year follow-up study of ventilatory function in adults with asthma. N Engl J Med 1998;339(17):1194–200.

9. Althuis MD, Sexton M, Prybylski D. Cigarette smoking and asthma symptom severity among adult asthmatics. J Asthma 1999;36(3):257–64.

10. Center for Disease Control and Prevention (CDC). Pneumococcal Vaccination: Who Needs It? 2015. Available at: http://www.cdc.gov/vaccines/vpd-vac/pneumo/vacc-in-short.htm. Accessed October 15, 2015.

11. Global Strategy for Asthma Management and Prevention, Global Initiative for Asthma (GINA). 2015.

12. Reddel HK, Bateman ED, Becker A, et al. A summary of the new GINA strategy: a roadmap to asthma control. Eur Respir J 2015;46(3):622–39.

13. National Asthma Education and Prevention Program. Expert Panel Report 3: Guidelines for the Diagnosis and Management of Asthma. Full Report 2007.

14. National Asthma Education Prevention Program. Expert Panel Report 3 (EPR-3): Guidelines for the Diagnosis and Management of Asthma-Summary Report 2007. J Allergy Clin Immunol 2007;120(5 Suppl):S94–138.

15. Pauwels RA, Lofdahl CG, Postma DS, et al. Effect of inhaled formoterol and budesonide on exacerbations of asthma. Formoterol and Corticosteroids Establishing Therapy (FACET) International Study Group. N Engl J Med 1997; 337(20):1405–11.

16. Faurschou P, Steffensen I, Jacques L. Effect of addition of inhaled salmeterol to the treatment of moderate-to-severe asthmatics uncontrolled on high-dose inhaled steroids. European Respiratory Study Group. Eur Respir J 1996;9(9): 1885–90.

17. Bateman ED, Boushey HA, Bousquet J, et al. Can guideline-defined asthma control be achieved? Am J Respir Crit Care Med 2004;170(8):836–44.

18. Nielsen LP, Pedersen B, Faurschou P, et al. Salmeterol reduces the need for inhaled corticosteroid in steroid-dependent asthmatics. Respir Med 1999; 93(12):863–8.

19. Nelson HS, Busse WW, Kerwin E, et al. Fluticasone propionate/salmeterol combination provides more effective asthma control than low-dose inhaled corticosteroid plus montelukast. J Allergy Clin Immunol 2000;106(6):1088–95.

20. O'Byrne PM, Bisgaard H, Godard PP, et al. Budesonide/formoterol combination therapy as both maintenance and reliever medication in asthma. Am J Respir Crit Care Med 2005;171(2):129–36.

21. O'Byrne PM. Acute asthma intervention: insights from the STAY study. J Allergy Clin Immunol 2007;119(6):1332–6.

22. Rabe KF, Atienza T, Magyar P, et al. Effect of budesonide in combination with formoterol for reliever therapy in asthma exacerbations: a randomised controlled, double-blind study. Lancet 2006;368(9537):744–53.

23. Stallberg B, Olsson P, Jorgensen LA, et al. Budesonide/formoterol adjustable maintenance dosing reduces asthma exacerbations versus fixed dosing. Int J Clin Pract 2003;57(8):656–61.

24. FitzGerald JM, Sears MR, Boulet LP, et al. Adjustable maintenance dosing with budesonide/formoterol reduces asthma exacerbations compared with traditional fixed dosing: a five-month multicentre Canadian study. Can Respir J 2003;10(8):427–34.

25. Leuppi JD, Salzberg M, Meyer L, et al. An individualized, adjustable maintenance regimen of budesonide/formoterol provides effective asthma symptom control at a lower overall dose than fixed dosing. Swiss Med Wkly 2003; 133(21–22):302–9.

26. Aalbers R, Backer V, Kava TT, et al. Adjustable maintenance dosing with budesonide/formoterol compared with fixed-dose salmeterol/fluticasone in moderate to severe asthma. Curr Med Res Opin 2004;20(2):225–40.

27. Buhl R, Kardos P, Richter K, et al. The effect of adjustable dosing with budesonide/formoterol on health-related quality of life and asthma control compared with fixed dosing. Curr Med Res Opin 2004;20(8):1209–20.

28. Canonica GW, Castellani P, Cazzola M, et al. Adjustable maintenance dosing with budesonide/formoterol in a single inhaler provides effective asthma symptom control at a lower dose than fixed maintenance dosing. Pulm Pharmacol Ther 2004;17(4):239–47.

29. Ind PW, Haughney J, Price D, et al. Adjustable and fixed dosing with budesonide/formoterol via a single inhaler in asthma patients: the ASSURE study. Respir Med 2004;98(5):464–75.

30. Busse WW, Shah SR, Somerville L, et al. Comparison of adjustable- and fixed-dose budesonide/formoterol pressurized metered-dose inhaler and fixed-dose fluticasone propionate/salmeterol dry powder inhaler in asthma patients. J Allergy Clin Immunol 2008;121(6):1407–14, 1414.e1–6.
31. Nelson HS, Weiss ST, Bleecker ER, et al, SMART Study Group. The Salmeterol Multicenter Asthma Research Trial: a comparison of usual pharmacotherapy for asthma or usual pharmacotherapy plus salmeterol. Chest 2006;129(1):15–26.
32. Nelson HS. Is there a problem with inhaled long-acting beta-adrenergic agonists? J Allergy Clin Immunol 2006;117(1):3–16 [quiz: 17].
33. Nelson HS. Long-acting beta-agonists in adult asthma: Evidence that these drugs are safe. Prim Care Respir J 2006;15(5):271–7.
34. FDA Drug Safety Communication: FDA requires post-market safety trials for Long-Acting Beta-Agonists (LABAs). Available at: http://www.fda.gov/Drugs/DrugSafety/ucm251512.htm. Accessed October 15, 2015.
35. Rodrigo GJ, Castro-Rodriguez JA. What is the role of tiotropium in asthma?: a systematic review with meta-analysis. Chest 2015;147(2):388–96.
36. McKeage K. Tiotropium Respimat(R): A Review of Its Use in Asthma Poorly Controlled with Inhaled Corticosteroids and Long-Acting beta2-Adrenergic Agonists. Drugs 2015;75(7):809–16.
37. Rodrigo GJ, Castro-Rodriguez JA. Tiotropium for the treatment of adolescents with moderate to severe symptomatic asthma: a systematic review with meta-analysis. Ann Allergy Asthma Immunol 2015;115(3):211–6.
38. Kerstjens HA, Engel M, Dahl R, et al. Tiotropium in asthma poorly controlled with standard combination therapy. N Engl J Med 2012;367(13):1198–207.
39. Bousquet J, Wenzel S, Holgate S, et al. Predicting response to omalizumab, an anti-IgE antibody, in patients with allergic asthma. Chest 2004;125(4):1378–86.
40. Humbert M, Beasley R, Ayres J, et al. Benefits of omalizumab as add-on therapy in patients with severe persistent asthma who are inadequately controlled despite best available therapy (GINA 2002 step 4 treatment): INNOVATE. Allergy 2005;60(3):309–16.
41. Hanania NA, Alpan O, Hamilos DL, et al. Omalizumab in severe allergic asthma inadequately controlled with standard therapy: a randomized trial. Ann Intern Med 2011;154(9):573–82.
42. Holgate ST, Djukanovic R, Casale T, et al. Anti-immunoglobulin E treatment with omalizumab in allergic diseases: an update on anti-inflammatory activity and clinical efficacy. Clin Exp Allergy 2005;35(4):408–16.
43. Lemanske RF Jr, Nayak A, McAlary M, et al. Omalizumab improves asthma-related quality of life in children with allergic asthma. Pediatrics 2002;110(5):e55.
44. Finn A, Gross G, van Bavel J, et al. Omalizumab improves asthma-related quality of life in patients with severe allergic asthma. J Allergy Clin Immunol 2003;111(2):278–84.
45. Busse W, Corren J, Lanier BQ, et al. Omalizumab, anti-IgE recombinant humanized monoclonal antibody, for the treatment of severe allergic asthma. J Allergy Clin Immunol 2001;108(2):184–90.
46. Hanania NA, Wenzel S, Rosen K, et al. Exploring the effects of omalizumab in allergic asthma: an analysis of biomarkers in the EXTRA study. Am J Respir Crit Care Med 2013;187(8):804–11.
47. Busse W, Spector S, Rosen K, et al. High eosinophil count: a potential biomarker for assessing successful omalizumab treatment effects. J Allergy Clin Immunol 2013;132(2):485–6.e11.

48. Bousquet J, Rabe K, Humbert M, et al. Predicting and evaluating response to omalizumab in patients with severe allergic asthma. Respir Med 2007;101(7): 1483–92.

49. Deniz YM, Gupta N. Safety and tolerability of omalizumab (Xolair), a recombinant humanized monoclonal anti-IgE antibody. Clin Rev Allergy Immunol 2005;29(1):31–48.

50. Cox L, Platts-Mills TA, Finegold I, et al. American Academy of Allergy, Asthma & Immunology/American College of Allergy, Asthma and Immunology Joint Task Force Report on omalizumab-associated anaphylaxis. J Allergy Clin Immunol 2007;120(6):1373–7.

51. Long A, Rahmaoui A, Rothman KJ, et al. Incidence of malignancy in patients with moderate-to-severe asthma treated with or without omalizumab. J Allergy Clin Immunol 2014;134(3):560–7.e4.

52. Busse W, Buhl R, Fernandez Vidaurre C, et al. Omalizumab and the risk of malignancy: results from a pooled analysis. J Allergy Clin Immunol 2012;129(4): 983–9.e6.

53. FDA. FDA Drug Safety Communication: FDA approves label changes for asthma drug Xolair (omalizumab), including describing slightly higher risk of heart and brain adverse events. Available at: http://www.fda.gov/Drugs/DrugSafety/ucm414911.htm. Accessed November 19, 2015.

54. Tan RA, Corren J. Safety of omalizumab in asthma. Expert Opin Drug Saf 2011; 10(3):463–71.

55. US National Institutes of Health. A Phase 1, Randomized, Placebo-controlled, Dose-escalation Safety Study of MEDI4212 in Subjects With IgE >= 30 IU/mL. Available at: https://clinicaltrials.gov/ct2/show/results/NCT01544348. Accessed October 20, 2015.

56. Cohen ES, Dobson CL, Kack H, et al. A novel IgE-neutralizing antibody for the treatment of severe uncontrolled asthma. Not Found In Database 2014;6(3): 756–64.

57. Ogirala RG, Aldrich TK, Prezant DJ, et al. High-dose intramuscular triamcinolone in severe, chronic, life-threatening asthma. N Engl J Med 1991;324(9): 585–9.

58. Leung DY, Szefler SJ. Diagnosis and management of steroid-resistant asthma. Clin Chest Med 1997;18(3):611–25.

59. Leung DY. Steroid-resistant asthma. West J Med 1995;163(4):367–8.

60. Cypcar D, Busse WW. Steroid-resistant asthma. J Allergy Clin Immunol 1993; 92(3):362–72.

61. Wang W, Li JJ, Foster PS, et al. Potential therapeutic targets for steroid-resistant asthma. Curr Drug Targets 2010;11(8):957–70.

62. Rowe BH, Spooner C, Ducharme FM, et al. Early emergency department treatment of acute asthma with systemic corticosteroids. Cochrane Database Syst Rev 2000;(2):CD002178.

63. Chapman KR, Verbeek PR, White JG, et al. Effect of a short course of prednisone in the prevention of early relapse after the emergency room treatment of acute asthma. N Engl J Med 1991;324(12):788–94.

64. Rowe BH, Keller JL, Oxman AD. Effectiveness of steroid therapy in acute exacerbations of asthma: a meta-analysis. Am J Emerg Med 1992;10(4):301–10.

65. Benatar SR. Fatal asthma. N Engl J Med 1986;314(7):423–9.

66. Fardet L, Kassar A, Cabane J, et al. Corticosteroid-induced adverse events in adults: frequency, screening and prevention. Drug Saf 2007;30(10):861–81.

67. Poetker DM, Reh DD. A comprehensive review of the adverse effects of systemic corticosteroids. Otolaryngol Clin North Am 2010;43(4):753–68.
68. Leatherman JW, Fluegel WL, David WS, et al. Muscle weakness in mechanically ventilated patients with severe asthma. Am J Respir Crit Care Med 1996;153(5): 1686–90.
69. Spears M, Donnelly I, Jolly L, et al. Effect of low-dose theophylline plus beclometasone on lung function in smokers with asthma: a pilot study. Eur Respir J 2009;33(5):1010–7.
70. Barnes PJ. Theophylline. Am J Respir Crit Care Med 2013;188(8):901–6.
71. Barnes PJ, Pauwels RA. Theophylline in the management of asthma: time for reappraisal? Eur Respir J 1994;7(3):579–91.
72. American Lung Association Asthma Clinical Research Centers. Clinical trial of low-dose theophylline and montelukast in patients with poorly controlled asthma. Am J Respir Crit Care Med 2007;175(3):235–42.
73. Kidney J, Dominguez M, Taylor PM, et al. Immunomodulation by theophylline in asthma. Demonstration by withdrawal of therapy. Am J Respir Crit Care Med 1995;151(6):1907–14.
74. Brenner M, Berkowitz R, Marshall N, et al. Need for theophylline in severe steroid-requiring asthmatics. Clin Allergy 1988;18(2):143–50.
75. Bisgaard H. Pathophysiology of the cysteinyl leukotrienes and effects of leukotriene receptor antagonists in asthma. Allergy 2001;56(Suppl 66):7–11.
76. Virchow JC Jr, Prasse A, Naya I, et al. Zafirlukast improves asthma control in patients receiving high-dose inhaled corticosteroids. Am J Respir Crit Care Med 2000;162(2 Pt 1):578–85.
77. Price DB, Swern A, Tozzi CA, et al. Effect of montelukast on lung function in asthma patients with allergic rhinitis: analysis from the COMPACT trial. Allergy 2006;61(6):737–42.
78. Price DB, Hernandez D, Magyar P, et al. Randomised controlled trial of montelukast plus inhaled budesonide versus double dose inhaled budesonide in adult patients with asthma. Thorax 2003;58(3):211–6.
79. Robinson DS, Campbell D, Barnes PJ. Addition of leukotriene antagonists to therapy in chronic persistent asthma: a randomised double-blind placebo-controlled trial. Lancet 2001;357(9273):2007–11.
80. Chauhan BF, Ducharme FM. Addition to inhaled corticosteroids of long-acting beta2-agonists versus anti-leukotrienes for chronic asthma. Cochrane Database Syst Rev 2014;(1):CD003137.
81. Dahlén SE, Malmstrom K, Nizankowska E, et al. Improvement of aspirin-intolerant asthma by montelukast, a leukotriene antagonist: a randomized, double-blind, placebo-controlled trial. Am J Respir Crit Care Med 2002; 165(1):9–14.
82. Israel E, Cohn J, Dube L, et al. Effect of treatment with zileuton, a 5-lipoxygenase inhibitor, in patients with asthma. A randomized controlled trial. Zileuton Clinical Trial Group. JAMA 1996;275(12):931–6.
83. Nelson H, Kemp J, Berger W, et al. Efficacy of zileuton controlled-release tablets administered twice daily in the treatment of moderate persistent asthma: a 3-month randomized controlled study. Ann Allergy Asthma Immunol 2007; 99(2):178–84.
84. Liu MC, Dube LM, Lancaster J. Acute and chronic effects of a 5-lipoxygenase inhibitor in asthma: a 6-month randomized multicenter trial. Zileuton Study Group. J Allergy Clin Immunol 1996;98(5 Pt 1):859–71.

85. Dahlén B, Nizankowska E, Szczeklik A, et al. Benefits from adding the 5-lipox-ygenase inhibitor zileuton to conventional therapy in aspirin-intolerant asth-matics. Am J Respir Crit Care Med 1998;157(4 Pt 1):1187–94.

86. Abramson MJ, Puy RM, Weiner JM. Injection allergen immunotherapy for asthma. Cochrane Database Syst Rev 2010;(8):CD001186.

87. Ross RN, Nelson HS, Finegold I. Effectiveness of specific immunotherapy in the treatment of asthma: a meta-analysis of prospective, randomized, double-blind, placebo-controlled studies. Clin Ther 2000;22(3):329–41.

88. Nelson HS. Multiallergen immunotherapy for allergic rhinitis and asthma. J Allergy Clin Immunol 2009;123(4):763–9.

89. James AL, Elliot JG, Jones RL, et al. Airway smooth muscle hypertrophy and hy-perplasia in asthma. Am J Respir Crit Care Med 2012;185(10):1058–64.

90. Panettieri RA Jr. Airway smooth muscle: immunomodulatory cells? Allergy Asthma Proc 2004;25(6):381–6.

91. Laxmanan B, Hogarth DK. Bronchial thermoplasty in asthma: current perspec-tives. J Asthma Allergy 2015;8:39–49.

92. Castro M, Rubin AS, Laviolette M, et al. Effectiveness and safety of bronchial thermoplasty in the treatment of severe asthma: a multicenter, randomized, double-blind, sham-controlled clinical trial. Am J Respir Crit Care Med 2010; 181(2):116–24.

93. Pavord ID, Cox G, Thomson NC, et al. Safety and efficacy of bronchial thermo-plasty in symptomatic, severe asthma. Am J Respir Crit Care Med 2007;176(12): 1185–91.

94. Cox G, Thomson NC, Rubin AS, et al. Asthma control during the year after bron-chial thermoplasty. N Engl J Med 2007;356(13):1327–37.

95. Pavord ID, Thomson NC, Niven RM, et al. Safety of bronchial thermoplasty in pa-tients with severe refractory asthma. Ann Allergy Asthma Immunol 2013;111(5): 402–7.

96. Thomson NC, Rubin AS, Niven RM, et al. Long-term (5 year) safety of bronchial thermoplasty: Asthma Intervention Research (AIR) trial. BMC Pulm Med 2011; 11:8.

97. Wechsler ME, Laviolette M, Rubin AS, et al. Bronchial thermoplasty: long-term safety and effectiveness in patients with severe persistent asthma. J Allergy Clin Immunol 2013;132(6):1295–302.

98. Long-term effects of budesonide or nedocromil in children with asthma. The Childhood Asthma Management Program Research Group. N Engl J Med 2000;343(15):1054–63.

99. Guilbert TW, Morgan WJ, Zeiger RS, et al. Long-term inhaled corticosteroids in preschool children at high risk for asthma. N Engl J Med 2006;354(19):1985–97.

100. Martinez FD, Chinchilli VM, Morgan WJ, et al. Use of beclomethasone dipropi-onate as rescue treatment for children with mild persistent asthma (TREXA): a randomised, double-blind, placebo-controlled trial. Lancet 2011;377(9766): 650–7.

101. National Heart, Lung, and Blood Institute, National Asthma Education and Pre-vention Program Asthma and Pregnancy Working Group. NAEPP expert panel report. Managing asthma during pregnancy: recommendations for pharmaco-logic treatment-2004 update. J Allergy Clin Immunol 2005;115(1):34–46.

102. Bain E, Pierides KL, Clifton VL, et al. Interventions for managing asthma in preg-nancy. Cochrane Database Syst Rev 2014;(10):CD010660.

103. Bakhireva LN, Schatz M, Jones KL, et al, Organization of Teratology Information Specialists Collaborative Research Group. Asthma control during pregnancy

and the risk of preterm delivery or impaired fetal growth. Ann Allergy Asthma Immunol 2008;101(2):137–43.
104. Blais L, Forget A. Asthma exacerbations during the first trimester of pregnancy and the risk of congenital malformations among asthmatic women. J Allergy Clin Immunol 2008;121(6):1379–84, 1384.e1.
105. Murphy VE, Gibson P, Talbot PI, et al. Severe asthma exacerbations during pregnancy. Obstet Gynecol 2005;106(5 Pt 1):1046–54.
106. Murphy VE, Gibson PG. Asthma in pregnancy. Clin Chest Med 2011;32(1): 93–110, ix.
107. Vatti RR, Teuber SS. Asthma and pregnancy. Clin Rev Allergy Immunol 2012; 43(1–2):45–56.
108. Park-Wyllie L, Mazzotta P, Pastuszak A, et al. Birth defects after maternal exposure to corticosteroids: prospective cohort study and meta-analysis of epidemiological studies. Teratology 2000;62(6):385–92.
109. Bracken MB, Triche EW, Belanger K, et al. Asthma symptoms, severity, and drug therapy: a prospective study of effects on 2205 pregnancies. Obstet Gynecol 2003;102(4):739–52.
110. Perlow JH, Montgomery D, Morgan MA, et al. Severity of asthma and perinatal outcome. Am J Obstet Gynecol 1992;167(4 Pt 1):963–7.
111. Schatz M, Zeiger RS, Harden K, et al. The safety of asthma and allergy medications during pregnancy. J Allergy Clin Immunol 1997;100(3):301–6.
112. American Academy of Pediatrics Committee on Drugs. Transfer of drugs and other chemicals into human milk. Pediatrics 2001;108(3):776–89.
113. Falt A, Bengtsson T, Kennedy BM, et al. Exposure of infants to budesonide through breast milk of asthmatic mothers. J Allergy Clin Immunol 2007;120(4): 798–802.
114. Gibeon D, Batuwita K, Osmond M, et al. Obesity-associated severe asthma represents a distinct clinical phenotype: analysis of the British Thoracic Society Difficult Asthma Registry Patient cohort according to BMI. Chest 2013;143(2): 406–14.
115. van Veen IH, Ten Brinke A, Sterk PJ, et al. Airway inflammation in obese and nonobese patients with difficult-to-treat asthma. Allergy 2008;63(5):570–4.
116. Beuther DA, Sutherland ER. Overweight, obesity, and incident asthma: a meta-analysis of prospective epidemiologic studies. Am J Respir Crit Care Med 2007; 175(7):661–6.
117. Boulet LP. Influence of obesity on the prevalence and clinical features of asthma. Clin Invest Med 2008;31(6):E386–90.
118. Heacock T, Lugogo N. Role of weight management in asthma symptoms and control. Immunol Allergy Clin North Am 2014;34(4):797–808.
119. Varraso R, Siroux V, Maccario J, et al. Asthma severity is associated with body mass index and early menarche in women. Am J Respir Crit Care Med 2005; 171(4):334–9.
120. Naqvi M, Tcheurekdjian H, DeBoard JA, et al. Inhaled corticosteroids and augmented bronchodilator responsiveness in Latino and African American asthmatic patients. Ann Allergy Asthma Immunol 2008;100(6):551–7.
121. Wechsler ME, Castro M, Lehman E, et al. Impact of race on asthma treatment failures in the asthma clinical research network. Am J Respir Crit Care Med 2011;184(11):1247–53.
122. Ortega VE, Meyers DA. Pharmacogenetics: implications of race and ethnicity on defining genetic profiles for personalized medicine. J Allergy Clin Immunol 2014;133(1):16–26.

123. Moore WC, Meyers DA, Wenzel SE, et al. Identification of asthma phenotypes using cluster analysis in the severe asthma research program. Am J Respir Crit Care Med 2010;181(4):315–23.
124. Campo P, Rodriguez F, Sanchez-Garcia S, et al. Phenotypes and endotypes of uncontrolled severe asthma: new treatments. J Investig Allergol Clin Immunol 2013;23(2):76–88 [quiz: 71 p. follow 88].

Emerging Biologics in Severe Asthma

Ian D. Pavord, FMedSci, DM, FRCP[a,b,*], Bart Hilvering, MD[a,b,c],
Rahul Shrimanker, MRCP[a,b]

KEYWORDS

- Severe asthma • Biomarkers • Type-2 cytokines • Anti-IL-5 • Anti-IL-13
- Anti-IL-4&13

KEY POINTS

- Patients with severe asthma have a large unmet need for better treatments.
- An important advance has been the recognition that severe asthma is heterogeneous with respect to clinical problems and the pattern of lower airway inflammation.
- Identification of eosinophilic inflammation in the airways is particularly important as biological agents blocking interleukin (IL)-5, IL-13, and both IL-4 and -13 are effective treatments in this subgroup.
- Effective use of these agents will require clinicians to think about airways disease differently and become familiar with new biomarkers and new ways of classifying airways disease.

INTRODUCTION

Asthma is a common chronic inflammatory disease of the airways that affects 300 million people worldwide.[1] Many patients achieve satisfactory control of the clinical manifestations of asthma with inhaled corticosteroids (ICS), but 5% to 10% have severe disease, requiring extensive treatment to control it or remaining uncontrolled despite extensive treatment.[2] This small subgroup accounts for most of the morbidity and mortality caused by asthma and 60% of the total health care costs attributable to asthma. Patients with a recent history of an asthma attack have particularly high annual health care costs, estimated to be $1740 (£1035; €1257), 3 times those of a patient with severe asthma and no history of an attack.[3]

Severe asthma is heterogeneous with respect to the clinical problem, the nature of the impairment of lung function, and the underlying abnormality.[4] It is often a complex

[a] Department of Respiratory Medicine, University of Oxford, Old Road, Oxford, OX3 7LE, UK; [b] Nuffield Department of Medicine, University of Oxford, Old Road Campus, Oxford, OX3 7FZ, UK; [c] Laboratory of Translational Immunology, Department of Respiratory Medicine, University Medical Center, Heidelberglaan 100, 3584 CX Utrecht, The Netherlands
* Corresponding author. Nuffield Department of Medicine, University of Oxford, NDM Research Building, Old Road Campus, Roosevelt Drive, Oxford OX3 7FZ, UK.
E-mail address: Ian.pavord@ndm.ox.ac.uk

Immunol Allergy Clin N Am 36 (2016) 609–623
http://dx.doi.org/10.1016/j.iac.2016.04.001   immunology.theclinics.com
0889-8561/16/$ – see front matter © 2016 Elsevier Inc. All rights reserved.

clinical problem because many patients have apparently severe asthma primarily because the diagnosis is incorrect, or because of issues with inhaler technique or treatment adherence; others have persistent asthma-like symptoms primarily driven by co-morbid factors. The recent international European Respiratory Society/American Thoracic Society (ERS/ATS) guidelines on severe asthma[2] acknowledge these difficulties and have produced what is likely to be the most widely accepted definition (**Box 1**). They suggest that the diagnosis of asthma is confirmed and comorbidities addressed before making a diagnosis of severe asthma. An important aspect of the ERS/ATS definition is that different criteria for uncontrolled asthma are suggested, and no assumptions about the involvement of similar pathophysiologic pathways are made.

The high level of morbidity, health care costs, and treatment-related side effects in severe asthma mean that there is a large unmet need for alternative therapies. New treatment should ideally target the pathophysiologic mechanism responsible for the morbidity and might therefore have to be adapted for each individual patient. One particularly fruitful area of development has been the use of monoclonal antibodies targeting T-helper (Th) 2-mediated airway inflammation. It is now known that anti-immunoglobulin E (IgE; Omalizumab) is only effective in patients with evidence of Th2 airway inflammation,[5] and several new approaches, including interleukin-4Rα (anti-IL-4Rα;Dupilumab, which blocks IL-4 and IL-13), anti-IL-13 (Lebrikizumab, Tralokizumab), and anti-IL-5 (Mepolizumab, Reslizumab, Benralizumab), are showing promise in patients with this feature. Among these, anti-IL-5 and specifically Mepolizumab have been most extensively investigated in clinical studies.

The clinical effects of Mepolizumab and other monoclonal antibodies targeting Th2 inflammation are strikingly consistent, showing a clinically important reduction in the frequency of asthma attack of around 50% and a small beneficial effect on symptoms

---

Box 1
European Respiratory Society/American Thoracic Society 2014 definition of severe asthma

Definition of severe asthma for patients 6 years old and older

Severe asthma is asthma that requires treatment with guidelines-suggested medications for GINA stages 4 to 5 asthma (high-dose inhaled CS[a] and LABA or leukotriene modifier/theophylline) for the previous year or systemic CS for $\geq$50% of the previous year to prevent it from becoming "uncontrolled" or from remaining "uncontrolled" despite this therapy.

- Uncontrolled asthma is defined as at least one of the following:
  - Poor symptom control: ACQ consistently greater than 1.5, ACT $\leq$19 (or "not well controlled" by NAEPP/GINA guidelines)
  - Frequent severe exacerbations: 2 or more bursts of systemic CSs (>3 days each) in the previous year
  - Serious exacerbations: at least one hospitalization, intensive care unit stay, or mechanical ventilation in the previous year
  - Airflow limitation: after appropriate bronchodilator, withhold FEV_1 less than 80% predicted (in the face of reduced FEV_1/forced vital capacity defined as less than the lower limit of normal)

- Controlled asthma that worsens on tapering of these high doses of inhaled CS or systemic CS (or additional biologics)

[a] The definition of high dose ICS is age-specific.
Abbreviations: ACT, asthma control test; CS, corticosteroids; GINA, Global Initiative for Asthma; NAEPP, National Asthma Education and Prevention Program.
From Chung KF, Wenzel SE, Brozek JL, et al. International ERS/ATS guidelines on definition, evaluation and treatment of severe asthma. Eur Respir J 2014;43:349; with permission.

and impaired lung function. These findings emphasize that symptoms and impaired lung function are to some extent dissociated from eosinophilic airway inflammation and the risk of asthma attacks (**Fig. 1**). This important conceptual advance has proven key in the successful clinical development of biological agent targeting Th2 cytokines. It means that eosinophilic, Th2 inflammation will need to be assessed in order to recognize patients suitable for these therapies. Several measures are available and suitable for use in clinical practice (**Table 1**). Whether different combinations of biomarkers are particularly related to the efficacy of different treatments is unclear; this is an important area for further study.

This article reviews the effectiveness and safety profile of anti-IL-5 drugs (Mepolizumab, Reslizumab, and Benralizumab), anti-IL-13 (Lebrikizumab, Tralokinumab), and anti-IL-4&13 (Dupilumab) for the treatment of patients with severe asthma. Biological treatment for non-Th2 asthma has been a less fruitful area. The authors briefly discuss potential biological treatments for this pattern of disease.

T-HELPER 2 CYTOKINES AS POTENTIAL TREATMENT TARGETS

Classically, eosinophilic airway inflammation is considered to be triggered by release of so-called type 2 cytokines (IL-5, IL-4, and IL-13) by allergens or parasites that come into contact and pass through the epithelial barrier (**Fig. 2**). Dendritic cells process antigens and trigger a response after binding to Th cells at regional lymphoid sites. CD4+ lymphocytes become Th2 cells and produce the cytokines IL-4, IL-5, IL-9, and IL-13. Allergens can also trigger an immediate bronchoconstrictor response as a result of triggering mast cell mediator release. Mast cells are also a potential source of type 2 cytokines.

IL-4 produced by Th2 cells causes a general shift in Th0 cells to differentiate into Th2 cells and an immunoglobulin class switch, resulting in IgE production by B cells. IgE subsequently binds to mast cells and eosinophils residing in the tissue, enabling them to release their toxic granules on antigen binding. IL-5 is a very important systemic regulator of eosinophil dynamics in humans because it leads to maturation and activation of eosinophils. Locally, it acts as a chemoattractant and causes migration of eosinophils to sites of damage. IL-5 functions also in combination with IL-9 to recruit mast cells and eosinophils to an affected tissue site. IL-13 acts with IL-4 in inducing IgE production by B cells, induces mucus production by goblet cells, causes goblet cell metaplasia, and increases airway hyperresponsiveness by a direct effect on airway smooth muscle.

Many patients with severe asthma and eosinophilic inflammation have adult-onset disease, are not atopic, and have normal serum IgE. This pattern of disease is typically associated with nasal polyposis and aspirin sensitivity; its presence implies that eosinophilic airway inflammation can be induced independent of exogenous allergens.

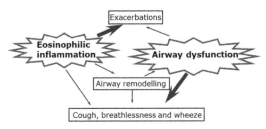

Fig. 1. Dissociation between airway inflammation, airway dysfunction, and clinical outcomes in severe asthma.

Table 1
Potential biomarkers of eosinophilic airway inflammation

Biomarker	Association with Treatment Response	Invasiveness	Comments
FeNO	Corticosteroids, anti-IL-13, anti-IL-4&13, anti-IgE	Noninvasive	Easy, quick, not specific, cheap, generally available
Serum IgE	Not associated	Minimal	Although recommended to measure, there is no clear association between IgE as a biomarker and treatment responses or clinical outcome
Serum periostin	Anti-IL-13[a]	Minimal	Effect shown with anti-IL-13, high costs, and limited availability currently
Blood eosinophil count	Anti-IL-5,[a] anti-IL4/13 (?)	Minimal	Generally available, high clinical impact, predicts anti-IL-5 response. Less clear predictor in anti-IL-4/13 treatment
Sputum eosinophil count	Corticosteroids, anti-IL-5	Moderate	Specialist centers, tissue specific, time-consuming

[a] Proven clinical efficacy in combination with this treatment.

A newly recognized class of cells called type 2 innate lymphoid cells (ILC2s) might be important in generating a Th2 response and persistent eosinophilic inflammation independent of allergens (see **Fig. 2**). ILC2s are able to produce large amounts of IL-5 and IL-13 but not IL-4, making them an attractive candidate for orchestrating the immune response in patients with nonatopic eosinophilic airway inflammation. The current paradigm for the role of ILC2s is that disruption of the epithelial barrier by an external trigger such as pollution or a virus causes epithelial damage and enhances production of IL-25, IL-33, and thymic stromal lymphopoietin by epithelial cells.[6] These cytokines cause ILC2 activation in the tissue and production of Th2 cytokines (see **Fig. 2**). Prostaglandin D2 and leukotriene E4 produced by recruited and activated eosinophils and mast cells might then enhance responsiveness of ILC2 cells leading to a perpetuating cycle.

T-HELPER 2 CYTOKINE BLOCKERS
Anti-Interleukin-5 or Anti-Interleukin-5R

Anti-IL-5 or Anti-IL-5R treatment influences eosinophil dynamics throughout the human immune system. Both basophils and eosinophils express the IL-5 receptor and can be targeted by blocking IL-5 or the IL-5 receptor. One of the first randomized controlled trials (RCT) with the IL-5 antagonist Mepolizumab in patients with asthma showed that a single dose of Mepolizumab (10 mg/kg) reduced blood eosinophil count for 16 weeks and sputum eosinophil count for up to 4 weeks.[7] Moreover, Mepolizumab was able to prevent blood eosinophilia during the late-phase response after allergen challenge. Although the biological effect was strong, no effect was seen on forced expiratory volume in the first second of expiration (FEV_1), airway responsiveness, or the airway response to allergen.

Two larger RCTs with Mepolizumab in patients with moderate asthma taking ICS confirmed the strong biological effect[8,9]; however, both were disappointing in respect to the clinical effect on airway responsiveness, lung function, asthma control

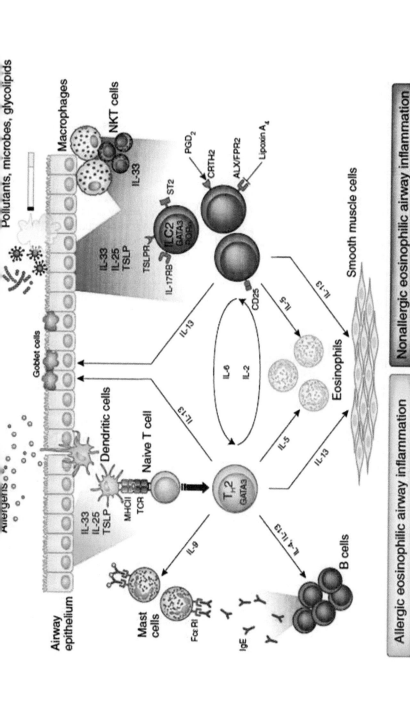

Fig. 2. Pathways leading to eosinophilic airway inflammation. PGD2, prostaglandin D2; TSLP, thymic stromal lymphopoietin. ALX/FPR2, N-formyl peptide receptor 2; CRTH2, chemokine receptor homologous molecule expressed on Th2 lymphocytes; FcεRI, Fc epsilon RI; NKT, Natural killer T cells; IL-17RB, IL-17 receptor B; TCR, T cell receptor. (*From* Brusselle GG, Maes T, Bracke KR. Eosinophils in the spotlight: eosinophilic airway inflammation in nonallergic asthma. Nat Med 2013;19:978; with permission.)

questionnaire (ACQ), or rescue medication use. Interestingly, in one study there was a nonsignificant trend in the reduction of asthma exacerbations after treatment with the highest dose of Mepolizumab,[9] although the study was neither long enough nor large enough to demonstrate such an effect definitively.

The fact that these studies did not clearly show a clinical effect led many to question whether eosinophilic inflammation is of any importance for the key clinical outcomes in asthma. The alternative possibility that treatment did not have a sufficiently large effect on eosinophilic airway inflammation was unlikely because the effects of treatment on sputum and airway biopsy eosinophil numbers were at least as great as that seen with corticosteroids.[10] A third possibility was that treatment failed because the treated population may not have had eosinophilic airway inflammation, and the outcome measures chosen were not responsive to change in response to reduction in eosinophilic airway inflammation. In support of this, airway inflammation, exacerbations, and symptom control are to some extent disconnected within patients and respond to treatment differently. Symptoms and lung function are more responsive to a long-acting β2-agonist, and exacerbations and eosinophilic airway inflammation are more responsive to a 4-fold increased dose of ICSs.[11] In addition, studies that have examined the clinical effects of a management strategy that controls eosinophilic airway inflammation as well as symptoms have shown a large reduction in exacerbation numbers but not much change in lung function and symptoms.[12,13] It is now clear that asthma symptoms and traditional physiologic tests of asthma are at best are weakly associated with the presence of eosinophilic airway inflammation. As many as 80% of patients with asthma who remain symptomatic despite ICSs have no evidence of eosinophilic airway inflammation[14] and are thus unlikely to respond to a treatment that targets this feature. A better model for eosinophilic airway inflammation and disordered airway inflammation is that these features are relatively independent and relate differently to different clinical outcomes (see **Fig. 1**).

These findings provided a strong basis for a more rigorous evaluation of the effects of blocking IL-5 with 2 important modifications to the clinical trial design:

i. Treating patients with evidence of active eosinophilic airway inflammation rather than an arbitrary and unrelated physiologic measure such as a large acute bronchodilator response

ii. Assessing the effect of treatment on asthma exacerbations, an outcome measure that is directly and potentially causally related to eosinophilic airway inflammation.

These studies provided strong validation to this model because monthly intravenous (IV) injections of 750 mg Mepolizumab had a large beneficial effect on exacerbations but a much smaller effect on asthma symptoms and lung function.[15] A clinically important oral steroid–sparing effect of Mepolizumab was also shown.[16]

In a subsequent large multicenter phase 2b trial, 75, 250, and 750 mg of Mepolizumab given monthly by intravenous injection was evaluated in 616 patients with eosinophilic asthma identified with more permissive criteria present on study entry or within the previous year: a blood eosinophil count greater than 0.3×10^9/L, a fraction of exhaled nitric oxide (FeNO) > 50 pbb, a sputum eosinophil count greater than 3%, and/or a prompt deterioration after a 25% or greater reduction in corticosteroid dose.[17] This study confirmed that treatment reduced asthma attacks by about 50% and showed no evidence of a dose-response relationship for this measure. The study had considerable power to investigate factors associated with treatment efficacy because the clinical effects were similar between doses and could therefore be combined. Of the many variables assessed, only the blood eosinophil count and the prior frequency of asthma attacks were associated with the beneficial effect of treatment. A multivariate analysis established that efficacy became apparent at a blood eosinophil count greater than 0.15×10^9/L and increased progressively with counts above this such that exacerbations were reduced by around 80% in patients with a baseline blood eosinophilia (count $>0.4 \times 10^9$/L). As with the initial proof-of-concept studies, this study showed no significant effect of Mepolizumab on asthma symptoms, quality of life, FeNO, or lung function.

The unexpected efficacy of the lowest dose of Mepolizumab meant that subcutaneous dosing was potentially feasible. Mepolizumab 100 mg given subcutaneously was evaluated in 2 phase 3 trials in patients with severe asthma, a blood eosinophil count greater than 0.15×10^9/L (and/or $>0.3 \times 10^9$/L within the last year), and 2 or more exacerbations in the past year. These studies confirmed that treatment reduced exacerbations by around 50%[18] but also found clear evidence of improvement in FEV_1, symptoms scores, and quality-of-life measures as well as a significant oral corticosteroid (OCS) sparing effect[19] and a clear decrease in exacerbation rate. The more complete effect of Mepolizumab in these phase 3 trials may reflect better selection of a responsive population as a result of using the blood eosinophil count to identify responsive patients. No particular safety issues have been identified with long-term use of Mepolizumab, and it is therefore a promising therapy.

Alternative Anti-Interleukin-5 Treatments

Reslizumab is a humanized IgG4 antibody targeting IL-5 that has also completed phase 3 trials[20] and has shown similar efficacy to Mepolizumab, albeit in a population that has a higher mean blood eosinophil count but rather less severe disease than those treated with Mepolizumab (**Tables 2** and **3**). Currently, Reslizumab has been given as a monthly intravenous injection with dosing based on weight, although a fixed-dose subcutaneous version is expected to follow.

Benralizumab is a humanized monoclonal antibody targeting the IL5-receptor α. It differs from Mepolizumab and Reslizumab in that it causes eosinophil cytotoxicity and has been shown to induce more profound and acute onset eosinopenia in a study with mild atopic asthmatics; it also depletes circulating basophils, which also express IL-5-receptor α. Whether these different biological effects translate into differences in clinical effects is unclear. One potential advantage of the acute effect on circulating eosinophil numbers is that Benralizumab might have an acute beneficial effect in patients presenting acutely with an exacerbation associated with an eosinophilia. Benralizumab has been evaluated in a phase IIb dose-ranging RCT in patients with eosinophilic and non-eosinophilic asthma.[21] The study showed a clear reduction in the rate of exacerbations in patients with asthma and a blood eosinophil count greater than 0.3×10^9/L but not in patients with non-eosinophilic asthma (see **Tables 2** and **3**). The effects of treatment were rather less clear in a population wherein eosinophilic asthma was defined according to an algorithm based on the eosinophil/lymphocyte and eosinophil/neutrophil (ELEN) index, which predicts sputum eosinophilia based on nonsputum parameters. Benralizumab has also been evaluated in patients with acute severe asthma, where it reduced the rate of repeat attacks, and in eosinophilic chronic obstructive pulmonary disease (COPD), where there was a strong and consistent trend for a beneficial effect against a variety of outcome measures in the subgroup with a blood eosinophil count greater than 0.3×10^9/L.[22]

The different anti-IL-5 approaches evaluated to date have very consistent beneficial clinical effects (see **Table 3**), appear to be safe, and have a well-defined and easily measured biomarker. They therefore represent a promising new approach to

Table 2
Summary of anti-interleukin-5 clinical trial programs

	Phase 3		Phase 2
	Mepolizumab (Anti-IL-5)	Reslizumab (Anti-IL-5)	Benralizumab (Anti-IL-5R)
Biomarker (cutoff)	Blood EOS ≥150/μL at initiation or 300/μL in previous 12 mo	Blood EOS (≥400/μL)	Weighted for eosinophilic based on proprietary index or FeNO >40 ppb
Baseline biomarker mean	290 ± 1050	590 (100–2300)	530–560
Background therapy	≥880 μg FP/d + another controller	≥440 μg FP/d ± another controller	High-/medium-dose ICS + another controller
Baseline patient demographics — Exacerbations required for inclusion (mean observed)	>2 (3.8 ± 2.7)	No requirement for FEV₁, study (55% ≥1 in past year)	2–6 in last year
FEV$_1$ pre-BD (mL)	1730 ± 660 (FEV₁ <80% predicted in adults)	2190	Not reported
Asthma symptoms (ACQ5/6)	2.26 ± 1.27	2.6	2.5–2.6
Asthma QOL (AQLQ)	Not reported	4.2	3.6–3.8
Maintenance OCS use % (mean dose, mg)	27% 12.6 (2–50)	Not reported	4%–11%
Age	≥12 y	≥12 y	≥18 y

Abbreviations: AQLQ, asthma quality of life questionnaire; EOS, eosinophils; FP, fluticasone propionate; QOL, quality of life.

Table 3
Summary of efficacy

	Phase 3		Phase 2
	Mepolizumab (Anti-IL-5)	Reslizumab (Anti-IL-5)	Benralizumab (Anti-IL-5R)
Exacerbation reduction relative to PBO	54% (subcutaneously [SC]) and 47% (IV) 80% at ≥500 blood EOS (SC)	50%–60% (top-line data) at 400 cut-off	57% for 20 mg dose in ≥300 cells/μL group
FEV$_1$ improvement (% FEV$_1$)	98 mL (6%) SC	160 mL (7%) and 270 mL (12%)[a]	0.23 L for ≥300 cells/μL group
Asthma symptoms (ACQ5/6)	0.44 0.75 in ≥500 PBO-corrected	0.36 PBO-corrected	0.44 PBO-corrected (>300 cutoff)
Asthma QOL	Unknown	Unknown	Not reported
Oral steroid sparing (min 5 mg/d prednisone)	50% median reduction in baseline OCS dose	No OCS sparing study	Unknown Planned for P3
Expected frequency and dosage	Every 4 wk 100 mg	Every 4 wk 3 mg/kg	3 × every 4 wk then every 8 wk (30 mg for P3)
ROA	SC lyophilized powder	IV	SC prefilled syringe
Safety	1 potential anaphylaxis case	1 case of anaphylaxis related to drug	Balanced

Abbreviations: ACQ, asthma control questionnaire; EOS, eosinophils; PBO, placebo; QOL, quality of life; ROA, route of administration.
[a] In subjects with high blood eosinophils

treatment of eosinophilic airways disease. Traditional variables used to stratify airways disease, such as bronchodilator responsiveness, severity of airflow obstruction, allergy, and age of onset, are not associated with a treatment response, whereas the presence of a raised blood eosinophil count and a past history of exacerbations are. New more coherent stratification methods for airways disease based on these measures are therefore likely to emerge when these treatments are introduced into the clinic.

Anti-Interleukin-13

The first trial in humans tested 2 anti-IL-13 compounds, using allergen challenge in mild atopic asthma; anti-IL-13 attenuated the drop in FEV$_1$ in the late phase.[23] A randomized controlled clinical trial of anti-IL-13 treatment (Lebrikizumab) in a cohort of moderate to severe asthma patients showed only a small improvement in FEV$_1$.[24] However, a post-hoc analysis of this study showed that patients with a serum periostin concentration above the median or a high FeNO had a greater FEV$_1$ improvement and a strong trend to reduced exacerbations with treatment. This finding is entirely plausible because both periostin and FeNO are known to be biomarkers of increased IL-13 activity within the airway and are both highly responsive to IL-13 blockade. Two subsequent phase 3 trials had to be stopped early on because of concerns about contamination occurring in the manufacturing process.[25] Analysis of the limited available findings suggested a large beneficial effect against asthma exacerbations in the population with serum periostin concentration above the median.

Another IL-13 monoclonal antibody, Tralokinumab, also showed an effect on FEV_1 but no effect on clinical markers.[26] This compound has shown rather less impressive effects in a phase 2b trial, although, in a post-hoc analysis, it was possible to identify a subgroup who were not treated with oral prednisolone, had high serum periostin, and had large acute bronchodilator reversibility that had a large response to treatment.[27] The anti-IL-13 compound, GSK679586, showed no clinical effect in a well-defined cohort of 198 patients with very severe asthma, even though the investigators retrospectively stratified the patients by periostin levels and by the presence of blood eosinophilia.[28] Collectively, these studies suggest that anti-IL-13 might be less effective in patients with more severe asthma.

Interleukin-4 Receptor-αBlockers

IL-13 is closely linked to IL-4 and exerts similar functions by binding and activating the α subunit of the IL-4 receptor. Blocking the α subunit of the IL-4 receptor will therefore inhibit both IL-4 and IL-13 signaling and may therefore produce a greater clinical benefit. The first trial with anti-IL-4-α blockers studied the effect of the fully human monoclonal antibody AMG 317 in patients with moderate to severe asthma and showed no beneficial effect on asthma symptoms assessed using the ACQ scores of the overall population.[29] However, it did show an effect in a subgroup that had high ACQ baseline scores. In a more recent trial of the anti-IL-4-α monoclonal antibody Dupilumab, more clear evidence of efficacy was seen in patients with persistent moderate-to-severe asthma who had blood eosinophilia greater than 0.3×10^9/L.[30] During the study, patients were withdrawn from long-acting-2 agonists (LABAs) followed by ICS, and exacerbation rates were compared. There was a significant difference in exacerbation rate observed after withdrawal, in favor of the dupilumab group. Secondary endpoints, such as FEV_1, improved significantly, and ACQ also dropped in the treatment arm with evidence of a treatment effect on these measures before LABA and ICS were withdrawn. Treatment reduced FeNO, IgE levels, TARC (thymus and activation-regulated chemokine), and eotaxin-3 levels, providing evidence of a biological effect of the drug. One concern with the main endpoint is the definition of an exacerbation, also described by the investigators. An exacerbation was defined as the need for systemic corticosteroids or doubling of the ICS dose, which differs from the current consensus statement in which greater than 3 days of OCS is used as a definition.

PROSPECTS FOR T-HELPER 2 LOW DISEASE

Prospects for modifying airway inflammation in Th2 low disease is much more uncertain because the patterns of airway inflammation and its likely causes are poorly understood. Some encouragement is provided by the beneficial effects of long-term low-dose macrolides in patients with non-eosinophilic asthma[31] and by preliminary evidence of a marked reduction of sputum neutrophil counts and clinical efficacy of a CXCR2 antagonist in patients with non-eosinophilic asthma.[32] Patients with COPD macrolides and CXCR2 antagonists have very different effects in smokers and ex-smokers, with the latter effectively reducing exacerbations in smokers but not ex-smokers, and the former having the opposite effect.[33,34] These findings suggest that there are at least 2 types of neutrophilic airway inflammation in patients with airway disease, differing in their relationship with smoking and airway infection.

Neutrophilic airway inflammation might also be driven by Th17-mediated processes. In a first clinical trial, Brodalumab, which blocks IL-17 signaling by inhibiting the IL-17 A receptor, did not improve ACQ scores (primary endpoint) in a group of moderate-to-severe asthmatics.[35] However, treatment did have beneficial effects in a subgroup with high reversibility to albuterol. A similar selective beneficial effect in bronchodilator-responsive patients with severe asthma has been reported with the tumor necrosis factor (TNF) -α antagonist Golimumab,[36] although this treatment was not pursued because there was a high incidence of malignancy in the treated population. Patient selection was not optimal in either anti-TNF or anti-IL-17 study because the presence of neutrophilic airway inflammation was not confirmed and there was no marker of TNF or IL-17 involvement included for selection. It remains possible that there is a definable subgroup of patients with severe asthma who derive net benefit from one or both of these treatments. More work is needed to understand the mechanisms and phenotypes of Th2 low asthma.

AN APPROACH TO ASSESSMENT OF PATIENTS WITH SEVERE ASTHMA POTENTIALLY SUITABLE FOR BIOLOGICAL TREATMENT

There are 2 important steps to the assessment of patients with severe asthma: establishing that asthma is the correct diagnosis and is responsible for morbidity; and determining the inflammatory pattern of disease.

Diagnosis

The diagnosis of asthma is based on recognition of typical symptoms (dyspnea, cough, and wheeze) in association with variable airflow obstruction. Although asthma is the most common cause of episodic wheeze, cough, and dyspnea, there are other potential causes, including dysfunctional breathing, vocal cord dysfunction, rhinitis, cough syndromes, and structural airway abnormalities. These conditions are prevalent in patients presenting to a severe asthma clinic[37] because symptoms do not respond to asthma treatments. The clinical assessment therefore has to be sufficiently rigorous to exclude these conditions with confidence.

The key step is to confirm that variable airflow obstruction is present. Convincing evidence is often available from retrospective review of the case notes, but if not, variable airflow obstruction can be demonstrated by the response to a bronchodilator (>12% improve of FEV_1); by demonstration of greater than 20% within day variability of peak expiratory flow (PEF); and/or by identification of airway hyperresponsiveness (ie, a provocative concentration of metacholine required to cause a 20% decrease in FEV_1 of <8 mg/mL). Abnormal PEF variability can occur independently of asthma,[38] and all the conditions listed above can coexist with asthma,[37] so assessment is not necessarily straightforward even if variable airflow obstruction has been demonstrated. Assessment of airway responsiveness and eosinophilic airway inflammation are generally more informative than more traditional tests.

COPD can be difficult to distinguish from severe asthma with confidence and can be associated with eosinophilic airway inflammation. However, this distinction may not be clinically important because treatment responses are likely independent of these labels. The authors' approach is to describe rather than categorize patients with shared features and focus the clinical assessment on identification of treatable aspects, such as eosinophilic airway inflammation.[4]

Asthma can also be apparently severe and treatment resistant in patients who have not mastered the basics of asthma management, such as treatment adherence, correct inhaler technique, and self-management. The clinical assessment should therefore include a thorough assessment of these aspects.

THE IDENTIFICATION OF THE PATTERN OF AIRWAY INFLAMMATION

After confirming the diagnosis of severe asthma, the next step is to identify the inflammatory pattern in order to direct treatment and risk-reduction strategies. Severe asthma is characterized by a marked dissociation between symptoms and disordered airway function on one hand and lower airway abnormality on the other, so it is necessary to assess both to get the full picture (see **Fig. 1**). Distinguishing eosinophilic inflammation from non-eosinophilic inflammation is important for several reasons:

i. Patients with eosinophilic airway inflammation are at high risk of severe attacks,[12] including episodes requiring ventilation[39];
ii. A treatment model based on identification and treatment of eosinophilic airway inflammation has been proven to reduce attacks[12];
iii. Prednisolone, Omalizumab,[5] and a number of new biological agents are highly active in patients with this pattern of lower airway inflammation.

Eosinophilic airway inflammation can be assessed directly by bronchoscopic techniques or by induced sputum or indirectly using the peripheral blood eosinophil count or FeNO. The pros and cons and measurement characteristics of these methods are summarized in **Table 1**.

SUMMARY

The success of the introduction of novel biological agents in asthma largely depends on the ability to select the appropriate asthma patients. All "successful" clinical studies that involved novel biological agents included a specific subgroup that was likely to be responsive to the treatment. Ideally, patients are selected by an easily measurable biomarker that is directly influenced by the treatment. It is interesting that existing data show that FeNO and serum periostin are good biomarkers of treatment response to Omalizumab[5] and biological agents targeting IL-13,[24] whereas the blood eosinophil count is most closely associated with a response to anti-IL-5.[17] Moreover, treatment with IL-5 reduces the blood eosinophil count but not FeNO, whereas the reverse is true for Omalizumab, anti-IL-13, and anti-IL-4&13 (**Table 4**). Whether these biomarkers can be used to identify subgroups of patients within the Th2 high population who are particularly suited to different cytokine blockade will be an important research question for the future. Another important priority is to understand the pathophysiology of asthma in patients with no evidence of Th2-mediated inflammation because patients with this phenotype of asthma have few treatment options.

Table 4
The effects of different cytokine blockers on clinical measures and biomarkers

	Effect on Clinical				Effect on Biomarkers			
	FEV$_1$	Symptoms	Exac	PC$_{20}$	Bl Eos	Sp Eos	FeNO	IgE
Oral steroids	+	+	++	++	↓↓	↓↓	↓↓	↓
Anti-IL-5	0/+	0/+	++	0	↓↓	↓↓	↔	↔
Anti-IL-13	+	+	++ (?)	0 (?)	↑	↓	↓↓	↓
Anti-IL-4/13	+	+	++ (?)	0 (?)	↑	↓	↓↓	↓↓
Anti-IgE	+	+	+	0	↔	↓	↓↓	↓

Abbreviations: (?), Not definitively proven; Bl, blood; Eos, eosinophils; Exac, exacerbations; Sp, sputum.

REFERENCES

1. 2014 GINA guidelines. From the Global Strategy for Asthma Management and Prevention, Global Initiative for Asthma (GINA) 2014. Available at: http://wwwginasthmaorg/. Accessed December 9, 2015.
2. Chung KF, Wenzel SE, Brozek JL, et al. International ERS/ATS guidelines on definition, evaluation and treatment of severe asthma. Eur Respir J 2014;43:343–73.
3. Ivanova JI, Bergman R, Birnbaum HG, et al. Effect of asthma exacerbations on health care costs among asthmatic patients with moderate and severe persistent asthma. J Allergy Clin Immunol 2012;129(5):1229–35.
4. Pavord ID. Complex airway disease: an approach to assessment and management. Lancet Respir Med 2013;1(1):84–90.
5. Hanania NA, Wenzel S, Rosen K, et al. Exploring the effects of omalizumab in allergic asthma: an analysis of biomarkers in the EXTRA study. Am J Respir Crit Care Med 2013;187(8):804–11.
6. Brusselle GG, Maes T, Bracke KR. Eosinophils in the spotlight: eosinophilic airway inflammation in nonallergic asthma. Nat Med 2013;19(8):977–9.
7. Leckie MJ, ten BA, Khan J, et al. Effects of an interleukin-5 blocking monoclonal antibody on eosinophils, airway hyper-responsiveness, and the late asthmatic response. Lancet 2000;356(9248):2144–8.
8. Flood-Page P, Menzies-Gow A, Phipps S, et al. Anti-IL-5 treatment reduces deposition of ECM proteins in the bronchial subepithelial basement membrane of mild atopic asthmatics. J Clin Invest 2003;112(7):1029–36.
9. Flood-Page P, Swenson C, Faiferman I, et al. A study to evaluate safety and efficacy of mepolizumab in patients with moderate persistent asthma. Am J Respir Crit Care Med 2007;176(11):1062–71.
10. Flood-Page PT, Menzies-Gow AN, Kay AB, et al. Eosinophil's role remains uncertain as anti-interleukin-5 only partially depletes numbers in asthmatic airway. Am J Respir Crit Care Med 2003;167(2):199–204.
11. Pauwels RA, Lofdahl CG, Postma DS, et al. Effect of inhaled formoterol and budesonide on exacerbations of asthma. Formoterol and Corticosteroids Establishing Therapy (FACET) International Study Group. N Engl J Med 1997;337(20):1405–11.
12. Green RH, Brightling CE, McKenna S, et al. Asthma exacerbations and sputum eosinophil counts: a randomised controlled trial. Lancet 2002;360(9347):1715–21.
13. Jayaram L, Pizzichini MM, Cook RJ, et al. Determining asthma treatment by monitoring sputum cell counts: effect on exacerbations. Eur Respir J 2006;27(3):483–94.
14. Green RH, Brightling CE, McKenna S, et al. Comparison of asthma treatment given in addition to inhaled corticosteroids on airway inflammation and responsiveness. Eur Respir J 2006;27(6):1144–51.
15. Haldar P, Brightling CE, Hargadon B, et al. Mepolizumab and exacerbations of refractory eosinophilic asthma. N Engl J Med 2009;360(10):973–84.
16. Nair P, Pizzichini MM, Kjarsgaard M, et al. Mepolizumab for prednisone-dependent asthma with sputum eosinophilia. N Engl J Med 2009;360(10):985–93.
17. Pavord ID, Korn S, Howarth P, et al. Mepolizumab for severe eosinophilic asthma (DREAM): a multicentre, double-blind, placebo-controlled trial. Lancet 2012;380(9842):651–9.
18. Ortega HG, Liu MC, Pavord ID, et al. Mepolizumab treatment in patients with severe eosinophilic asthma. N Engl J Med 2014;371(13):1198–207.
19. Bel EH, Wenzel SE, Thompson PJ, et al. Oral glucocorticoid-sparing effect of mepolizumab in eosinophilic asthma. N Engl J Med 2014;371(13):1189–97.

20. Castro M, Zangrilli J, Wechsler ME, et al. Reslizumab for inadequately controlled asthma with elevated blood eosinophil counts: results from two multicentre, parallel, double-blind, randomised, placebo-controlled, phase 3 trials. Lancet Respir Med 2015;3(5):355–66.

21. Castro M, Wenzel SE, Bleecker ER, et al. Benralizumab, an anti-interleukin 5 receptor alpha monoclonal antibody, versus placebo for uncontrolled eosinophilic asthma: a phase 2b randomised dose-ranging study. Lancet Respir Med 2014;2(11):879–90.

22. Brightling CE, Bleecker ER, Panettieri RA Jr, et al. Benralizumab for chronic obstructive pulmonary disease and sputum eosinophilia: a randomised, double-blind, placebo-controlled, phase 2a study. Lancet Respir Med 2014;2(11):891–901.

23. Gauvreau GM, Boulet LP, Cockcroft DW, et al. Effects of interleukin-13 blockade on allergen-induced airway responses in mild atopic asthma. Am J Respir Crit Care Med 2011;183(8):1007–14.

24. Corren J, Lemanske RF, Hanania NA, et al. Lebrikizumab treatment in adults with asthma. N Engl J Med 2011;365(12):1088–98.

25. Hanania NA, Noonan M, Corren J, et al. Lebrikizumab in moderate-to-severe asthma: pooled data from two randomised placebo-controlled studies. Thorax 2015;70(8):748–56.

26. Piper E, Brightling C, Niven R, et al. A phase II placebo-controlled study of tralokinumab in moderate-to-severe asthma. Eur Respir J 2013;41(2):330–8.

27. Brightling CE, Chanez P, Leigh R, et al. Efficacy and safety of tralokinumab in patients with severe uncontrolled asthma: a randomised, double-blind, placebo-controlled, phase 2b trial. Lancet Respir Med 2015;3(9):692–701.

28. De Boever EH, Ashman C, Cahn AP, et al. Efficacy and safety of an anti-IL-13 mAb in patients with severe asthma: a randomized trial. J Allergy Clin Immunol 2014;133(4):989–96.

29. Corren J, Busse W, Meltzer EO, et al. A randomized, controlled, phase 2 study of AMG 317, an IL-4Ralpha antagonist, in patients with asthma. Am J Respir Crit Care Med 2010;181(8):788–96.

30. Wenzel S, Ford L, Pearlman D, et al. Dupilumab in persistent asthma with elevated eosinophil levels. N Engl J Med 2013;368(26):2455–66.

31. Brusselle GG, VanderStichele C, Jordens P, et al. Azithromycin for prevention of exacerbations in severe asthma (AZISAST): a multicentre randomised double-blind placebo-controlled trial. Thorax 2013;68(4):322–9.

32. Nair P, Gaga M, Zervas E, et al. Safety and efficacy of a CXCR2 antagonist in patients with severe asthma and sputum neutrophils: a randomized, placebo-controlled clinical trial. Clin Exp Allergy 2012;42(7):1097–103.

33. Rennard SI, Dale DC, Donohue JF, et al. CXCR2 antagonist MK-7123-A phase 2 proof-of-concept trial for chronic obstructive pulmonary disease. Am J Respir Crit Care Med 2015;191(9):1001–11.

34. Han MK, Tayob N, Murray S, et al. Predictors of chronic obstructive pulmonary disease exacerbation reduction in response to daily azithromycin therapy. Am J Respir Crit Care Med 2014;189(12):1503–8.

35. Busse WW, Holgate S, Kerwin E, et al. Randomized, double-blind, placebo-controlled study of brodalumab, a human anti-IL-17 receptor monoclonal antibody, in moderate to severe asthma. Am J Respir Crit Care Med 2013;188(11):1294–302.

36. Wenzel SE, Barnes PJ, Bleecker ER, et al. A randomized, double-blind, placebo-controlled study of tumor necrosis factor-alpha blockade in severe persistent asthma. Am J Respir Crit Care Med 2009;179(7):549–58.

37. Heaney LG, Robinson DS. Severe asthma treatment: need for characterising patients. Lancet 2005;365(9463):974–6.
38. Hunter CJ, Brightling CE, Woltmann G, et al. A comparison of the validity of different diagnostic tests in adults with asthma. Chest 2002;121(4):1051–7.
39. Wenzel SE, Schwartz LB, Langmack EL, et al. Evidence that severe asthma can be divided pathologically into two inflammatory subtypes with distinct physiologic and clinical characteristics. Am J Respir Crit Care Med 1999;160(3):1001–8.

Printed and bound by CPI Group (UK) Ltd, Croydon, CR0 4YY

07/10/2024

01040500-0001